D1766036

Human Airway Inflammation

METHODS IN MOLECULAR MEDICINE™

John M. Walker, SERIES EDITOR

METHODS IN MOLECULAR MEDICINE™

4716050

Human Airway Inflammation

*Sampling Techniques
and Analytical Protocols*

Edited by

Duncan F. Rogers

and

Louise E. Donnelly

National Heart and Lung Institute, Imperial College, London, UK

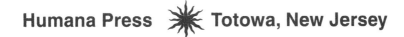

Humana Press ✳ **Totowa, New Jersey**

The content and opinions expressed in this book are the sole work of the authors and editors, who have warranted due diligence in the creation and issuance of their work. The publisher, editors, and authors are not responsible for errors or omissions or for any consequences arising from the information or opinions presented in this book and make no warranty, express or implied, with respect to its contents.

This publication is printed on acid-free paper. ∞
ANSI Z39.48-1984 (American Standards Institute) Permanence of Paper for Printed Library Materials.

Cover design by Patricia F. Cleary

For additional copies, pricing for bulk purchases, and/or information about other Humana titles, contact Humana at the above address or at any of the following numbers: Tel: 973-256-1699; Fax: 973-256-8341; E-mail: humana@humanapr.com or visit our Website at www.humanapress.com

Cover illustrations: Background is Fig. 4 from Chapter 10, "Airway Epithelial Cells (Primaries vs. Cell Lines)" by Louis E. Donnelly; foreground is Fig. 1 from Chapter 13, "Isolation and Culture of Human Airway Smooth Muscle Cells" by Aili L. Lazaar and Reynold A. Panettieri, Jr.

Printed in the United States of America. 10 9 8 7 6 5 4 3 2 1

Library of Congress Cataloging in Publication Data

Main entry under title:

Methods in molecular medicine™.

Human airway inflammation: smapling techniques and analytical protocols / edited by Duncan F. Rogers and Louise E. Donnelly.
     p.;cm.—(Methods in molecular medicine; 56)
     Includes bibliographic references and index.
     ISBN 0-89603-923-4 (alk. paper)
     1. Airway (Medicine)–Inflammation–Diagnosis. 2. Asthma–Diagnosis. 3. Lungs–Diseases, Obstructive Diagnosis. 4. Molecular diagnosis. I. Rogers, D. F. (Duncan F.), 1953–II. Donnelly, Louise E. III. Series
     [DNLM: 1. Asthma–physiopathology, 2. Gene Expression Regulation. 3. Inflammation–diagnosis. 4. Lung Diseases, Obstructive–pathophysiology. WF 553 H918 2001]
     RC732.H85 2001
     616.2'38075–dc21   00-058136

Preface

Rubor (redness), tumor (swelling), calor (heat), and dolor (pain) are the classical signs of inflammation. These features are obvious in the skin, where injury or disease causes flare, wheal, and painful burning sensations. Vasodilatation underlies the flare and heat, plasma exudation the swelling, and activation of sensory nerves relays pain. In chronic conditions, skin biopsies show inflammatory cell infiltrate. Inflammation is not unique to the skin and contributes to disease and repair processes in other organ systems in the body. From the viewpoint of this volume, lung inflammation is now recognized as central to the pathophysiology of a number of severe respiratory conditions, the two most common being asthma and chronic obstructive pulmonary disease (COPD). In asthma, and to a lesser extent COPD, there is evidence of vasodilatation, with congestion of blood vessels accompanied by reddening of the airway mucosa, and of plasma exudation, leading to swelling of the airway wall. Similarly, although less pronounced than in the skin, there is evidence of pain, for example, the unpleasant chest sensations associated with asthma attacks. Understanding the pathogenesis of airway inflammation will enable rational design of drugs to effectively treat conditions such as asthma and COPD. However, whereas immediate access to the skin facilitates investigation of disease processes, the lung, although "open to atmosphere," is much less accessible. Consequently, the investigation of lung inflammation is usually indirect. Thus, a wide variety of research techniques are used.

Human Airway Inflammation: Sampling Techniques and Analytical Protocols attempts to draw together many of the important methodologies and protocols for assessing inflammation in human airways. We start with techniques for the collection of samples. These can be such airway liquids as sputum or exhaled gases as nitric oxide (NO). Once collected, the samples can be used for the isolation and characterization of cells or for the measurement of markers of inflammation. Techniques to isolate and analyze all of the major inflammatory cells associated with lung inflammation are given. Similarly, protocols to measure many of the inflammatory mediators and enzymes released during lung inflammation are detailed herein. In an attempt to be inclusive and to attract both experienced researchers and the novice, we have included specialized chapters (for example, on tracing intracellular mediator storage), mixed with

v

more general chapters (for example, on Northern blotting). We wanted our volume to have something for everyone interested in assessing lung inflammation.

To achieve our aim, we are indebted to our authors for sharing their methodological secrets. As we all know, following the published "recipe" does not always (some would say ever) reproduce the data presented. To that end, the "Methods" series includes the authors "Notes." These are the tips and nuances that convert abject failure into a successful experiment. Our contributors have been most forthcoming on their methods, most of which were painstakingly developed over long periods of time. Another factor that increases the impact of the book is the inclusion of color figures in some of the chapters. We are most grateful to Astra Zeneca and Boehringer Ingelheim, UK for sponsoring color reproduction. Finally, we wish to thank John Walker and Thomas Lanigan for inviting us to put this volume together—it has been an invaluable learning experience for us all.

Duncan F. Rogers
Louise E. Donnelly

Contents

Contributors

JENNIFER R. ALLPORT • *Vascular Research Division, Department of Pathology, Brigham and Women's Hospital, Boston, MA*

MORGAN ANDERSSON • *Department of Otorhinolaryngology, Head and Neck Surgery, University Hospital, Lund, Sweden*

PETER J. BARNES • *Department of Thoracic Medicine, National Heart and Lung Institute, Imperial College School of Science, Technology and Medicine, London, UK*

DARREN BAYLEY • *Department of Respiratory Medicine, Queen Elizabeth Hospital, Birmingham, UK*

SHANNON A. BRYAN • *Royal Brompton Clinical Studies Unit, National Heart and Lung Institute, Imperial College School of Science, Technology and Medicine, London, UK*

C. M. BURKE • *Department of Respiratory Medicine, James Connolly Memorial Hospital, Blanchardstown, Dublin, Ireland*

BRIAN W. CHRISTMAN • *Center for Lung Research, Vanderbilt University Medical Center, Nashville, TN*

PAUL COFFER • *Department of Pulmonary Diseases, University Hospital, Utrecht, The Netherlands*

SARAH V. CULPITT • *Department of Thoracic Medicine, National Heart and Lung Institute, Imperial College School of Science, Technology and Medicine, London, UK*

LOUISE E. DONNELLY • *Department of Thoracic Medicine, National Heart and Lung Institute, Imperial College School of Science, Technology and Medicine, London, UK*

RYSZARD DWORSKI • *Division of Allergy, Pulmonary, and Critical Care Medicine, Vanderbilt University School of Medicine, Nashville, TN*

ANN EFTHIMIADIS • *Firestone Regional Chest and Allergy Unit, St. Joseph's Hospital, Ontario, Canada*

MADELEINE ENNIS • *Department of Clinical Biochemistry, Institute of Clinical Science, The Queen's University of Belfast, Belfast, UK*

AXEL FISCHER • *Allergy Research Group, Humboldt University, Charité, Berlin, Germany*

GUILLERMO GARCIA-CARDEÑA • *Vascular Research Division, Department of Pathology, Brigham and Women's Hospital, Boston, MA*

BERNHARD F. GIBBS • *Department of Dermatology, Medical University of Lübeck, Lübeck, Germany*

SIMON GOMPERTZ • *Department of Respiratory Medicine, Queen Elizabeth Hospital, Birmingham, UK*

LENNART GREIFF • *Department of Otorhinolaryngology, Head and Neck Surgery, University Hospital, Lund, Sweden*

EL-BDAOUI HADDAD • *Department of Pharmacology, Discovery Biology, Aventis Pharma, Dagenham, UK*

TREVOR T. HANSEL • *Royal Brompton Clinical Studies, National Heart and Lung Institute, Imperial College School of Science, Technology, and Medicine, London, UK*

FREDERICK E. HARGREAVE • *Firestone Regional Chest and Allergy Unit, St. Joseph's Hospital, Ontario, Canada*

ADELE HARTNELL • *Leukocyte Biology Section, Biomedical Sciences Division, Imperial College School of Science, Technology and Medicine, London, UK*

ADAM HILL • *Department of Respiratory Medicine, Queen Elizabeth Hospital, Birmingham, UK*

STEPHEN T. HOLGATE • *Medical Specialities, Southhampton General Hospital, Southhampton, UK*

GAVIN JENKINS • *Royal Brompton Clinical Studies Unit, National Heart and Lung Institute, Imperial College School of Science, Technology and Medicine, London, UK*

RIJN JÖBSIS • *Department of Pediatrics/Pediatric Respiratory Medicine, Sophia Children's Hospital, Rotterdam, The Netherlands*

JOHAN C. DE JONGSTE • *Department of Pediatrics/Pediatric Respiratory Medicine, Sophia Children's Hospital, Rotterdam, The Netherlands*

A. BARRY KAY • *Allergy and Clinical Immunology, National Heart and Lung Institute, Imperial College School of Science, Technology and Medicine, London, UK*

VERA M. KEATINGS • *Department of Medicine, Education and Research Centre, St. Vincent's Hospital, Elm Park, Dublin, Ireland*

DIANE KELLEY • *Barnes-Jewish Hospital, St. Louis, MO*

MARGARET M. KELLEY• *Firestone Regional Chest and Allergy Unit, St. Joseph's Hospital, Ontario, Canada*

SERGEI A. KHARITONOV • *Department of Thoracic Medicine, National Heart and Lung Institute, Imperial College School of Science, Technology and Medicine, London, UK*

DALE KOBAYASHI • *Barnes-Jewish Hospital, St. Louis, MO*

Leo Koenderman • *Department of Pulmonary Diseases, University Hospital, Utrecht, Utrecht, The Netherlands*

Paige Lacy • *Pulmonary Research Group, Department of Medicine, University of Alberta, Alberta, Canada*

Aili L. Lazaar • *Pulmonary and Critical Care Division, University of Pennsylvania, Philadelphia, PA*

Margaret J. Leckie • *Royal Brompton Clinical Studies, National Heart and Lung Institute, Imperial College School of Science, Technology and Medicine, London, UK*

Yaw-Chyn Lim • *Vascular Research Division, Department of Pathology, Brigham and Women's Hospital, Boston, MA*

Jan van der Linden • *Department of Pulmonary Diseases, University Hospital, Utrecht, Utrecht, The Netherlands*

Francis W. Luscinskas • *Vascular Research Division, Department of Pathology, Brigham and Women's Hospital, Boston, MA*

Salahaddin Mahmudi-Azer • *Pulmonary Research Group, Department of Medicine, University of Alberta, Alberta, Canada*

Redwan Moqbel • *Pulmonary Research Group, Department of Medicine, University of Alberta, Alberta, Canada*

Robert Newton • *Department of Thoracic Medicine, National Heart Institute, Imperial College School of Science, Technology and Medicine, London, UK*

Julia A. Nightingale • *Department of Thoracic Medicine, National Heart and Lung Institute, Imperial College School of Science, Technology and Medicine, London, UK*

Reynold A. Panettieri, Jr. • *Pulmonary and Critical Care Division, University of Pennsylvania, Philadelphia, PA*

Paolo Paredi • *Department of Thoracic Medicine, National Heart and Lung Institute, Imperial College School of Science, Technology and Medicine, London, UK*

Carl G. A. Persson • *Department of Clinical Pharmacology, University Hospital, Lund, Sweden*

Leonard W. Poulter • *Department of Clinical Immunology, Royal Free Hospital School of Medicine, London, UK*

Kelly Pritchard • *Department of Thoracic Medicine, National Heart and Lung Institute, Imperial College School of Science, Technology and Medicine, London, UK*

H. Rolien Raatgeep • *Department of Pediatrics/Pediatric Respiratory Medicine, Sophia Children's Hospital, Rotterdam, The Netherlands*

DUNCAN F. ROGERS • *Department of Thoracic Medicine, National Heart and Lung Institute, Imperial College School of Science, Technology and Medicine, London, UK*

JONATHAN ROUSELL • *Department of Clinical Ophthalmology, Institute of Ophthalmology, London, UK*

IAN SABROE • *Leukocyte Biology Section, Biomedical Sciences Division, Imperial College School of Science, Technology and Medicine, London, UK*

MARINA SAETTA • *Istituto di Medicina del Lavoro, Università di Padova, Padova, Italy*

JOACHIM SEYBOLD • *Medizinische Klinik m.S. Infektiologie, Charité, Humboldt-Universität, Berlin, Germany*

STEVEN D. SHAPIRO • *Barnes-Jewish Hospital, St. Louis, MO*

JAMES R. SHELLER • *Center for Lung Research, Vanderbilt University Medical Center, Nashville, TN*

ALINKA K. SMITH • *Department of Thoracic Medicine, National Heart and Lung Institute, Imperial College School of Science, Technology and Medicine, London, UK*

YANNIS SOTSIOS • *Department of Pharmacy and Pharmacology, University of Bath, Bath, UK*

JOCHEN SPRINGER • *Allergy Research Group, Humboldt University Charité, Berlin, Germany*

KARL J. STAPLES • *Department of Thoracic Medicine, National Heart and Lung Institute, Imperial College School of Science, Technology and Medicine, London, UK*

ROBERT STOCKLEY • *ADAPT, Bayer Lung Resource, Queen Elizabeth Hospital, Birmingham, UK*

NORBERT SUTTORP • *Medizinische Klinik m.S. Infektiologie, Charité, Humboldt-Universität, Berlin, Germany*

TERESA D. TETLEY • *Respiratory Medicine, Charing Cross Hospital, Imperial College School of Science, Technology and Medicine, London, UK*

GRAZIELLA TURATO • *Istituto di Medicina del Lavoro, Università di Padova, Padova, Italy*

LAURIEN ULFMAN • *Department of Pulmonary Diseases, University Hospital, Utrecht, Utrecht, The Netherlands*

E. HAYDN WALTERS • *Department of Respiratory Medicine, Alfred Hospital and Monash University Medical School, Victoria, Australia*

CHRIS WARD • *Department of Respiratory Medicine, Alfred Hospital and Monash University Medical School, Victoria, Australia*

STEPHEN G. WARD • *Department of Pharmacy and Pharmacology, University of Bath, Bath, UK*

SALLY E. WENZEL • *National Jewish Medical and Research Center, Denver, CO*

JAY Y. WESCOTT • *National Jewish Medical and Research Center, Denver, CO*

TIMOTHY J. WILLIAMS • *Leukocyte Biology Section, Biomedical Sciences Division, Imperial College of Science, Technology and Medicine, London, UK*

IAN R. WITHERDEN • *Respiratory Medicine, Charing Cross Hospital, Imperial College School of Science, Technology and Medicine, London, UK*

SUN YING • *Allergy and Clinical Immunology, National Heart and Lung Institute, Imperial College School of Science, Technology and Medicine, London, UK*

1

Airway Inflammation and Remodeling in Asthma

Current Concepts

Stephen T. Holgate

1. Introduction

Asthma is a heterogeneous disorder of the airways with intermittent airflow obstruction frequently accompanied by increased responsiveness of the bronchi to a wide variety of exogenous and endogenous stimuli. A number of different types of asthma have been described, based largely on the clinical manifestations of, or factors precipitating, the airflow obstruction. As the disease becomes more severe and chronic, it is suggested that the airflow obstruction may progressively lose some of its reversibility and, in this respect, resemble some aspects of chronic obstructive pulmonary disease (COPD). However, in a small proportion of patients with life-threatening asthma, the airways are highly labile on account of greatly enhanced bronchial hyperresponsiveness. At the other end of the disease severity spectrum there are many patients with mild intermittent asthma whose disease only manifests when exposed to particular sensitizing allergens to which they are sensitive (e.g. outdoor allergens during the pollen season).

Over the last 50 yr, the prevalence of asthma and allied allergic disorders have progressively increased on a worldwide scale, in both developed and developing countries. In addition to an increase in asthma-related symptoms, there is evidence of increased medication usage and a rise in hospital admissions for asthma. The reasons for these rising trends may be multiple. Suggestions include:

From: *Methods in Molecular Medicine, vol. 56:*
Human Airway Inflammation: Sampling Techniques and Analytical Protocols
Edited by: D. F. Rogers and L. E. Donnelly © Humana Press Inc., Totowa, NJ

1. Increased allergen exposure (especially within the domestic setting).
2. Reduced exposure to childhood infections.
3. Changes to the diet (e.g., reduced antioxidant and δ 13 polyunsaturated fatty acids).
4. Alterations to the lung or gastrointestinal flora possibly linked to increased antibiotic prescribing in infancy.

Whatever the underlying causes for these rising trends, asthma has now become a public health issue. Therefore, it is of the utmost importance that a clear understanding is obtained of underlying cell and molecular mechanisms in order that appropriate biomarkers are identified that can be used to detect the disease earlier and follow its outcome. In childhood and early adulthood, asthma occurs in association with atopy, which is characterized by elevated circulating allergen-specific IgE and positive skin prick test responses to allergen extracts. However, asthma in adults tends to lose its close association with atopy, particularly in those patients with late onset and chronic disease. Recent estimates suggest that approx 50% of asthma can be linked to immunological mechanisms associated with atopy. Compelling epidemiological evidence indicates that atopy alone (i.e., the genetic susceptibility to generate allergen-specific IgE) is insufficient for the development of asthma and, what is also required is a susceptibility of the airways to express and respond to localized inflammatory responses. With the recent description of a subtype of asthma manifesting as intermittent cough (cough-variant asthma) in which there is airway inflammation in the absence of bronchial hyperresponsiveness, it would seem that inflammation alone is also insufficient to produce the variable airflow obstruction and accompanying symptoms of chronic asthma. It would appear that some alteration to the airway structure (airway wall remodeling) upon which the inflammatory response is acting is also required.

2. The Epidemiology of Asthma and the Role of IgE

Although atopy is the single strongest risk factor for the development of asthma increasing the risk up to 20-fold, only about one-fifth of atopic subjects progress to develop chronic asthma requiring regular therapy. Both in childhood and in adults, epidemiological associations have been shown between asthma and IgE, whether assessed as total serum IgE or as allergen-specific IgE. In many parts of the world it is exposure to indoor allergens that appears to drive the expression of atopy linked to asthma and specifically exposure to dust mite, cat, and fungal antigens. Domestic exposure in early life to the major dust mite allergen *der P₁* levels of >2 µg/g of house dust has been shown to significantly increase the risk of initial allergen sensitization and the development of asthma. Exposure to levels in excess of 10 µg/g of dust increases the risk of acute exacerbations of preexisting disease. Exposure to *Alternaria* allergens has been linked to acute life-threatening attacks of asthma, whereas other allergens including animal dander, insect dust, grass pollen, and molds have also been linked to asthma exacerbations. Epidemics of asthma, as occurred in Barcelona or following thunderstorms in the United Kingdom, have also been linked to exposure to high concentrations of allergens. These incidents have been attributed, respectively, to the unloading of soy bean in Barcelona harbor and the release of pollen fragments into the air following osmotic lysis of pollen grains at the peak of the pollen season.

3. The Pathological Features of Asthma

Asthma is classically an inflammatory disorder of the airways with infiltration of the submucosa and adventitia of both the large and small airways with activated mast cells, tissue macrophages, eosinophils, and, in certain cases, neutrophils. In acute severe asthma that may be provoked by respiratory virus infections, the airways become infiltrated with neutrophils in addition to eosinophils, an observation that has also been described in patients dying suddenly of their disease. A second important characteristic of asthma is damage to the ciliated stratified epithelium with a deposition of interstitial collagens (types I, III, and V) as well as laminin and tenascin C beneath the true epithelial basement membrane, which has been linked to the proliferation of subepithelial myofibroblasts. The epithelium in asthma also undergoes metaplasia with the acquisition of a repair phenotype and an increase in the number of goblet cells, especially in chronic disease. A third pathological characteristic of chronic asthma is hyperplasia of the formed elements of the airway, including microvessels, afferent neurons, and smooth muscle as well as deposition of matrix proteins and proteoglycans (versican, fibromodulin, biglycan, and decorin) in the submucosa and outside the airway smooth muscle. Taken together, the inflammatory response is superimposed on a remodeled airway, and it is this that gives rise to clinical heterogeneity so characteristic of asthma.

Although once considered as purely a disease of airway smooth muscle, asthma is now known to be a chronic inflammatory disorder of the airways, orchestrated by $CD4^+$ lymphocytes. There is evidence to support the view that the asthmatic airway inflammation is driven by the persistence of chronically activated T cells of a memory phenotype ($CD45RO^+$) with a proportion of these being directed to allergenic, occupational, or viral antigens. This is supported by a large number of studies using BAL and bronchial mucosal biopsies from subjects with asthma. These studies revealed increased transcription and product release of a discrete set of cytokines encoded on the long arm of chromosome $5q_{31-33}$, which includes interleukin (IL)-3, IL-4, IL-5, IL-9, IL-13, and granulocyte macrophage colony stimulating factor (GM-CSF). In more severe asthma and some cases of occupational asthma, $CD8^+$ as well as $CD4^+$ T cells are the source of these cytokines.

Although many of the cytokines associated with the Th-2 phenotype have pleiotropic functions, there are specific aspects of each one that are worth highlighting when linking their function to airway pathology in asthma. In most types the predominant inflammatory cell infiltrating the airway wall is the eosinophil that is derived from $CD34^+$ precursor cells, which are present in the bone marrow, recruited from the circulation, and located in the airway wall itself. Under the influence of IL-3, IL-5, and GM-CSF, eosinophils acquire a mature phenotype with the capacity to secrete a range of preformed and newly generated mediators. Interleukin-4 and IL–13 are intimately involved in the isotype switching of B cells from IgM to IgE and also in the upregulation of a specific adhesion molecule, vascular cell adhesion molecule-1 (VCAM-1), involved in the recruitment of basophils, eosinophils, and Th2-like T cells. Following allergen exposure, it is the interaction of the inflammatory cell integrin VLA-4 with VCAM-1 that plays a key role in the recruitment of eosinophils, basophils, and Th-2 cells from the circulation into the airways. An additional property of IL-4 (which is not shared by IL-13) is the ability of this cytokine to support the development of Th-2 T cells and enhance their survival. Two IL-4 and two IL-13 receptors have been described on a variety of cell types with subtle differences in their ability to initiate intracellular activation mechanisms. These involve the transcription factor signal transducer and activator of transcription (STAT)-6 and insulin receptor substrate (IRS)-1/2 that are involved in IL-4/IL-13 induced gene transcription and cell proliferation, respectively. Bronchial epithelial cells and fibroblasts also express IL-4 and IL-13 receptors and are highly responsive to these cytokines in vitro. In vivo overexpression of IL-13 into the bronchial epithelium of transgenic mice not only leads to increased IgE production but also goblet cell metaplasia, subepithelial fibrosis, and bronchial smooth muscle hyperplasia, linked to the acquisition of bronchial hyperresponsiveness.

A Th-2 cytokine that is gaining importance in asthma is GM-CSF, which serves as a growth factor for eosinophils, basophils, macrophages, and dendritic cells and is also a key cytokine for rescuing eosinophils from programmed cell death (apoptosis).

4. An Important Role for Chemokines in Asthma

Apart from Th-2 cytokines, a second group of low-molecular-weight proteins are required for the recruitment of inflammatory cells into the asthmatic airway — the chemokines. At the transcriptional and protein levels, both C-C and C-X-C chemokines are generated by asthmatic airways but, of particular relevance, are the C-X-C chemokines regulated on activation normal T cell expressed and secreted (RANTES), eotaxin, and monocyte chemoattractant protein (MCP)-1, -3, and -4. These five chemokines interact with the CCR-3 receptor that is expressed in high numbers on eosinophils, basophils, and a subset of Th-2 cells. Besides promoting local migration of leukocytes within the airway wall, the same chemokines are also involved in the release of eosinophils and their precursors from the bone marrow when appropriate signals are received from the lung via the circulation.

Although both immune and inflammatory cells have the capacity to release CCR-3 ligands, the most abundant sources of these chemoattractants are the formed airway elements: the bronchial epithelium, microvascular endothelium, and myofibroblast/fibroblast. There is also in vitro evidence to suggest that proliferation of airway smooth muscle can generate chemokines as well as a number of other cytokines, including those encoded in the IL-4 gene cluster.

5. Antigen Processing and Presentation: The Role of Dendritic Cells

Activation of the mucosal immune response involving $CD4^+$ T cells is a central feature of chronic asthma. In order for mucosal T cells to either proliferate and/or generate appropriate cytokines, they require activation usually via the T-cell receptor, CD3. Uptake of antigen by dendritic cells, in allergic disease, is enhanced by the ability of these cells to express both high and low affinity IgE Fc receptors that increase the efficiency of allergen capture by 50–1000-fold. On internalization, a peptide sequence is selected and presented in the groove of major histocompatibility complex (MHC) class II to the T-cell receptor (signal 1). However, in order for T cells to respond to this antigen-specific stimulus, engagement of a second signal is required involving both the costimulatory molecules B7.1 (CD80) or B7.2 (CD86) that engage the homodimeric molecule CD28 on the T-cell (signal 2). In contrast to peripheral blood mononuclear cells that preferentially utilize CD86 for Th-2 cytokine production, CD28 on T cells in the bronchial mucosa of asthmatics engage either CD80 or CD86 in augmenting local Th-2 cytokine production. In the presence of IL-4, a monomeric adhesion molecule CTLA-4 is induced on T cells that has an increased affinity for both CD80 or CD86 and is able to "steal" the CD28 signal from the B7 ligands, thereby rendering the T-cell anergic or initiate its programmed cell death.

Dendritic cells are characterized by their cell surface expression of CD1, high density of MHC class II, and costimulatory molecules. They form a network within the bronchial epithelium and submucosa. On chronic exposure to antigen, the number of dendritic cells increases, thereby enhancing mucosal responsiveness to sensitizing antigens. These cells are seen to be obligatory for the development of primary allergen-specific airway responses, although, once sensitization has occurred, there are other cells in the airways including B cells and possibly epithelial cells, that may also provide an antigen-processing and -presenting function.

There are strong genetic determinants for the development of Th-2 polarization within the lower airways. Not only do antigen-presenting cells provide T cells with antigen and costimulatory signals, but also soluble signals that polarize their subsequent differentiation (signal 3). The Th-2 biased responses observed in atopic diseases appear to be associated with a decreased IL-12/prostaglandin (PG)-E_2 ratio and, as a consequence, downregulation of Th-2 cytokine production. The presence of interferon-γ (IFN-γ) enhances the ability of immature dendritic cells to produce IL-12, which in turn creates the environment for preferential Th-1 T cell maturation. In contrast, PGE_2 primes for a reduced IL-12, producing ability and consequently, biasing T-cell development in favor of a Th-2 phenotype. Thus, it is suggested that antigens provoke either a Th-1 or Th-2 response by inducing the production of a pattern of inflammatory dendritic cell mediators with the capacity to direct at the local site of exposure. This concept may be of particular relevance to the early life origins of allergic disease because, in children destined to develop atopic disorders, their cord blood mononuclear cells have an impaired capacity to respond to IL-12 and, as a consequence, to generate IFN-γ efficiently. Because IFN-γ provides such a strong negative signal to Th-2 development, its impaired production may predispose the infant to persistence into postnatal life of Th-2 responsiveness that in normal infants shuts down efficiently prior to birth. It has been shown that the impaired production of T-cell IFN-γ production in atopic children persists into late childhood providing further evidence that reduction in this inhibitory pathway rather than enhancement of the excitatory is responsible for the persistence of the Th-2 phenotype linked to the allergic phenotype.

6. The Role of IgE

The identification of the passive sensitizing agent "reagin" as immunoglobulin E has provided the immunological basis for type I hypersensitivity disorders. Immunoglobulin-E directed to specific allergens is generated by B cells and plasma cells through an interaction with antigen-specific T cells in the presence of IL-4 or its homolog (IL-13) together with engagement of the costimulatory molecules CD40 on B cells and CD40 ligand on T cells. Immunoglobulin E binds to both high-affinity Fc receptors ($\alpha_1,\beta_1,\gamma_2$: Fc$\epsilon$R1) expressed on mast cells, basophils, dendritic cells, and eosinophils and also to monomeric low-affinity receptors (FcϵR2 or CD23) expressed on a wide variety of cell types including epithelial cells, B cells, monocytes, T cells, neutrophils, and eosinophils. Although the role of IgE in the manifestation of many allergic diseases such as anaphylaxis and rhinoconjunctivitis is without dispute, there is considerable debate over the role of this signaling molecule and its receptors in asthma. The availability of a fully humanized blocking monoclonal antibody against IgE (E25) has provided considerable insight into the role of IgE-mediated mechanisms in allergic asthma.

This humanized monoclonal antibody was directed to that part of IgE that, under normal circumstances, binds with high affinity to the α chain of the tetrameric FcεR1 receptor. Thus, following a single injection of Mab E-25, there occurs a >90% decrease in circulating levels of IgE with a composite increase in IgE/E25 complexes. These small complexes are rapidly cleared by the reticuloendothelial system and, so far, have not been associated with any adverse immune complex deposition effects. Over periods of 9–12 wk the regular administration of Mab E25 produced profound attenuation of both the early and late phase bronchoconstrictor responses following allergen provocation of the airways of patients with atopic asthma, as well as causing a reduction in allergen-induced acquired bronchial hyperresponsiveness (BHR). A clinical trial involving over 300 patients in whom E25 was administered over a period of 12 wk has demonstrated improvement in all parameters of asthma, including the requirement of inhaled and oral corticosteroids. Not all patients responded equally to this treatment, although there appear to be no particular features that identify "responders" from "nonresponders."

Although IgE has been classically associated with asthma of the atopic extrinsic type, in patients with intrinsic nonallergic asthma Th-2 development in the bronchial mucosa is also accompanied by an increase in the number of cells bearing the FcεR1 receptor. This indicates that local IgE production may contribute to this form of the disease. The putative role of local airway IgE synthesis is further supported by the increased expression of ε germ line transcripts (Iε) and mRNA for ε heavy chain of IgE in bronchial biopsies from both atopic and nonatopic asthmatics. However, in the latter case the initiating antigen or antigens have yet to be identified. It has been suggested that the inflammatory response in nonatopic asthma is preferentially promoted by the activation of IgE receptors on monocytes/macrophages rather than mast cells and involves putative "autoimmune" processes.

7. The Role of the Mast Cell in Asthma

Immunoglobulin-E-dependent activation of mast cells provides the basis for the early asthmatic response. Crosslinkage of FcεR1 on the surface of sensitized mast cells by allergen results in the noncytotoxic secretion of both preformed and newly generated mediators. In addition to preformed histamine and heparin, the mast cell secretory granule also contains a range of enzymes, including exoglycosidases, endoglycosidases, and serum proteases. The mucosal type mast cell (MC_T) that predominates in the asthmatic airway contains the unique four-chained neutral protease tryptase that is stabilized by heparin. Tryptase has the capacity to cleave a number of soluble substrates, but in asthma its main function may well be to activate protease-activated receptors (specifically PAR-2), through cleavage of a small peptide from the tethered ligand. This enables the receptor to stimulate cell proliferation and cytokine production. PAR-2 receptors are found on bronchial epithelial, endothelial, neural ganglia, smooth muscle, and fibroblast cells and their function may be to initiate and maintain airway wall remodeling. Activation of PAR-2 receptors in the epithelium and endothelium leads to the release of chemokines such as RANTES and IL-8, which may provide one mechanism for chemokine release when sensitized airways are exposed to allergen.

In addition to releasing granule-associated preformed mediators, activated mast cells have the capacity to generate an array of newly generated products including the cysteinyl leukotriene LTC_4 and PGD_2. The combination of LTC_4, LTD_4, LTE_4 (together comprising slow reacting substance of anaphylaxis; SRS-A), histamine, and PGD_2 accounts for the majority of the early asthmatic response following allergen challenge. Thus, inhibitors of receptor activation or mediator synthesis, either by themselves or, more effectively, in combination, or mast cell stabilizers, such as sodium cromoglycate and nedocromil sodium, attenuate the early asthmatic response. The same mediators are also implicated in the pathogenesis of exercise-induced asthma. The most popular prevailing hypothesis to explain exercise-induced asthma is that increased ventilation impacts on a damaged epithelium resulting in water loss from the airway lining fluid that is inadequately replaced and, as a consequence, causes activation of primed mast cells by a hyperosmolar environment. Bronchoconstriction provoked by isocapnic ventilation, cold dry air, and hypertonic sodium chloride (or mannitol) aerosols is produced by a similar mast cell-dependent mechanism. Similarly, in asthma, adenosine generated by mast cells (and also by other cells) interacts with adenosine A_{2B} receptors on primed mast cells leading to autacoid release. H_1-antihistamines and mast cell suppressor drugs (e.g., sodium cromoglycate and nedocromil sodium) can also inhibit this early response.

A characteristic feature of asthma associated with known environmental sensitizing agents is the occurrence of delayed bronchoconstriction 4–24 h following inhalation exposure, which is accompanied by a progressive increase in bronchial hyperresponsiveness that may last up to 3 wk following challenge. This late asthmatic response is, in part, mast cell dependent because it is also inhibited by sodium cromoglycate and nedocromil sodium and also by nonanaphylactogenic antihuman IgE. The most likely explanation for the onset of a late asthmatic response is the release of cytokines from activated mast cells, specifically TNFα, IL-4, IL-5, GM-CSF, and chemokines active at the CCR3 receptor. Human mast cells store small quantities of cytokines within their secretory granules that can be released rapidly. In addition, activation of their IgE receptors in the presence of stem cell factor (a mast cell growth factor) leads to increased cytokine transcription with subsequent product release that may persist for up to 48–72 h. Mast cell-derived histamine and leukotrienes express the preformed adhesion molecule P selectin on endothelial cells resulting in leukocyte "rolling." TNFα upregulates the expression of the adhesion molecules E-selectin, intercellular adhesion molecule-1 (ICAM-1), and VCAM-1, the latter also requiring either IL-4 or IL-13 for stabilization of expression. By interacting with their complementary ligands on neutrophils, eosinophils, basophils, T cells, and monocytes, these adhesion molecules enable leukocytes to be recruited selectively into the airway wall.

There is strong evidence that cytokine release from T cells also contributes to the latter period of the late phase bronchoconstrictor response and the accompanying increase in BHR. Antigen specific T cells have the capacity to be selectively recruited into exposed airways, possibly involving novel chemokine and epithelial homing receptors.

8. The Eosinophil

The presence of eosinophils in the walls and lumen of the conducting airways is a characteristic feature of chronic asthma and has placed this cell at the center of the mediator cascade in all types of asthma irrespective of etiology. The extent of airway eosinophilia is closely linked to epithelial damage and disease severity, as reflected by eosinophil counts and the presence of granule proteins in lavage fluid, mucosal tissue, and induced sputum. In chronic asthma increased eosinophil survival by locally produced GM-CSF, IL-3, and IL-5 is at least as important in maintaining airway eosinophilia as is the recruitment of new cells from the circulation. More recently, the identification of CD3[+] leukocyte precursors in the airway wall bearing receptors for the same eosinophilopoietic cytokines suggests that part of the tissue eosinophilia may be locally generated.

The eosinophil granules contain a number of arginine rich proteins (major basic protein [MBP]; eosinophil cationic protein [ECP]; eosinophil, derived neurotoxin [EDN]; and eosinophil peroxidase [EPO]). At high concentrations these proteins are cytotoxic to the bronchial epithelium whereas when present in smaller amounts they activate epithelial stress signaling pathways and have the capacity to interfere with muscarinic neurotransmission. It has been suggested that MBP and possibly ECP are responsible for the epithelial disruption in asthma. However, there is also evidence that detachment of columnar cells from basal cells occurs through weakening of cell adhesion complexes, possibly mediated by an altered epithelial phenotype, proteolytic attack, or increased apoptosis. Eosinophils and neutrophils are rich sources of the metalloproteinase MMP-9 whose inhibition by the endogenous tissue inhibitor TIMP-1 has been shown to be impaired in chronic asthma. MMP-9 is also induced in epithelial cells when they are engaged in a repair response.

Human eosinophils have the capacity to generate large quantities of the cysteinyl leukotriene LTC_4, which, through extracellular peptide cleavage, is rapidly converted to LTD_4 and subsequently to LTE_4, the terminal product in humans. During the first phase of the allergen-induced late phase response, when neutrophils then eosinophils are recruited in large numbers, cysteinyl leukotrienes are produced that are responsible for much of the smooth muscle contraction and airway wall edema that underpins the bronchoconstriction. Thus, cysteinyl LT_1 receptor antagonists inhibit a substantial portion of the allergen-provoked late-phase response. When combined with a selective H_1 antagonist, inhibition of the late phase response is almost total, suggesting that histamine (possibly from basophils) and cysteinyl leukotrienes account for most of the disordered airway function during this period. Eosinophils release substantial quantities of prostanoids, specifically PGE_2, PGI_2 and thromboxane A_2 (TxA_2), 15-hydroxyeicosatetranoic acid (15-HETE), and platelet-activating factor (PAF), which, in combination, may contribute to the ability of these cells to cause smooth muscle contraction, microvascular leakage, and mucus secretion. Like the mast cell, eosinophils are also an important source of cytokines, including IL-1β, IL-3, IL-4, IL-5, IL-6, IL-16, TNFα, GM-CSF, IFN-γ, and transforming growth factors (TGF) α and β. However, their capacity to secrete these cytokines as soluble mediators into the extracellular milieu may be limited.

It has been widely held that the mechanism whereby eosinophils are recruited into the asthmatic airway following allergen exposure is IL-5 dependent. This supposition has been based on the greatly increased production of IL-5 found in association with the late-phase response and on antibody blocking and gene manipulation studies in animal models. Allergen-induced eosinophilic inflammation is first associated in the peripheral circulation with a decrease, then an increase in eosinophil and basophil progenitors recruited from the bone marrow through upregulation of the IL-5 receptor on progenitors and their increased response to this cytokine. This has led to the suggestion that the effect of inhaled corticosteroids on allergen-induced airway responses is mediated through preventing their maturation in the bone marrow or release of mature cells into the circulation. Recently, the pivotal role of IL-5 in mediating the late-phase allergen response has been brought into question following studies using a humanized blocking monoclonal antibody directed to IL-5. A single injection of this antibody produces a progressive decrease in circulating eosinophil counts to a nadir of approx 80% of the starting value and also abolishes the allergen-provoked increase in circulating and sputum eosinophils. Thus, in atopic asthmatic subjects, both before and after allergen provocation, the circulating and tissue eosinophilia are in large part IL-5-dependent. However, in contrast to its abbrogating effect on eosinophils, anti-IL-5 failed to inhibit either the early- or late-phase airway response to allergen or basal bronchial hyperresponsiveness, or the increase in hyperresponsiveness postallergen challenge. Using a similar experimental design, human recombinant IL-12, with its potent and specific effect of inducing IFN-γ production when given to atopic asthmatic patients in increasing doses over 8 wk, also caused a progressive decline in blood and sputum eosinophils. However, this treatment again failed to attenuate either the early- or the late-phase allergen response, although, in this case, there was a small significant reduction in bronchial hyperresponsiveness. Overall, these experiments cast some doubt over the role of the circulating eosinophil in mediating the late-phase response. However, it is still possible that eosinophils and their precursors already resident in the airways could still respond to IgE-dependent stimulation because it has recently been demonstrated that tissue, as opposed to circulating eosinophils, exhibit functional FcϵR1. If eosinophils are not the only source of the cysteinyl leukotrienes during late-phase responses, then tissue macrophages and basophils deserve further attention.

9. Monocytes and Macrophages

Apart from their capacity to differentiate into phagocytic or antigen-presenting cells, tissue macrophages are an important source of proinflammatory mediators, including PGE$_2$, reactive oxygen species, cysteinyl leukotrienes, and a range of cytokines (IL-1β, TNF-α, IL-6, IL-8, IL-10, IL-12, GM-CSF, IFN-γ, and TGFβ). Tissue macrophages may be especially important in driving the inflammatory response in nonatopic and corticosteroid-resistant asthma. However, macrophages recovered by BAL are generally relatively ineffective in their capacity to present antigen to T lymphocytes and appear to have predominantly an immunosuppressive role in the lung. Indeed, in the DO10.11 transgenic mouse whose T-cell receptors recognize 16 amino acids of ovalbumin, repeated aerosol exposure to ovalbumin leads to loss of the eosinophilic airway inflammatory response in parallel with loss of antigen-specific lung T-cell responsiveness in vitro. In contrast, T cells isolated from the draining lymph nodes or spleen maintain their capacity to proliferate. Because removal of macrophages from the tolerant lung tissue results in restoration of antigen-induced T-cell proliferation, these cells may be particularly important in downregulating airway responses to allergens as occurs in human subjects who express atopy but not asthma. Phenotypically, these "inhibitory" macrophages share many features in common with dendritic cells (enriched in MHC class II and costimulatory molecules) but through cell contact they provide a negative rather than a positive signal to T cells. In active asthma, the increased expression of CD80 and CD86 on macrophages recovered by lavage might indicate that in disease these costimulatory molecules are under separate local regulation in order to enhance the antigen presenting capacity of these cells.

10. The Bronchial Epithelium as a Regulator
of Airway Inflammation

Although at one time thought to be a passive barrier between the external and internal airway environments, the bronchial epithelium is now considered to play a dynamic role in regulating both the inflammatory and remodeling processes in asthma. The epithelium is a source of a range of proinflammatory agents, including those derived from arachidonic acid (15-HETE, PGE_2, and lipoxins), nitric oxide (NO), endothelin-1, and a range of cytokines (IL-1β, IL-5, IL-6, IL-11, GM-CSF, IL-16, IL-18), chemokines (IL-8, GROα, MCP-1, MCP-3, RANTES, MIP1α, MIP2, eotaxin, and eotaxin-2), and proliferative growth factors (EGF, TGFβ_1, TGFβ_2, platelet derived growth factor — [PDGF], insulin-like growth factor — [IGF-1], and basic fibroblast growth factor — [b-FGF]).

Inflammatory cells recruited into the airways release a number of cytokines and tissue-damaging proteases and cationic proteins that are considered important in disturbing the structure and function of the epithelium. Mast cell-derived serum proteases, such as tryptase and MMP-3 (stromolysin), together with MMP-9 derived from eosinophils and neutrophils, are capable of disrupting epithelial integrity by breaking cell adhesion complexes. These proteases are also able to initiate epithelial cell transcription of cytokines and mediator-generating enzymes as well as increasing the expression of cell-surface adhesion molecules. Allergens with proteolytic activity (e.g., the house dust mite allergens Der p_1, a cysteinyl protease, and Der p_6, a serine protease) can directly stimulate cytokine and chemokine release and increase ICAM-1 expression by bronchial epithelial cells, possibly through activation of PARs. The ability of many allergens to either exhibit protease activity or be delivered along with proteases has recently been shown to disrupt epithelial tight junctions through cleavage of the protein occludin. Disruption of the epithelial barrier by allergens or proteases derived from inflammatory cells would facilitate the passage of allergens and other environmental stimuli to antigen-presenting cells resident in the submucosa, thereby accentuating activation of the mucosal Th-2 directed immune system.

In chronic asthma, there is evidence that the epithelium is phenotypically altered toward a repair phenotype with increased expression of CD44. The epithelial isoform (v3) of CD44 is enriched with acidic glycosoaminoglycans, which bind and concentrate at the cell surface specific growth factors, including heparin binding epidermal-like growth factor (HB-EGF).

11. The Epithelial–Mesenchymal Trophic Unit in Asthma

The epithelium, as an important formed element of the airway, may not be alone in orchestrating inflammatory and repair responses characteristic of asthma. A unique and highly characteristic feature of asthma is the deposition of interstitial collagens secreted by myofibroblasts beneath the basement membrane. The bronchial epithelium and subepithelial mesenchymal cells are intimately involved in the fetal development of the lung with signaling between these cells promoting airway growth and branching. Key cytokines involved in this signaling include members of the epidermal growth factor family (EGF itself, amphiregulin, HB-EGF, β cellulin, and epiregulin), b-FGF, endothelin-1, PDGF, and IGF-1. In the reverse direction, myofibroblasts and fibroblasts are important sources of keratinocyte growth factor (KGF), acid fibroblast growth factor (a-FGF), and PDGF. Both epithelial cells and myofibroblasts/fibroblasts generate GMCSF stem cell factor (ckit ligand) and nerve growth factor (NGF). It seems that this *"epithelial–mesenchymal trophic"* unit becomes activated or reactivated in asthma with increased cross talk between epithelial cells and the underlying mesenchyme.

Although the molecular mechanisms controlling these events are not yet clearly understood, it seems that in asthma the epithelium has a reduced capacity to restitute itself following injury produced by infiltrating inflammatory cells, allergens, pollutants, or respiratory virus infection. In chronic disease, there occurs greatly enhanced epithelial cell-surface expression of the EGF receptor (EGFR) c erb B1 but no change to c erb B2 or c erb B3 that are also expressed by airway epithelial cells. Because expression of EGFR is induced by injury to the epithelium as a "repair" response, these findings indicate that in asthma the epithelium is permanently subjected to an ongoing injury-repair response. The majority of the EGFR ligands (EGF, HB-EGF, TGFα, and amphiregulin) generated by the airway in response to injury derives from the epithelium itself, acting in an autacoid fashion. This involves activation of the EGFR tyrosine kinase and crossphosphorylation of tyrosine residues on the adjacent monomers of EGFR. Thus, inhibition of EGFR signaling by the selective tyrphostin EGFR tyrosine kinase inhibitor, AG1478, not only slows epithelial restitution in vitro but also enhances profibrogenic growth factor (e.g., TGF β_2 production). It follows that, if the bronchial epithelium is "held" in a repair state, it becomes a continuous source of proliferative and profibrogenic cytokines, the situation observed in chronic asthma. Using decreased expression of proliferating cell nuclear antigen (PCNA) as a marker of cell proliferation and increased expression of $P_{21}{}^{waf}$ as one of the cell cycle inhibitors, in chronic asthma, it appears that the epithelium is impaired in its ability to proliferate. The molecular mechanisms of this impairment are likely to be fundamental to the airway wall remodeling, which occurs through the enhanced secretion of proliferative and profibrogenic cytokines from the activated epithelial mesenchymal trophic unit.

12. An Integrated Model for the Development and Progression of Asthma

Based on the above considerations, for asthma to persist there is a requirement for two cellular processes, the first involving polarization of T cells toward enhanced production of cytokines of the IL-4 gene cluster and, the second, reactivation of the epithelial–mesenchymal trophic unit. These two events are likely to interact. Products from epithelial cells, such as PGE_2, IL-18, and TGFβ, are important mediators for inducing dendritic cells to polarize T-cell development, whereas cytokines and mediators from activated T cells and recruited inflammatory cells are able to interact with the epithelium and underlying mesenchyme to initiate inflammatory and repair cascades. One example of this duality of function is the ability of IL-4 and IL-13 to:

1. Act on immunocompetent cells to enhance eosinophil-mediated inflammation.
2. Modify epithelial repair.
3. Increase cytokine production.
4. Promote epithelial goblet cell metaplasia.
5. Stimulate fibroblast proliferation.
6. Convert fibroblasts to a myofibroblast phenotype.
7. Enhance secretion of collagen and other matrix molecules.

13. Susceptibility Genes in Asthma

The last 25 yr has seen asthma pass through the complete cycle, beginning with the concept of an abnormality in smooth muscle passing through the era of airway inflammation and now back to remodeling. T-cell polarization toward a Th-2 phenotype and activation of the bronchial epithelial–mesenchymal trophic unit are essential prerequisites for the development of asthma, leading to sustained airway inflammation and airway wall remodeling. These processes are likely to be under strong genetic influences. Although a number of candidate genes have been suggested to account for a small proportion of the allergy or asthma phenotype, as yet no single gene of megaphenic effect has yet been described. Whole genome searches and positional cloning are being used in an attempt to identify novel genes that may be contributing to the genetic predisposition for developing asthma. Candidate chromosomal regions where linkage has been shown in different populations are located on chromosome 5q, 6p, 11q, 12q, 13p, and 16p. The most difficult task will be to identify within these relatively large chromosomal regions which candidate genes account for the significant positive linkage. This task may be made easier when differential RNA expression arrays are used to identify disease-related genes being specifically expressed in asthmatic tissue.

14. Concluding Comments

The challenge for the future will be to bring together the various methodological approaches for studying airway inflammation and remodeling in asthma toward a common objective of identifying novel gene products which underpin asthma susceptibility and disease progression engaging both altered mucosal immune responses, inflammation, and airway wall remodeling. These will not only provide potential targets for therapeutic interaction, but also form the basis for novel biomarkers that can be used to predict the course and natural history of the disease.

15. Suggested Readings

Chung KF, Barnes PF. Cytokines in asthma. Thorax 1999; 54:825–857.

Cookson W. The alliance of genes and environment in asthma and allergy. Nature. 1999; 402 (6760 Suppl):B5–11.

Gilliland FD, Berhane K, McConnell R, Gauderman WJ, Vora H, Rappaport EB, Avol E, Peters JM. Maternal smoking during pregnancy, environmental tobacco smoke exposure and childhood lung function. Thorax. 2000; 55: 271–276.

Hirst SJ. Airway smooth muscle culture: application to studies of airway wall remodeling and phenotype plasticity in asthma. Eur Respir J 1996; 9:808–820.

Holgate ST, Davies DE, Lackie PM, Wilson SJ, Puddicombe SM, Lordan JL. Epithelial-mesenchymal interactions in the pathogenesis of asthma. J Allergy Clin Immunol 2000; 105:193–204.

Holgate ST. Genetic and environmental interactions in allergy and asthma. J Allergy Clin Immunol 1999; 104:1139-1146.

Holgate ST. The epidemic of allergy and asthma. Nature 1999; 402 (Suppl.):B2–B4.

ISAAC Steering Committee. Worldwide variation in prevalence of symptoms of asthma, allergic rhinoconjunctivitis and atopic eczema: ISAAC. Lancet 1998; 351:1225–1232.

Kips JC, Pauwels RA. Airway wall remodeling: does it occur and what does it mean? Clin Exp Allergy 1999; 29:1457–1466.

Laitinen A, Karjalainen E-M, Altraju A, Laitinen L. Histopathologic features of early and progressive asthma. J Allergy Clin Immunol 2000; 105 (pt.2):S509–S513.

Mosmann TR, Coffman RL. Th1 and Th2 cells: different patterns of lymphokine secretion lead to different functional properties. Ann Rev Immunol 1989; 7:145–173.

Postma DS, Gerritsen J (eds). The link between asthma and COPD. Clin Exp Allergy 1999; 29 (Suppl.2):3–128.

Rosi E, Scano G. Association of sputum parameters with clinical and functional measurements in asthma. Thorax 2000; 55:235–238.

Sears MR. Descriptive epidemiology of asthma. Lancet 1997; 350 (Suppl.II):1–4.

Sont JK, Willens LNA, Bel EH, van Kreiken JHJM, Vandenbroncke JP, Sterk PJ and the AMPUL Study Group. Clinical control and histopathological outcome of asthma when using airway hyperresponsiveness as additional guide to long term treatment. Am J Respir Crit Care Med 1999; 159:1043–1051.

Sterk PJ, Buist SA, Woolcock AJ Marks GB, Platts-Mills TA, von Mutius E, Bousquet J, Frew AJ, Pauwels RA, Ait-Khaled N, Hill SL, Partridge MR. The message from the World Asthma meeting 1998. Eur Respir J 1999; 14:1435–1453.

Tattersfield AE. Limitations of current treatment. Lancet 1997; 350 (Suppl.II):24–27.

Von Hertzen LC, Haahtela T. Could the risk of asthma and atopy be reduced by a vaccine that induces a strong T-helper Type 1 response? Am J Respir Cell Mol Biol 2000; 22:139–142.

Warner JO, Pohunek P, Marguet C, Roche WR, Clough JB. Issues in understanding childhood asthma. J Allergy Clin Immunol 2000; 105 (pt.2): S473–S476.

I

SAMPLE COLLECTION

INVASIVE TECHNIQUES

2

Biopsy Techniques

Optimization for Collection and Preservation

Marina Saetta and Graziella Turato

1. Introduction

Fiberoptic bronchoscopy provides a good tool to investigate bronchial biopsies, transbronchial biopsies, and bronchoalveolar lavage (BAL) in chronic inflammatory diseases such as asthma and chronic obstructive pulmonary disease (COPD) *(1–8)*. The advantage of bronchial biopsies over other sampling techniques, such as induced sputum or BAL, is that they give anatomical information on airway morphology, therefore allowing the examination of the different compartments of the bronchial wall such as epithelium, subepithelium, smooth muscle, and glands.

Bronchial biopsies can be examined with light microscopy using histochemical and immunohistochemical methods or *in situ* hybridization (ISH). Histochemical methods provide simple and inexpensive staining, which allows identification of some common cell types (e.g., eosinophils, mast cells, goblet cells) *(1)* and of some tissue components (e.g., collagen, smooth muscle) *(2)*. Immunohistochemical methods are used to identify cell types and their subsets, markers of activation, cytokines, adhesion molecules, and a variety of other tissue components of interest *(3)*. ISH has been used to localize messenger ribonucleic acid (mRNA) transcripts *(4)*.

Light microscopic analysis can be performed either directly using an appropriate magnification (400–1000×) or by enlarging the image and transferring it to a screen or monitor and making the assessment with the aid of a computerized image system.

From: *Methods in Molecular Medicine, vol. 56:*
Human Airway Inflammation: Sampling Techniques and Analytical Protocols
Edited by: D. F. Rogers and L. E. Donnelly © Humana Press Inc., Totowa, NJ

Table 1
Advantages and Disadvantages of the Different Techniques
for Processing Bronchial Biopsies for Light Microscopic Analysis[a]

Procedure	Advantages	Disadvantages
Snap-freezing without prior fixation	-immunoreactivity for all antibodies -ISH can be performed	-bad morphology -limited duration of immunoreactivity
Paraformaldehyde fixation and freezing	-good morphology -immunoreactivity for increasing number of antibodies -ISH can be performed	-not all antibodies are reacting
Formalin fixation and paraffin-embedding	-good morphology -immunoreactivity for increasing number of antibodies -ISH can be performed	-not all antibodies are reacting
Fixation and GMA-embedding	-good morphology -very thin sections - immunoreactivity for increasing number of antibodies	-not all antibodies are reacting -expensive instruments for cutting ultrathin sections.

[a]GMA, glycol-methacrylate; ISH, *in situ* hybridization.

There are various methods of processing biopsy samples for light microscopic analysis:

1. Snap-freezing without prior fixation.
2. Paraformaldehyde fixation and freezing.
3. Formalin fixation and paraffin-embedding.
4. Fixation and glycol-methacrylate (GMA)-embedding (*see* **Table 1**).

Bronchial biopsies can also be examined by electron microscopy *(9)*. Although the amount of tissue that can be examined with this technique is very small, electron microscopy allows analysis of cell ultrastructure. This is a crucial analysis, because unequivocal identification of certain cell types (e.g., myofibroblasts) and their degranulation state (e.g., eosinophils) rely on their ultrastructural characteristics.

Bronchial biopsies have also been used for study of polymerase chain reaction (PCR) *(10)* or for cell culture and cell cloning *(11)*.

Although the advent of the flexible fiberoptic bronchoscope has provided a relatively safe method for sampling of the bronchial wall, bronchoscopy still remains an invasive technique. In order to maximize the information derived from each sample, it is essential to ensure that good quality biopsies are obtained. Because the method chosen for the processing of bronchial biopsies needs to be compatible with the specific objective and question of each study, careful planning and agreement of the aims and specific objectives need to be agreed on well before the study commences. The design of the study should be agreed on by all the investigators including the histopathologist, and the number of patients and biopsies should be determined in order to assess the power of the study in the detection of the differences of interest *(12)*.

In this chapter we will describe the procedures for 1) bronchial biopsy collection and 2) bronchial biopsy preservation for light microscopic analysis. In addition, typical procedures to perform immunohistochemical analysis will be shown.

2. Materials

2.1. Snap-Freezing Without Prior Fixation

1. Thermo-flask (nitrogen-proof).
2. Optimum cutter temperature (OCT) compound: e.g., Tissue-Tek (Miles, Elkart, IN, USA).
3. Cork embedding disks.
4. Phosphate buffered saline (PBS) (Sigma P-4417): dissolve 1 PBS tablet in 200 mL distilled water to obtain 0.01 M PBS, pH 7.4 (*see* **Note 1**). PBS can be stored at room temperature for 2–3 d.
5. Isopentane (Aldrich).
6. Liquid nitrogen.

2.2. Paraformaldehyde Fixation and Freezing

All materials listed in **Subheading 2.1.** including PBS. In addition:

1. 2% paraformaldehyde (Sigma P-6148): heat PBS to 58–60°C on a hotplate stirrer, add preweighed paraformaldehyde powder (Sigma P-6148) to the heated PBS (2 g/100 mL) (in fumehood to avoid fumes), and stir for 60–90 min until dissolved. Cool solution and, if necessary, filter. Use the same day or store overnight at 4°C and use the day after (*see* **Note 2**).
2. 15% sucrose/PBS: add. 15 g suncrose (Sigma S9378) and 0.01 g sodium azide (Merck 6688) 15% sucrose for every 100 mL PBS and mix; this mixture can be stored at room temperature for 2 or 3 d.

2.3. Formalin Fixation and Paraffin Embedding

1. PBS. *See* **Subheading 2.1.4.**
2. 10% formalin (approx 4% formaldehyde). Add 100 mL 37% formaldehyde (Sigma F-1635) to 900 mL PBS and mix. 10% formalin can be stored at 4°C.
3. 70% ethanol: add 70-mL absolute ethanol (Sigma) to 30-mL distilled water and mix. 70% ethanol can be stored at room temperature.
4. Ethanol 90%: add 90-mL absolute ethanol (Sigma) to 10-mL distilled water and mix. 90% ethanol can be stored at room temperature.
5. A safety-approved clearing medium, e.g., K Clear (Kaltek).
6. Paraffin wax (Merk).
7. Base tissue molds (Kaltek).
8. Tissue cassettes (Kaltek)

2.4. Fixation and GMA Embedding

1. Acetone (Merk).
2. Phenylmethyl sulfonyl fluoride (Sigma P-7626).
3. Iodoacetamide (Sigma I-6125).
4. Methyl benzoate (Merk 29214 4L).
5. Embedding resin: JB4 embedding kit (Park Scientific 0226), which includes GMA solution A (GMA monomer), GMA solution B, and benzoyl peroxide. GMA solution A is required more often and can be bought separately (Park Scientific 0226A).
6. Embedding capsules (TAAB C094).

3. Methods

3.1. Biopsy Collection

1. Premedicate patients with intravenous atropine (0.5–1 mg) and fentanyl (0.15–0.30 mg).
2. Spray lidocaine solution 2% onto the base of the tongue, pharynx, and nasal passages for topical anesthesia.
3. A flexible bronchoscope is introduced transorally or transnasally with the patient in a supine position and passed through the larynx.
4. Up to 10 mL of 2% lidocaine are instilled through the bronchoscope channel to provide anesthesia for the airways below the vocal cords (*see* **Notes 3–5**).
5. Take one to eight bronchial biopsies through the bronchoscope from the subcarina of a basal segmental bronchus of the right lower lobe (*see* **Notes 6–9**).

3.2. Biopsy Preservation

The biopsies obtained by bronchoscopy should be gently extracted from the forceps and immediately prepared for microscopic analysis. There are various methods of processing biopsy samples:

1. Snap-freezing without prior fixation (*3*).

2. Paraformaldehyde fixation and freezing *(13)*.
3. Formalin fixation and paraffin-embedding *(14)*.
4. Fixation and GMA-embedding *(15,16)*.

   Bronchial biopsies are potentially hazardous human material, and the same precautions as used in handling blood samples must apply before tissue is fixed.

3.2.1. Snap-Freezing Without Prior Fixation

1. Place biopsy in PBS.
2. Cool isopentane in a polypropylene beaker by immersing it in liquid nitrogen kept in a Dewar thermo-flask until the lower aspects and edges appear frozen and white.
3. Label the back of each cork embedding disk with information about the biopsy.
4. Put a drop of OCT compound on the cork to form a base.
5. Place the biopsy on the OCT base with a further covering drop of OCT.
6. Holding the disk with a pair of long forceps, immediately plunge the disk with the OCT-covered biopsy into the liquid nitrogen-cooled isopentane and hold it there until the tissue and medium is frozen (i.e., turns white).
7. Wrap in tin foil (with information about tissue source and so on appended) and store in a well-labeled container at –80°C until use (*see* **Note 10**).

3.2.2. Paraformaldehyde Fixation and Freezing

1. Place biopsy samples in freshly prepared 2% paraformaldehyde for 2 h at 4°C (in this and in the following steps use a 20-mL vial to hold the biopsies) (*see* **Note 11**).
2. Transfer biopsy samples to 15% sucrose/PBS for 1 h at 4°C (*see* **Note 12**).
3. Change into 15% sucrose/PBS overnight at 4°C.
4. Snap-freeze following the procedure described in **Subheading 3.2.1.**
5. This method can be modified for study of gene expression by ISH (*see* **Note 13**).

3.2.3. Formalin Fixation and Paraffin Embedding

1. Melt paraffin wax in a stove at 58°C.
2. Place biopsy samples in 10% formalin for 4 h at 4°C (in this and in the following steps use a 20-mL vial to hold the biopsies).
3. After fixation, dehydrate the biopsies by passing them through a graded series of ethanol (70%, 90%, 100%, 100%, 100%) at room temperature, 15 min each.
4. After dehydration, pass the biopsies in three changes of a safety-approved clearing medium (15 min between changes) at room temperature.
5. Place biopsies in liquid paraffin wax at 58°C for 1 h.
6. Place each biopsy in a tissue base mold containing liquid paraffin, cover with a tissue cassette, add liquid paraffin, and allow to "refresh."
7. Remove paraffin-embedded biopsies from the tissue base mold.
8. Paraffin-embedded biopsies may be stored at room temperature for several years.
9. This method can be modified for study of gene expression by ISH (*see* **Note 13**).

3.2.4. Fixation and GMA Embedding

1. Place biopsies immediately into ice cold acetone containing 2 m*M* phenylmethyl sulfonyl fluoride (35 mg/100 mL) and 20 m*M* iodoacetamide (370 mg/100 mL).
2. Fix overnight at –20°C.
3. Transfer to acetone at room temperature for 15 min.
4. Immerse in methyl benzoate at room temperature for 15 min.
5. Pass in three changes of GMA monomer (GMA solution A) containing 5% methyl benzoate at 4°C, 2 h each.
6. Prepare GMA embedding resin: GMA solution A 10 mL, GMA solution B 250 mL, benzoyl peroxide 45 mg.
7. Embed biopsy in freshly prepared GMA embedding resin in a Taab flat bottomed capsule, placing biopsy in the bottom of the capsule and filling to the brim with resin and closing lid to exclude air.
8. Polymerize overnight at 4°C.
9. Blocks can be stored in airtight container at –20°C.
10. **Steps 4–7** must carried out under a fume extraction hood.

3.3. Advantages and Disadvantages of the Different Methods to Preserve Bronchial Biopsies

Snap-freezing without prior fixation provides samples for immunohistochemical analysis of certain antigen expression, which fixation tends to mask. Moreover, sections obtained from these biopsies, after fixation in freshly prepared paraformaldehyde, can be used for subsequent studies of gene expression by ISH. A disadvantage of snap-freezing without prior fixation is that tissue structure is not well-preserved for morphometric analysis (*see* **Table 1**).

Immediate fixation in freshly prepared paraformaldehyde and subsequent freezing preserves good morphology and facilitates subsequent molecular analysis, but does not allow for immunohistochemical analysis of certain antigens, such as cell-surface adhesion molecules. In addition, fixation in paraformaldehyde has the advantage that these biopsies can also be used for ISH (*see* **Note 13** and **Table 1**).

One advantage of paraffin embedding is that it provides excellent morphology and allows for a preliminary overview of the extent of mucosal inflammation using histochemical methods. A disadvantage of the technique is that it does not allow for extensive cell phenotyping by immunohistochemical means, and many of the required surface epitopes may be masked by the processing of the tissue. During fixation, formalin denatures proteins by reacting primarily with basic amino acids of the epitope to form crosslinking "methylene bridges." Therefore, after formalin fixation, some antigens are masked and cannot be easily demonstrated. Several of these can be revealed after proteolytic digestion with trypsin (*17*), microwaving (*18,19*), or autoclaving (*20*) (*see* **Table 1**).

The advantage of GMA-embedding technique is the relative thinness of the section (1–2 μm), which gives a greater resolution or "clarity" compared with a 5-μm thick section. This is because of the thin section having fewer focal planes through which the light microscope must focus. In addition, thinness allows the possibility of more than one cut through a single cell using adjacent sections. This enables staining of two distinct epitopes on the same cell. In paraffin-embedded sections, "double labeling" techniques can be applied for the same effect, although these procedures are less easy to control (*see* **Table 1**).

3.4. Immunohistochemical Analysis of Bronchial Biopsies

Immunohistochemistry applied to biopsy sections is usually performed using immunoenzymatic-staining methods that give colored end-product reactions. Other methods such as fluorescence can be applied to snap frozen sections, but tissue morphology is not easily visible without phase contrast microscopy. Furthermore, fluorochromes are usually short-lived and should be captured photographically to ensure a record is kept. However, a distinct advantage of the fluorescence technique is in the form of double-labeling methods that can be applied, where red and green fluorochromes may be separately seen using selected filter blocks. By a procedure of photographic double exposures, those cells that are double-labeled appear in a resultant mixture of color (i.e., yellow) *(17)*.

There are a number of immunoenzymatic staining methods that include "direct" and "indirect" immuno-methods. Direct methods are now used only rarely and have been superseded by indirect methods, which include avidin–biotin methods and soluble enzyme immune-complex methods. Both are indirect three-stage methods. In both procedures the first stage utilizes the immunochemical properties of the antibody to combine specifically with the antigen. The unconjugated primary antibody applied to sections in this stage may be polyclonal, generally raised in rabbit, or monoclonal, mainly raised in mouse. There are numerous advantages of monoclonal antibodies in immuno-histochemistry over their polyclonal counterparts. These include high homo-geneity, absence of nonspecific reaction, and negligible lot-to-lot variability. However, the end reaction intensity may be relatively weak compared with polyclonal antibodies. The second stage of the avidin–biotin method comprises an antibody (link antibody) labeled with the vitamin biotin that has been raised against the animal species of the primary antibody. Biotin is used as the label as it has a specific chemical affinity (not immunological) for either avidin, a gly-coprotein of egg white, or streptavidin, a protein isolated from the bacterium *Streptomyces avidii*. The third stage comprises a complex of either avidin or streptavidin labeled with an enzyme-like horseradish peroxidase or alkaline phosphatase that will bind to the biotin of the second stage. These sites are then visualized by reacting with a chromogenic substrate. In the soluble enzyme immune complex methods the general procedure differs from that for avidin–biotin methods in respect of the following:

1. An unconjugated antibody directed against immunoglobulins from the species used for the primary antibody is applied to the sections as the link antibody. The link antibody is added in excess, so one of its two binding sites (Fab sites) remains free.
2. The enzyme immune complex consists of an enzyme (peroxidase or phosphatase) and an antibody directed against the enzyme itself. The antibody of the enzyme immune complex and the primary antibody must be raised in the same species. So that, when the enzyme immune complex is added to the sections, the second free binding site of the link antibody will bind the enzyme immune complex.

For all the immunohistochemical procedures listed above, appropriate positive and negative controls must be included in each staining run. As positive controls, use can be made of tissue sections known to be positive for the antigen under study, for example, tonsil or clones producing specific cytokines or cells transfected with copy deoxyribonucleic acid (cDNA) encoding specific human cytokines. This method can also be implemented to assess the specificity of the primary antibody. To confirm the specificity, use can be made of tissue sections known to be negative for the antigen under study. Affinity absorption of the primary antibody with highly purified antigen provides the ideal negative control for differentiating specific from non-specific staining. As negative controls, use can be made of sections of the tissue under study incubated either without primary monoclonal antibody or with isotype and species-matched irrelevant primary monoclonal antibodies.

4. Notes

1. PBS may be obtained using different procedures. However, it is mandatory to use the same kind of PBS to collect all the samples of the study.
2. 2% paraformaldehyde may be frozen in 20-mL aliquots at –80°C and stored at –80°C until needed.
3. The first studies on airway inflammation in asthma used rigid bronchoscopy. Although rigid bronchoscopy has been performed under local anesthesia, it usually requires general anesthesia, and its use in research has been very limited because of considerable discomfort to the patient. In contrast, fiberoptic bronchoscopy, which can be easily performed under local anesthesia, using premedication with bronchodilators and mild sedation, has been much more acceptable in the clinical and research setting *(21)*.
4. Premedication and sedation vary. Most investigators use premedication with bronchodilators such as salbutamol by metered dose or other inhaler, or nebu-

lizer followed by intravenous atropine, which reduce bronchial secretions and cough during the procedure. Sedation is often used during bronchoscopy in the hope that it will reduce stress level and cough and that it will induce analgesia, euphoria, and amnesia, altering the subject's perception of discomfort. The drugs used include either midazolam or diazemuls intravenously *(22,23)*.

5. Various bronchoscopes have been used, with various biopsy forceps. Some investigators used cupped forceps or alligator forceps. Clearly bigger broncho-scope channels and bigger forceps will give more tissue. Some investigators think that relatively new forceps give better biopsies. It is prudent to have several sets of forceps available at the time of bronchoscopy as this covers the possibility of malfunction *(21)*.

6. Biopsies should be taken under direct bronchoscopic vision from segmental and subsegmental carinae. Studies that have compared different airway levels *(24,25)* did not find differences in immunohistochemistry, so that samples can be pooled. When taking repeated biopsies from the same subject over time, one should avoid previous biopsy sites. Video recording of the procedure may be helpful.

7. Many protocols combine bronchial biopsies with BAL, almost always with BAL performed first. This approach has the advantage of sampling large and small airways, but prior BAL may make biopsies more difficult to obtain (in the face of residual lavage fluid or local bronchospasm associated with BAL).

8. Fiberoptic bronchoscopy in association with endobronchial biopsies is usually well tolerated and does not induce significant long-term clinical sequelae. Caution has been exercised when performing bronchoscopy in asthmatic subjects because of concern about its safety in patients with hyperresponsive airways. However, several studies have reported that fiberoptic bronchoscopy can be conducted safely in asthma although caution must be exercised in those with very responsive airways because of the possibility of bronchoconstriction *(21)*.

9. It is essential that skilled bronchoscopists carry out research bronchoscopies to expedite the procedure and, if severe patients are to be studied, this should be performed in centers with considerable experience. Resuscitation equipment (for intubation, electrocardiographic monitoring, and defibrillation) together with necessary drugs (salbutamol, adrenaline, hydrocortisone) should be available, and the subject should have an existing cannula. The procedure should be preferably in a facility dedicated to bronchoscopy *(23)*.

10. The freezing procedure itself is a knack that once learned is not difficult. However, it must be taught and practiced in order to avoid the common (and often published) artifact of ice-crystal damage. The result of such damage is a peppering of the tissue with artifactual spaces that do not allow adequate and reliable quantification of inflammatory cells. The importance of good quality starting material and fast freezing rates cannot be overemphasized for successful results.

11. Some investigators use 4% paraformaldehyde to fix bronchial biopsies.

12. Prior soaking of the tissue in cryoprotectants such as 15% sucrose buffer can help to prevent ice-crystal formation during the freezing procedure. 0.01% sodium azide should be added to inhibit bacterial contamination and growth.

13. This method can be modified to collect bronchial biopsies for study of gene expression by ISH. Modifications are necessary to prevent RNAse contamination and include:

    i. Gloves must be worn during the handling of the reagents. Glassware used for preparation of solutions must be backed at 200°C for 2 h. Disposable weighing boats and baked lab weighing spoons must be used.

    ii. Distilled water should be replaced with diethyl pyrocarbonate (DEPC)-treated water obtained as follows:

        a. Add 2-mL DEPC, (Sigma D-5758) to every 2000 mL of double distilled water and let the solution stir for a minimum of 2 h in a fumehood.

        b. Pour the solution in DEPC labeled bottles and autoclave for 25 min in order to destroy the DEPC.

References

1. Saetta, M., Maestrelli, P., Di Stefano, A., De Marzo, N., Milani, G. F., Pivirotto, F., Mapp, C. E., and Fabbri, L. M . (1992) Effect of cessation of exposure to toluene diisocyanate (TDI) on bronchial mucosa of subjects with TDI-induced asthma. *Am. Rev. Respir. Dis.* **145,** 169–174.
2. Chu, H. W., Halliday, J. L., Martin, R. J., Leung, D. Y.M., Szefler, S. J., and Wenzel, S.E. (1998) Collagen deposition in large airways may not differentiate severe asthma from milder forms of the disease. *Am. J. Respir. Crit. Care Med.* **158,** 1936–1944.
3. Di Stefano, A., Maestrelli, P., Roggeri, A., Turato, G., Calabro, S., Potena, A., Mapp, C.E., Ciaccia, A., Covacev, L., Fabbri, L.M., and Saetta, M. (1994) Upregulation of adhesion molecules in the bronchial mucosa of subjects with chronic obstructive bronchitis. *Am. J. Respir. Crit. Care Med.* **149,** 803–810.
4. Hamid, Q., Azzawi, M., Sun, Ying, et al. (1991) Expression of mRNA for Il-5 in mucosal bronchial biopsies from asthma. *J. Clin. Invest.* **87,** 1541–1546.
5. Lacoste, J.Y., Bousquet, J., Chanez, P., Van Vyve, T., Simony-Lafontaine, J., Lequeu, N., et al. (1993) Eosinophilic and neutrophilic inflammation in asthma , chronic bronchitis and chronic obstructive pulmonary disease. *J. Allergy Clin. Immunol* **92,** 537–548.
6. Bradding, P., Roberts, J. A., Britten, K. M., Montefort, S., Djukanovic, R., Mueller, R., et al. (1994) Interleukin-4,-5, and -6 and tumor necrosis factor-a in normal and asthmatic airways: evidence for the human mast cell as a source of these cytokines. *Am. J. Respir. Cell Mol. Biol.* **10,** 471–480.
7. Wenzel, S. E., Szefler, S. J., Leung, D. Y. M., Sloan, S. I., Rex, M. D., and Martin, R. J. (1997) Bronchoscopic evaluation of severe asthma. *Am. J. Respir. Crit. Care Med.* **156,** 737–743.
8. Kraft, M., Djukanovich, R., Torvik, J., et al. (1995) Evaluation of airway inflammation by endobronchial and transbronchial biopsy in nocturnal and non-nocturnal asthma. *Chest* **107,** 162S.
9. Laitinen, L.A., Laitinen, A., and Haahtela, T. 1993. Airway mucosal inflammation even in patients with newly diagnosed asthma. *Am. Rev. Respir. Dis.* **147,** 697–704.

10. Frew, A. J., Li, D., Jeffery, P. K. (1998) In situ hybridization and the polymerase chain reaction. *Eur. Respir. J.* **11,** 30S–32S.
11. Maestrelli, P., Del Prete, G. F., De Carli, M. (1994) CD8 T-cell clones producing interleukin-5 and interferon –gamma in bronchial mucosa of patients with asthma induced by toluene diisocyanate. *Scand. J. Work Environ. Health* **20,** 376–381.
12. Saetta, M., Jeffery, P. K., Maestrelli, P., Timens, W. (1998) Biopsies: processing and assessment. *Eur. Respir. J.* **11,** 20S–25S
13. O'Shaughnessy, Ansari, T. W., Barnes, N. C., and Jeffery, P. K.(1997) Inflammation in bronchial biopsies of subjects with chronic bronchitis: inverse relationship of CD8+ T lymphocytes with FEV$_1$. *Am. J. Respir. Crit. Care. Med.* **155,** 852–857.
14. Di Stefano, A., Turato, G., Maestrell,i P., Mapp, C. E., Ruggieri, M. P., Roggeri, A., et al. (1996) Airflow limitation in chronic bronchitis is associated with T-lymphocyte and macrophage infiltration of the bronchial mucosa. *Am. J. Respir. Crit. Care. Med.* **153,** 629–632.
15. Britten, K. M., Howarth, P. H., and Roche, W. R. (1993) Immunohistochemistry on resin sections: a comparison of resin embedding techniques for small mucosal biopsies. *Biotechnic. and Histochemistry* **68,** 271–279.
16. Wenzel, S. E., Schwartz, L. B., Langmack, E. L., Halliday, J. L., Trudeau, J. B., Gibbs, R. L., and Chu, H. W. (1999) Evidence that severe asthma can be divided pathologically into two inflammatory subtypes with distinct physiologic and clinical characteristics. *Am. J. Respir. Crit. Care. Med.* **160,** 1001–1008.
17. Huang, S., Minassian, H., and More, J. D. (1976) Application of immunofluorescent staining improved by trypsin digestion. *Laboratory Investigation* **35,** 383–391.
18. Shi. S., Key, M., and Kalra, K. (1991) Antigen Retrieval in formalin fixed, paraffin embedded tissues; an enhancement method for immunohistochemical staining based on microwave oven heating of tissue sections. *J. Histochem. Cytochem.* **39,** 741–748.
19. Arleen, E., Hollema, H., Suurmeyer, A., Koudstaal, J. (1994) A modified method for antigen retrieval MIB-1 staining of valvular carcinoma. *Eur. J. Morphol.* **32,** 335S–336S.
20. Arleen, E., Hollema, H., and Koudstaal, J. (1994) Autoclave heating: an alternative method for microwaving. *Eur. J. Morphol.* **32,** 337S–340S.
21. Djukanovic, R., Wilson, J. W., Lai, C. K. W., Holgate, S. T., and Howarth, P. H. (1991) The safety aspects of fiberoptic bronchoscopy, bronchoalveolar lavage and endobronchial biopsy in asthma. *Am. Rev. Respir. Dis.* **143,** 772–777.
22. Robinson, D. S., Faurschou, P., Barnes, N., and Adelroth, E. (1998) Biopsies: bronchoscopic technique and sampling. *Eur. Respir. J.* **11,** 16S–19S.
23. Djukanovic, R., Dahl, R., Jarjour, N., and Aalbers, R. (1998) Safety of biopsies and bronchoalveolar lavage. *Eur. Respir. J.* **11,** 39S–41S.
24. Jeffery, P. K., Wardlaw, A. J., Nelson, F. C., Collins, J. V., and Kay, A. B. (1989) Bronchial biopsies in asthma: an ultrastructural, quantitative study and correlation with hyperreactivity. *Am. Rev. Respir. Dis.* **140,** 1745–1753.
25. Bradley, B. L., Azzawi, M., Jacbson, M., et al. (1991) Eosinophils, T-lymphocytes, mast cells, neutrophils and macrophages in bronchial biopsy specimens from atopic subjects with asthma. *J. Allergy. Clin. Immunol.* **88,** 661–674.

3

Bronchoalveolar Lavage (BAL)

Critical Evaluation of Techniques

Chris Ward and E. Haydn Walters

1. Introduction

In the late 19th century, the rigid bronchoscope was pioneered by Chevalier Jackson and employed for the performance of bronchial lavage to wash purulent secretions from the airways of subjects with bronchiectasis in order to achieve symptomatic relief *(1,2)*. The impetus of this work was rapidly advanced in the late 1960s by the development of fiberoptic technology and its application in the flexible fiberoptic bronchoscope by Ikeda *(3)*. This instrument transformed the ease and convenience of bronchoscopy, opened it up for research procedures even in volunteers, and allowed development of novel sampling methods, including bronchoalveolar lavage (BAL).

During bronchoscopy, a fiberoptic scope is passed into a subsegmental airway until it is "wedged" (i.e., it tightly fits and seals off the distal segment). A known amount of saline is instilled, via the suction channel of the bronchoscope, into the intubated subsegment of the tracheobronchial tree and is subsequently aspirated. The technique is a safe means of directly sampling cells, pathogens, and solutes from the human lung in health and disease. The reported complication rate attributed to BAL is less than 5% with the large majority of these complications being minor (i.e., mainly mild, transient fever, requiring no treatment *(4)*). The study of cellular and soluble mediators in BAL is used both in clinical practice and in medical research and has made significant contributions to both areas of medicine *(4–7)*. More rarely, large volume BAL is also used therapeutically, most particularly in alveolar proteinosis *(8)*, but also experimentally in other conditions such as silicosis *(9)*.

From: *Methods in Molecular Medicine, vol. 56:*
Human Airway Inflammation: Sampling Techniques and Analytical Protocols
Edited by: D. F. Rogers and L. E. Donnelly © Humana Press Inc., Totowa, NJ

BAL is useful diagnostically in assessment of lower respiratory infections and has been particularly useful in immunocompromised patients *(10)*. The technique is also used clinically in oncology and especially in the diagnosis of peripheral lung cancer *(11)*. The use of BAL in diagnosing infection or cancer will not be discussed further in this chapter, and is extensively covered elsewhere (e.g., European Respiratory Monograph: Pulmonary Endoscopy and Biopsy Techniques. Strausz, J. Ed. Munksgaard, Copenhagen, Denmark, or on the Internet, http://bioscience.org/1998/v3/e/baughman/e1-12.htm reviews the role of BAL in diagnosing infection). The focus of this chapter is the description of the sampling methods used in the assessment of cells and solutes relevant to the study of "airway and lung inflammation".

Despite the established significance of the BAL technique, there is an increasing recognition that in order for BAL to realize its true potential, both in the clinical and research setting, there needs to be greater standardization of some basic methodological issues *(12)*. This is a necessary prerequisite to the effective use of BAL in individual centers, as well as comparison of results between laboratories. To facilitate this, it is important that journal editors insist on the inclusion of the precise details of how BAL was performed and how the products were processed and analyzed. Unfortunately, this is frequently not the case.

BAL and biopsy techniques should not be regarded as alternative or rival procedures, but as complementary to each other. They frequently provide quite a different picture and perspective on a condition. Ideally, both BAL and biopsy methods should be done in bronchoscopic research studies *(5)* (*see* **Notes 1–4**).

A successful BAL requires a technically adequate clinical procedure, which then has to be quantified for cellular indices/analytes of interest. The end result of the BAL and the usefulness of information that is gained are affected by variables at both the clinical and laboratory ends of the procedure. Details that require standardization are often basic, but nonetheless fundamental. Hence the results of a procedure will be compromised if the instilled BAL volume is not standardized, no matter how sophisticated and standardized the subsequent laboratory procedures. Similarly, basic information such as the differential cell count is a function of both how the estimation is performed and BAL is obtained, as well as any "real" clinical or experimental characteristic.

The advent and subsequent widespread use of the fiberoptic bronchoscope made BAL simple and safe to perform. It also represented an opportunity to adopt a standard technique for its performance, which would have advantages for the comparison of results from different centers. Unfortunately, considerable variation in procedural technique across centers developed, making comparison of data problematical (*see* **Notes 5** and **6**). The volume of fluid instilled even for similar research purposes has varied considerably from 20 mL *(13)* to 300 mL *(14)*, and the site of BAL has also varied from major bronchi *(15)* to subsegmental airways *(16)*. In addition, the volume, strength *(17)* and route *(18)* of local anesthesia has also varied considerably, despite evidence that shows that the instilled anesthetic is potentially cytotoxic to the sample recovered at BAL as well as being potentially dangerous to the subject. Thus, it should be noted that methodological practice also has important implications for the safety of the overall bronchoscopic procedure (*see* **Notes 7–11**).

2. Materials

2.1. Reagents

UK details are given. Internet contacts are included where possible, to allow sourcing of suppliers in other countries.

1. Glass Tissue culture bottles (e.g., Schott): British Drug Houses (BDH) Ltd, Poole, Dorset, UK (http://www.bdh.com) or Sigma, Poole, Dorset, U.K (http://www.sigma.sial.com).
2. Sterile phosphate buffered saline (PBS) for BAL: Should be prepared by a hospital pharmacy department, who can validate its suitability for human procedures. An alternative is normal physiological saline, buffered with sodium bicarbonate.
3. Filtration: 200 μm^2 stainless steel mesh: George Bopp and Co., London, U.K.
4. Neubauer counting chamber (BDH).
5. Trypan blue (Sigma).
6. Acridine orange/ethidium bromide (Sigma): Dissolve 15 mg acridine orange and 50 mg ethidium bromide in 1 mL 95% (v/v) ethanol (BDH), made to 50 mL in water. Freeze as 1 mL aliquots. Dilute 1:100 for use, and store for 1 month in brown bottle.
7. PBS tablets (Sigma).
8. Diff Quik reagent: Australian Laboratory Supply, Victoria, Australia (or BDH).
9. Carnoys fluid: 10 mL glacial acetic acid (BDH), 60 mL 100% ethyl alcohol (BDH), 30 mL chloroform (BDH).
10. Toluidine blue (for staining mast cells): 0.3% in 3% acetic acid (Sigma).
11. Lysing reagents: Ortho mune lysing solution (Johnson and Johnson, Ortho-Diagnostic Co, NJ USA).
12. Virkon biocidal disinfectant: Antec International, Sudbury, Suffolk, UK (http://www.antec.org/hh/)

2.2. Apparatus

1. Cytocentrifuge; Shandon cytospin III, Shandon, Astmoor, Runcorn, Cheshire UK (http://www.shandon.com).
2. Polypropylene 50-mL tubes, Sarstedt Ltd, Beaumont Leys Leicester UK. (http://www.sarstedt.com).
3. Cryotubes; Sarstedt.

3. Methods

A successful BAL analysis depends upon the interface between a technically adequate clinical procedure and subsequent laboratory processing. Even though a BAL may be regarded as a straightforward procedure, the bronchoscopist must be experienced, and accredited to perform the task. Two attending clinicians should be available for the procedure where practicable. Because the technical aspects of the bronchoscopy and BAL procedure are at least as important as the subsequent laboratory process some guideline notes are given relating to the clinical part of the procedure. The following is a guide only, based on reviewing current practice. Precise details of clinical procedures may vary according to circumstances and it is up to the clinicians responsible for the medical procedure to satisfy themselves that appropriate, safe procedures are followed. It is the responsibility of the supervising physician to consider a risk/benefit assessment. In general BAL might be considered inappropriate in patients with severely compromised lung function (e.g., FEV_1 <1.5 L) (*see* **Note 7**).

The minimum sample requirements for BAL are:

1. Analyses performed on the pooled return from a 180mL BAL would be consistent with obtaining "alveolar" return (*see* **Notes 12** and **13**). Splitting or discarding aliquots (e.g., for "airway" vs "peripheral wash") is not generally recommended. This practice complicates matters and is predicated on a number of assumptions for which evidence is rather poor (*see* **Note 13**).
2. Preferably >33% of instilled volume should be required to be aspirated as a minimally satisfactory procedure. One should usually obtain >50% of the instilled volume in the return in most circumstances, apart from significantly obstructed patients.

3.1. Preparation of the Subject

1. Subjects should be asked to give consent specifically for BAL.
2. Lung function results should be available. Record patient's smoking habits.
3. Absence of respiratory infection >4 weeks prior to bronchoscopy (with the obvious exception of instances where current infection is the indication for this procedure) (*see* **Note 14**).
4. Subjects should be "nil by mouth" 10 h before procedure.
5. Premedication: atropine 0.6 mg and diazepam 10–20mg IV, 15 min before procedure (or equivalent sedation). If deeper sedation is required, an anesthetist should be present.
6. Apply lignocaine spray (4%) to oropharynx and nose.
7. β_2-agonist (e.g., salbutamol) inhalation 15 min before if asthma present or suspected.
8. Lignocaine 4% sterile solution is used for local anesthesia above the vocal chords.

9. Below the chords 2% lignocaine sterile solution in 2-mL aliquots instilled during procedure via the biopsy channel of bronchoscope (we use an upper limit of 16 mL × 2% lignocaine; the maximal safe systemic plasma level of lignocaine is <5mg/L or 22μmol/L *(19)* and total dose given into the airways must not exceed 400 mg *[18]*).
10. Perform routine endobronchial examination before lavage.
11. Oxygen at 4 L/min during procedure and for at least 60 min after (via nasal cannulae).
12. Monitor electrocardiogram (ECG) and arterial oxygen saturation with pulse oximetry.

3.2. Bronchoscopy

1. Wedge bronchoscope firmly in subsegment (*see* **Note 15**). In general, the middle lobe is standard as it provides good access and ease of wedging.
2. Attach a large sputum trap in the form of a siliconised glass bottle (e.g., 250-mL tissue culture Schott bottle), in series with the bronchoscope aspiration channel and vacuum source.
3. Instill 60 mL sterile phosphate buffered saline (prewarmed to 37°C) using steady hand pressure on the syringe applied by the operator.
4. Immediately apply suction until fluid return ceases. Reduce suction pressure to the minimum that is consistent with steady, visible BAL return (*see* **Note 16**). Standardize to 50–80 mmHg negative aspiration pressure. The use of an adjustable vacuum source (e.g., compressor pump), which can be set to the required aspiration pressure, is recommended.
5. The operator watches down the scope to ensure that the wedge is maintained. If possible the return should come back in an unbroken stream, with a steady aspiration rather than a "pulsatile" suction applied by the operator. The return volume from the first aspirate will be less than for the second and third. A graduated bottle helps the operator to keep track of returns.
6. After completion of the aspiration, which may take up to 3 min, do not "blindly aspirate" with the suction. The BAL should all be in the context of a good wedge. A measured and steady approach to aspiration will optimize returns.
7. Repeat the above with two further aliquots of 60-mL saline.
8. The sample should be sent directly for laboratory processing. Preferably, the scientist responsible for subsequent BAL processing should collect the sample immediately after the procedure. The sample should be processed as soon as possible and stored at 4°C for no longer than 4 h. Long-term storage is not appropriate for unprocessed BAL.

3.3. Processing of the BAL Sample

Any work involving the use of biological samples should be performed in a Class II laminar flow hood where practicable. All liquid waste is disposed of into an appropriate biocidal agent (e.g., Virkon) and sluiced down a designated laboratory sink. Solid waste is disposed of in the appropriate waste bins, and "sharps" including pipet tips in a standard sharps box. Although the technique of BAL is widely used to investigate the pathophysiology of lung disease, there is a lack of consensus regarding BAL processing, including basic analytical methodology, such as the most accurate method of producing the widely quoted BAL differential cell count. Differences in techniques used for BAL procedures and subsequent processing are probably a major potential obstacle to the universal acceptance of BAL as a clinical and research tool, and more importantly confound the comparison of results between centers (*see* **Note 5**). This limits the generalization of data. The following suggestions regarding BAL processing methods are evidence-based as far as possible, and also stem from our specific practical experiences and formal, published evaluation work:

1. Any processing (filtration, cell washing/centrifugation) will alter the total and differential cell counts. This effect can be profound (*see* **Notes 17** and **18**). This protocol is, therefore, based around generating total and differential cell counts on cells that have not been processed (i.e., "raw" BAL aspirate). This is a practicable working protocol and should be feasible in most (>90%) specimens. An obvious exception is when the technical quality of the clinical BAL specimen is inadequate (e.g., where a central airway wash, or overt bleeding has occurred). As already stated, good BAL data are a product of a technically adequate clinical procedure and follow-up by a laboratory with the necessary technical expertise and infrastructure and consistently poor BAL specimens might indicate a requirement to improve this vital interface, as well as the technical expertise at both ends of the procedural process.

2. Individual priorities and specific requirements may mean that this protocol is changed to suit specific circumstances (e.g., cell function or culture studies may require the rapid washing and resuspension of cells in specific media).

   a. The scientist responsible for subsequent BAL processing should ideally collect the sample immediately after the procedure. This individual can provide continuity and quality control for the procedure, which may be especially useful if the clinician is junior, or not part of a designated research team. If the sample is delivered through "routine" hospital means there is a strong possibility of sample processing being delayed and compromised.

   b. Note BAL identification information and demographic details on results form, which should also be used for primary data such as return volumes and cell counts. Record patient's smoking history. Anything else relevant, which might assist in the subsequent follow-up of data, should be included. This may seem an obvious step, but is frequently poorly performed and can cause a great deal of wasted effort later on.

   c. Measure BAL return with an appropriate sized polyethylene or polycarbonate measuring cylinder. Note this on the results form that has accompanied the BAL sample to the laboratory for performance of a total cell count (*see* **Subheading 3.4.**).

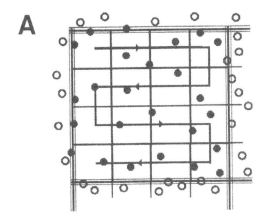

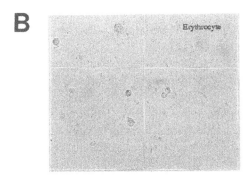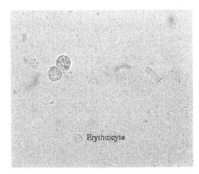

Fig. 1. Counting BAL cells using a Neubauer chamber. (**A**) A diagrammatic view of one of the four outer squares of the chamber is shown. The filled circles represent the cells that would be included in the count (i.e. 25 cells). (**B**) The realities of performing a BAL total cell count in a stable lung transplant recipient. The first image (Dage 3 chip video camera, Image Pro Plus analysis software) is taken using a 20X objective. The second uses a 40X objective. In the latter image three BAL cells can clearly be differentiated from erythrocytes/debris. Red blood cells appear reddish, have no nucleus, are sensitive to osmotic challenge, and have the classic "doughnut" appearance when the operator varies the plane of focus. Accurate BAL cell counts require experience with the use of an adequate microscope objective (at least 40X), especially important.

d. The remainder of the BAL sample is passed through a 200-μM gauze filter to remove coarse contaminants and mucus.

e. Decant filtrate into appropriate number of polypropylene 50 mL tubes.

f. Centrifuge for 15 min at 42g and 4°C.

g. Decant and retain supernatant and aliquot into 20 × 1.8 mL cryotubes (*see* **Subheading 3.7.**).

h. Store cryotubes at –80°C. Fill out the details in the freezer and sample log.

    i. Resuspend BAL cell pellet in PBS or preferred cell medium (dependent on what subsequent work is required, e.g., *see* Chapter 16).

3.4. BAL Total Cell Counts (Tcc) (see Fig. 1)

The Neubauer counting chamber is a quick and relatively simple means of performing a total cell count that can also be used for cell viability determinations. In setting up a preparation care should be taken that the chamber is not overfilled and a fine transfer pipet or micropipet should be used. Overfilling will result if the side channels fill up.

1. Fill the chamber carefully with ~15 µL undiluted BAL aspirate, using a 1–20 µL pipet.
2. Counting should be performed using at least a 40X objective lens. At least 100 cells need to be counted which should be achievable by counting the four large outer squares of the counting chamber. The Tcc should be performed in duplicate, with repeat counts if there is undue (>15%) variation.
3. The count should be performed in duplicate, at least.
4. A simple rule when working out the Tcc from a Neubauer counting chamber is that if 100 cells were counted in one of the large outer quadrants, this would indicate a count of 1×10^6/mL or 1×10^9/L in the BAL aspirate. Hence, if a total of 120 were counted in the four chambers then the BAL cell count would be 3×10^5/mL (0.3×10^6/mL). This arithmetic for the Tcc may vary depending on the type of counting chamber used, and this needs to be specifically checked.

3.5. Scoring of Cell Viability

3.5.1. Trypan Blue Method

1. Mix an aliquot of cells with an equal volume of 0.2% trypan blue (Sigma) and incubate at 37°C for 3 min (the plasma membrane of an intact cell does not allow uptake of the dye; hence dead cells are denoted by dye uptake).
2. Scoring is performed using a Neubauer counting chamber, as above in **Subheading 3.4.**, under bright field or phase contrast illumination.

3.5.2. Acridine Orange/Ethidium Bromide Method

This is preferable to trypan blue but requires access to a fluorescence microscope.

1. Mix a 250 µL aliquot of cells with 250 µL of solution of acridine orange/ethidium bromide.
2. Cells are scored under dim brightfield illumination using a Neubauer counting chamber and then under mercury lamp illumination visualized through a 495 nm primary and 515 nm secondary filter (live cells fluoresce green with acridine orange and dead cells can be positively identified by orange fluorescence with ethidium bromide).

Following the Tcc/viability estimation the BAL cells are aliquoted appropriately, depending upon subsequent analysis. For example:

1. 1×20–30-mL aliquot, depending on the cell count for RNA/DNA archival (e.g., we use such a sample in reverse transcriptase polymerase chain reaction (RT-PCR) determinations of cytokine mRNA and quantification of DNA viral load). Centrifuge for 15 min at $42g$ at 4°C. Decant supernatant and snap-freeze the cell pellet in liquid nitrogen.
2. 1×6 mL of unprocessed ("Pre") BAL aspirate is required for basic cytological assessment: 0.8 mL for cytospins. ($4 \times 200\mu$L spots); 0.2 mL for Neubauer counts and viability estimation; 5 mL for stored cytospin preparations.

3.6. Differential Cell Counts

The preparation of a differential cell count is a deceptively simple undertaking and there is controversy about whether the widely used cytospin is an optimal method (*see* **Notes 19–21**). The cytospin can give a differential count that is acceptable and basically this method has gained the most favor and is likely to be the most frequently used method in the foreseeable future. It is particularly unfortunate, however, that cytospin differentials continue to be confounded by simple, well-described artefacts (*see* **Note 20**). In particular, adequate spin speeds, use of an unmodified aspirate in making slides, as well as good basic staining and counting practice are important when making an accurate differential cell count.

3.6.1. Cytospin Slide Preparation and Storage

1. To save time, clearly label slides before brochoscopy.
2. With the cytospin slide clip opened, fit labeled glass slide, filter card, and sample chamber against the cytoclip slide clip (*see* **Fig. 2**). Secure in place (two retaining hooks on Cytospin III). Assemble six slide clips to make slides for differential cell counts.
3. Carefully pipet 200 µL unfiltered aspirate from a 3x60 mL BAL into the bottom of the sample chambers (Tcc above 5×10^5/ mL may need dilution or less raw BAL fluid).
4. The cytocentrifuge should be programmed for a spin speed of 850 rpm (81.57 g) for 2 min (*see* **Note 20**).
5. Air-dry the slides and stain with Diff Quik reagent. Use of the alternative May Grunwald Giemsa stain (BDH Ltd.) aids differentiation of neutrophils and eosinophils (bright orange cytoplasmic granules: *see* **Fig. 3**).
6. Slides should be coverslipped using a permanent mounting medium (e.g., crystal mount).
7. The remaining slides should be used for any further cytological staining required (e.g., fixation in Carnoys fluid followed by toluidine blue staining for 10 s for identification of metachromatic mast cells).

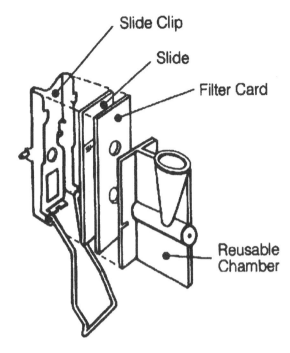

Fig. 2. Schematic diagram of a cytospin slide clip, assembled with a microscope slide, cytospin filter card, and cytospin sample chamber.

8. Following the preparation of slides for differential cell counts, it is convenient to make 12 double cytospin spots as above in **Subheading 3.6.1., steps 2–4,** for storage. For this procedure the slide and filter need to be carefully taken out of the holder and turned around by 180°. Slides should be wrapped in pairs, back-to-back, in labeled foil packets and stored at −80°C. Fill out freezer log and store in an organized archive.

3.6.2. Scoring Differential Cell Counts

Differential cell counts and cytological scoring should be performed by an experienced observer (*see* **Note 22,** and **Figs. 3** and **4**). Five hundred cells should be counted, with duplicate counts performed. For mast cells, an estimated 5000 cells should be assessed using a field scanning technique: i.e., calculate number of cells in an average high power field (hpf; using a 40X objective lens) by counting the number of cells in at least 10 hpfs and calculating the mean. Assess the number of hpf that are consistent with sampling an estimated 5000 cells for mast cell staining (i.e., 5000/mean cell number in hpf= the number of hpf that need to be surveyed).

3.7. Measurement of BAL Solutes

Measurements of solutes in BAL supernatants represent a valuable strategy for quantitative research (*see* **Table 1**). Analyses that are now possible range

Table 1
Expected Values of BAL Solutes in Healthy Never Smokers

Variable	Mean ± SEM	5th Centile [†]	95th Centile [‡]
IgG, μg/mL**	5.9 ± 0.5	1.6	14.5
IgA, μg/mL**	6.2 ± 0.6	1.1	15.3
IgM, μg/mL**	0.2 ± 0.02	0.03	0.6
Albumin, μg/mL**	34.2 ± 1.7	15.7	59.3
Total protein, μg/mL**	78.2 ± 4.0	39.5	140.7

** 240 mL lavage fluid instilled, † 5th Centile of the study population
‡ 95th Centile of the study population.
(Adapted after *6*).

from simple protein determinations (e.g., BAL albumin), through to measurement of cytokines and parameters of oxidative stress *(9)*. Direct assays on raw BAL supernatants are preferable to assays that require concentration steps, which can cause artefacts at a number of levels. If concentration is necessary then particular attention should be made to validating methods with regard to sample recovery and possible matrix effects (e.g., the affect of any increase in salt concentrations on the assay).

Direct assays on unconcentrated BAL supernatants are increasingly practicable with the very sensitive detection systems that are now routinely available (e.g., chemiluminescent, enzyme-linked immunosorbent assay (ELISA) systems allowing detection of pg concentrations of cytokines). The usefulness of such measurements are again absolutely dependent on the correctness of the clinical parts of the procedure (e.g., standardized and uniform instilled volumes are especially important). Several aliquots of BAL supernatant should be stored for subsequent solute measurements (*see* **Subheading 3.3, step g**) and archival details promptly filled out in the freezer and sample log.

The major problem with measuring solutes in BAL fluid is that there is currently no acceptable "denominator" of dilution which takes into account the complex and variable dilution factors that are inherent to the sampling method (*see* **Notes 23** and **24**). In particular the measurement of epithelial lining fluid (ELF) volume by the so called "urea method" should not be used *(12)* (*see* **Note 25**). BAL solutes are best represented per mL of BAL aspirate or per total return, determinants which at least make few unfounded presumptions.

4. Notes

1. BAL and biopsy techniques should be regarded as complementary to each other *(5)*. Ideally, both BAL and biopsy methods should be used in bronchoscopic

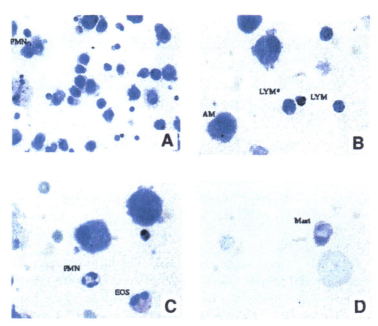

Fig. 3. BAL cytospins captured using Image Pro Plus image analysis software with brief "cell recognition notes" , to facilitate cell identification. Alveolar macrophages (AM) are present in a broad range of sizes from small monocyte-like cells to large mature macrophages (*see* **panels a and b**). Nuclei are indented, convoluted or oval in shape, with chromatin being less dense than in lymphocytes. The AM cytoplasm contains vacuoles and has a characteristic foamy and opaque appearance. Lymphocytes (LYM) also vary widely in their size and appearance (*see* **panel b**), with the overlap in appearance between a large activated T lymphocyte and a small monocyte-like AM representing a particular problem for observers. Small lymphoctes are characterized by small round nuclei, dense chromatin and scant cytopasm. Cytoplasm can appear as a crescent especially in larger lymphocytes where the nucleus is often eccentrically placed, with pale granules present in the perinuclear area of the cell. Remaining cytoplasm is characteristically transparent. Neutrophils (PMN) are recognizable by the distinct lobulations of the nucleas with most having 3 or 4 lobes (*see* **panel c**). Lobulation increases with the age of the cell. The cytoplasm is transparent and contains granules. Eosinophils (EOS) are identified by intense eosinophilic granule staining in the cytoplasm (*see* **panel c**). The nucleus usually has a distinct bi-lobed appearance. Airway epithelial cells (particularly ciliated columnar cells) are very easy to score. Some observers do not include these cells in differentials, but given that epithelial shedding may be a part of a pathology under investigation this would seem to be paradoxical and we believe that this information should be part of the differential cell count. **Mast cells**: Mast cells are rare (<0.5% in most BALs) and need to be identified through specific staining methods following appropriate fixation, since these cells exhibit differential sensitivity to fixatives. A standard method is metachromatic staining of the mast cell with toluidine blue on cells fixed in Carnoys fluid (*see* **panel d**; Mast).

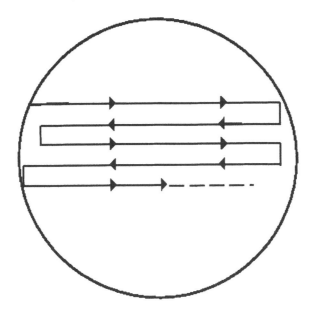

Fig. 4. Suggested pattern for evaluating a differential cell count on a cytospin preparation that ensures that cells are not counted on multiple occasions. At least 500 cells should be counted on duplicate cytospins, using at least a 40X objective lens (typically 400X final magnification, assuming 10X eyepieces).

research studies. Insufficient work has been done to adequately compare and contrast the cell data obtained from biopsy samples and BAL and more extended comparative studies are needed.

2. When BAL and endobronchial biopsies have been compared in asthma, the "signal" of disease activity (e.g., increase in eosinophil number) was much the same, but with some distinct differences *(5,20)*, e.g., endobronchial biopsies are small in size (~2 mm^3), and are limited to sampling the central airways. Consequently, they have the potential problem of sampling bias. Furthermore, there is a significant chance of damage in collection or processing. BAL on the other hand, has the potential to sample from a large epithelial surface area within the bronchopulmonary segment, including large, medium, and small airways. Large numbers of cells (10–20 million) are obtained in suspension in a conventional full BAL procedure, and these can be cultured or investigated for activity, and the supernatant fluid can be studied for solute content. The precise origin of the BAL sample cannot be defined, however, unlike biopsies, which are taken with direct visualization.

3. We have published data comparing the results of BAL, endobronchial biopsy (EBB), and transbronchial lung biopsy (TBB) in 18 lung transplant recipients. BAL gave strong signals and allowed quantitative assessment of inflammation *(21)*. Our results also indicated a possible role for EBB in surveillance bronchoscopies of lung allograft recipients, which proved especially suitable for reliably sampling inflamed large airways in the transplant recipients, with inflammatory

cells present in all samples. In contrast TBB gave information about parenchymal lung tissue and small airways but airway material could only be evaluated in 78% of the samples and inflammation, if present, could only be estimated semiquantitatively. These results underline the fact that BAL can be used in assessment of airway as well as lung parenchymal pathologies, and gives valuable information that can be better than, and complementary to, endobronchial or transbronchial biopsy.

4. Sample size: we found that the reproducibility of cellular data obtained from stable asthma patients using BAL and endobronchial biopsies is comparable (*22,23*). Such data is necessary to calculate the "power" of drug studies in asthma which involve assessment of changes in pathology and suggest that an adequate parallel group study in asthma should include 12—15 patients in each limb. It is of interest that a number of BAL studies have used substantially smaller numbers than these and lack of power in studies may be a reason for equivocal findings in the literature (*24*), which may reflect "Type II" statistical errors.

5. We have recently undertaken a questionnaire survey of active BAL centers regarding their current practice (*see* **Table 2**). This was carried out under the auspices of the European Respiratory Society (ERS) BAL task force, which has been charged with investigating standardization issues (*12*). These are not yet fully published, but selected results are worth considering. In 1998 we surveyed BAL researchers in Europe, USA, and Australia, based on a database held by the ERS BAL task force. The questionnaire was developed by our center, but in collaboration with leading members of the BAL task force. Where possible a "closed and coded" design of questions was adopted.

   Some salient results from the questionnaire study were:

   a. Of 90 questionnaires sent, there were 32 responding centers (response rate 36%).

   b. The median BAL volume instilled by the responding centers was 150 mL, with a range of 100–300 mL.

   c. There was a diverse range of practice in how this volume was instilled, including the following number of aliquot and volumes (mL): 5×20, 6×20, 7×20, 3×50, 3×60, 15×20.

   d. 57% of responders analyzed aliquots separately and 30% discarded the first aliquot return.

   e. 61% of responders performed total and differential cell counts on filtered and "washed" BAL cells, 28% filtered without a wash and only 6% used the unprocessed aspirate.

   f. Cytospins were used by all but two responders, but spin speeds ranged between $22.86g$ and $112.9g$.

   g. There was a wide range of normal BAL total and differential cell counts reported (*see* **Tables 3–5**).

   h. There was a wide range of normal BAL lymphocyte subset data reported with a wide range of methods for performing subset analysis used, including: flow cytometry, cytospins, and smears as well as other slide-based methods (e.g., adhesion slides) (*see* **Tables 6–8**).

Table 2
Sample Questions from BAL Questionnaire on Technical Details and the
Generation of Normal BAL Reference Data

Section A: Bronchoscopic Procedure

1.   Please give details of the premedication regime you are using for the BAL procedure:

    ....

2.   Please give details of the local anaesthetic (including % concentration)
    regime you are using for BAL Procedure:

    ....

3(a). What type of bronchoscope(s) are you using for Bronchoscopy/BAL procedures?

    ....

   (b).   For each of the bronchoscopes named in (a) please state:

        (i) outer diameter (mm) ....

        (ii) inner suction channel diameter (mm) ....

4.   Are the subjects most often supine 1 ☐ or upright 2 ☐?

5.   In which lobe is a sub segment most often lavaged?
    (Tick one option only)

        1 ☐ RML   2 ☐ LINGULA   3 ☐ RLL
        4 ☐ LLL   5 ☐ RUL   6 ☐ LUL

6.   What medium is used for BAL?
    (Tick one option only)

        1 ☐ 0.9 % Saline   2 ☐ phosphate buffered saline
        3 ☐ other, please specify:..

7.   What temperature is the medium at?   ....°C

8.   What volume and number of BAL aliquots is used?
    (e.g., 5 × 20ml aliquots)

    ....

9.   How is instillation carried out?
    (Tick one option only)

        1 ☐ hand pressure on syringe
        2 ☐ other, please specify:...

10.   How long is the "dwell time" (i.e., time in minutes between instillation and aspiration of the
    fluid) for the procedure?
    (If nil, please state)

Table 3
Normal Values for BAL Cellular Indices using a 180 mL Wash

VARIABLE	MEDIAN (RANGE)
% Recovery of lavagate	68 (41–74)
Total cell count ($\times 10^3$/mL)	146 (49–306)
% Macrophages	79 (25–95)
% Lymphocytes	17 (3–46)
% Neutrophils	2 (0.1–7)
% Eosinophils	0.3 (0.1–4.2)
% Mast cells	0.08 (0.02–0.54)

Data are derived from 180 mL BAL samples. These were taken from 26 normal, unmedicated volunteers (median age 21 yr; range 20–26), without any history of respiratory disease. There were 15 males and 9 were atopic (Adapted after *20*).

Table 4
Expected Values of BAL Cellular Constituents in Healthy Never Smokers

Variable	Mean ± SEM	5th Centile [†]	95th Centile [‡]
% recovery of lavagate	63.4 ± 1.1	40.8	80.3
Total cells, $10^{6 \S}$	18.1 ± 1.9	5.2	33.1
Total cells/mL, $10^{4 \S}$	12.9 ± 2.0	3.1	35.1
Macrophages, %§	85.2 ± 1.6	54.6	97.1
Macrophages/mL, $10^{4 \S}$	9.9 ± 0.8	2.7	27.5
Lymphocytes, %§	11.8 ± 1.1	1.9	34.3
Lymphocytes/mL, $10^{4 \S}$	1.5 ± 0.25	0.2	4.9
Neutrophils, §	1.6 ± 0.7	0.0	3.1
Neutrophils/mL, $10^{4 \S}$	1.2 ± 1.1	0.0	0.4
Eosinophils, %§	0.2 ± 0.06	0.0	1.1
Eosinophils/mL, $10^{4 \S}$	0.02 ± 0.007	0.0	0.2

† 5th percentile of the study population
‡ 95th percentile of the study population.
§ $n = 77$.
(Adapted after *6*).

    i. 82% of responders felt that increased standardization was practicable, which presumably means they would cooperate if an authoritative body laid down precise guidelines for best practice, and indeed 97% would welcome further guidelines.

The above data has been presented to the ERS BAL task force and is currently undergoing further analysis prior to submission for full publication. The current position of the BAL working group is that the continuing usefulness of BAL requires greater knowledge of, and consensus on, standardization issues. This

Table 5
Normal Questionnaire Results

AM	LYM	PMN	EOS	EPITH.	MAST
92	7	1	0.3	0.6	0.036
(68–95)	(5–22)	(0–8)	(0–3)	(0–2)	(0–0.1)

The median values (all %) of the BAL differential means reported for normals by centers responding to a BAL questionnaire on how data are obtained. The range of the means reported is in brackets and indicates the wide variation in BAL normal differential values even in the best centers.

AM=Alveolar macrophages, LYM=Lymphocytes, PMN=Neutrophils, EOS=Eosinophils, EPITH.=Epithelial cells, MAST=Mast cells.

Table 6
Normal Values for BAL Lymphocyte Subsets using a 180 mL BAL

VARIABLE	MEDIAN (AND RANGE)
% Recovery of lavagate	68 (41–74)
Total cell count ($\times 10^3$/mL)	146 (49–306)
% T helper cells*	39 (4–69)
% T-suppressor cells*	58 (32–100)
% DR +ve T cells*	40 (9–66)
% CD25 +ve T cells*	18 (4–43)

* Expressed as % of CD3 positive lymphocytes

Data are derived from 180-mL BAL samples. These were taken from 26 normal, un-medicated volunteers (median age 21 yr; range 20–26), without any history of respiratory disease. There were 15 males and 9 were atopic (Adapted after).

need is illustrated in the results of this survey. Future developments may include a broadened availability of training courses, through the ERS, building on the courses already available prior to the annual scientific conferences. The continued role of an active BAL task force (*see* **Table 9**), which Professor Ulrich Costabel chairs, is an important component of this strategy. In addition, "between center" quality assurance schemes are under active consideration.

6. Given that other sections of this chapter have stressed the problems associated with lack of standardization, it might seem paradoxical to discuss variations in procedure. Such variations should be the domain of centers that are trying to address very specific questions and the methods are therefore not recommended for the majority of users wanting to obtain and analyze traditional BAL samples.

Table 7
Expected Values of BAL T-Cell Subsets Constituents
in Healthy Never Smokers

Variable	Mean ± SEM	5th Centile [†]	95th Centile [‡]
% recovery of lavagate	63.4 ± 1.1	40.8	80.3
Total cells, $10^{6§}$	18.1 ± 1.9	5.2	33.1
Total cells/mL, $10^{4§}$	12.9 ± 2.0	3.1	35.1
T cells, %§	70.3 ± 3.6	25.6	94.9
T-helper cells, %§	44.4 ± 3.7	7.6	83.5
T-suppressor cells, %§	20.7 ± 2.2	6.6	49.4
Helper/suppressor ratio§	2.6 ± 0.3	0.5	6.4
B cells, %§	3.2 ± 0.9	0.0	17.1

    † 5th Centile of the study population
    ‡ 95th Centile of the study population, § n = 77, ① n = 30.
    (Adapted after *6*).

Table 8
Normal Questionnaire Results

CD3 (T cells)	CD4 (Helper/Inducer)	CD8 (Suppressor/cytotoxic)	CD25/CD3 (Activated T cells)	HLADR/CD3 (Activated T cells)
73 (36–100)	42 (24–58)	31 (7–32)	3 (1–18)	32 (4–40)

Normal values for BAL Lymphocyte subsets reported by responders to the BAL questionnaire. The median values in percentages are given, with the range of the means reported in brackets.

It is perhaps worth reiterating that use of these technical variations do not change some of the basic considerations that need to be borne in mind when performing BAL. Hence clinical and laboratory standardization remains vitally important and the basic physics of the process (e.g., potential diffusional changes in solutes and artefactual ELF determinations remain). On this topic it is worth mentioning attempts to isolate a segment of large airway with a balloon catheter to obtain a more defined central airway wash, using the technique of catheter lavage *(25)*. In the Intensive Care Unit (ICU), this technique has been extended to diagnosing lower respiratory tract infections, when a 40-mL catheter lavage was used with a 12-gauge Foley balloon tipped catheter *(26)*. In an ICU the catheter lavage does not require bronchoscopic expertise, and has therefore been commended by some centers for this specific application, where a speedy

Table 9
Useful Contacts Regarding Technical Aspects of BAL

	Email /html	Comment
Prof Haydn Walters	Haydn.walters@med.monash.edu.au Http://www.med.monash.edu.au/medicine/ Alfred/research/respiratory_medicine/	Senior author of this chapter. Member ERS BAL task force.
Prof Ulrich Costabel	Erj.costabel@t-online.de	European BAL Task Force Chairmen
Dr Theo Out	t.a.out@AMC.UVA.NL	Contact for Dutch BAL group.
Dr Henk Kaufman	h.f.kauffman@int.azg.nl	Contact for Dutch BAL group.
Dr Leif Bjermer	Leif.bjermer@medisin.ntnu.no	Contact for Norwegian contact
Prof Stavros Constantopoulos	University of Ioannina Medical School, Ioannina, Greece. Fax 0651 67860 97582.	Contact for Greek BAL Group.
Dr Pat Haslam	p.haslam@ic.ac.uk	UK Contact for European BAL Task Force.
Dr Len Poulter	Royal Free Hospital School of Medicine, London, UK Fax 0171 431 0879	UK Contact for European BAL Task Force.
Dr Bob Baughman	Baughmrp@alpha.che.uc.edu Http://bioscience.org/1998/v3/e/baughman/e1-12.htm	USA contact on BAL issues. Member ERS BAL task force. URL reviews a BAL diagnostic role.
Dr Steve Rennard	Srennard@MAIL.UNMC.EDU	USA contact on BAL issues. Member ERS BAL task force.
Prof H Klech	KLECH_HEINRICH@lilly.com	Contact for European BAL Task Force.
Dr Michael Pirozynski	m.pirozynski@igichp.edu.pl	Organisers BAL 2000 Conference, Krakow, Poland.
Dr Ryszard Kurzawar	r.kurzawa@zpigichp.edu.pl	
BAL 2000 conference	http://www.igichp.edu.pl/Bal2000/bal2000.htm	
BAL 2002	Dr Carlo Albera, University of Turin Albera@sluigi.unito.it	Organiser BAL 2002 Turin Italy
BAL 2004	Dr Elizabet Fireman Fireman@post.tau.ac.il	Organiser BAL 2004 Tel Aviv, Israel
BAL 2006	Professor Carlos Robalo Cordeiro e-mail: crobalo@mail.telepac.pt	Organiser BAL 2006 Portugal
Dr Gerdt Riise	Gerdt.riise@hjl.gu.se	Contact for Swedish BAL centres (incl. BAL solutes).
Mr Chris Ward	Chris.ward@med.monash.edu.au	Executive author of this chapter, member of ERS BAL task force.
NIH Clinical Center Nursing Department	Http://www.cc.nih.gov/nursing/bronchos.html	National Institute of Health Guidelines: Procedure: Assisting with Bronchoscopy

characterization of organisms can be vital. For quantitative cell and solute studies such techniques would seem to have all the pitfalls of other small volume
lavage procedures, and we would not recommend them unless there is a specific need for this type of sample.

7. Extensive guidelines exist for bronchoscopic and BAL-based research in
    asthma and these are useful when considering safety issues in this and other
    patient groups *(27)*. The procedure has been safely performed in asthmatic
    patients with an FEV_1 as low as 37% predicted *(28)*. In our own institution
    many hundreds of asthma patients have undergone bronchoscopy for purely
    research purposes, but we have an informal lower cutoff limit for FEV_1 post
    bronchodilator of 1.5 L for inclusion.

8. Oxygen desaturation and bronchospasm are usually not a major problem during
    the bronchoscopic procedures in asthma, but this is not predictable *(29,30)*. We
    routinely give intravenous atropine (0.6 mg) and sufficient midazolam to make
    the patient comfortable during the procedure. In addition, nebulized salbutamol
    is usually given to asthmatics and should be used routinely unless for some
    reason the research protocol does not allow this. The latter should be the excep-
    tion, and bronchoscopy should not be undertaken without the use of a bron-
    chodilator if the patient is in any way symptomatic. If salbutamol is being used
    pre-bronchoscopy in a study, then we feel it should be given to all, including to
    any controls (even if normal) to prevent any confounding in case the salbutamol
    itself has an effect on the indices of interest.

9. Local anesthetic (lignocaine) is given to the vocal cords and airways. We use
    4% lignocaine above the vocal chords and 2% solutions thereafter, with a maxi-
    mal instilled volume of 16 mL. Higher lignocaine concentrations may affect the
    viability and morphology of the cells harvested *(31)* with a threshold at around 2
    m*M*. Lignocaine use at bronchoscopy has also been associated with significant
    clinical adverse events, including epileptic fitting, and a fatality attributable to
    lignocaine toxicity in a normal volunteer undergoing a research bronchoscopy
    has been reported *(19)*. The maximal safe blood concentration is <5mg/L or
    22μmol/L. The maximum total dose given to the airway should not exceed 400
    mg *(18)* and with the regime advocated, blood levels can be kept to levels that are
    well within the limits recommended. We find that patients can usually be kept
    quite comfortable throughout the bronchoscopy and BAL and airway biopsies
    obtained without undue coughing. With adequate midazolam there is frequently
    little if any memory of the procedure.

10. We routinely give 2 L/min oxygen throughout by nasal or oral cannulae although
    still monitoring oxygen saturation with a pulse oximeter, and allow the patient to
    recover over 2 to 3 h before discharge home. The subject is kept "nil by mouth"
    until complete recovery from pharyngeal local anesthetic, to avoid aspiration,
    and we usually suggest a period of at least 4 h.

11. Adverse sequelae to the research bronchoscopy are unusual. More severe asth-
    matic patients may experience an increase in nonspecific airway responsiveness
    (32) but this does not seem to be the rule *(33,34)* and deterioration in clinical

asthma is rare. A flu-like syndrome with malaise and pyrexia may occur after a few hours and can be associated with pleuritic chest pain in the area of lavage. We usually suggest paracetamol 4 hourly if this occurs, and the condition almost always resolves quickly.

12. The "3 × 60mL aliquot BAL protocol." Our suggested protocol represents a choosing of "middle ground" from published studies, and we would suggest this as a standard method. Unfortunately, there remains considerable variation between centers. Commonly, centers employ a lobar or segmental lavage of the lingula or middle lobe using 100–240 mL sterile saline warmed to 37°C. Largely based on empirical descriptions of changes in returned cytological profiles, especially increases in polymorphs, groups have concluded that a low volume BAL (<60 mL) yields a wash of central airways *(35)*, whereas a greater instilled volume may allow the sampling of "alveoli" *(36,37)*. Thus, the routine discarding of the "early" part of the aspirate has been advocated, although the actual evidence for such a neat dichotomy is limited.

13. There have been few studies focusing on the vexed question of the distribution of BAL infusate and the anatomic origin of the lavage aspirate and it is difficult to know precisely what area of the bronchopulmonary segment BAL best samples. In a radiographic study using a computerized digital subtraction imaging technique, our research group demonstrated that BAL fluid containing radiopaque Niopam did indeed reach the periphery of the lung segment *(38)*. However, aspiration of the first 60-mL aliquot caused fluid movement toward the bronchoscope only in the proximal airways, whereas with aspiration of subsequent aliquots of the BAL there was more uniform movement of fluid, throughout the lung segment, back toward the proximally placed bronchoscope tip. However, the study could not really contribute to telling us whether the actual sampling of fluid was uniform. A subsequent pilot study in which each aliquot of a 3 × 60 mL BAL was differentially "labeled", indicated that the degree of mixing between aliquots may be substantially less than is generally supposed and that much of each aspiration included predominantly from the aliquot just introduced *(38)*. New and larger studies are needed in this important area, but the data that exists would suggest that a traditional large volume BAL is quite suitable for the study of airways disease, and has distinct advantages over a smaller volume approach. This type of data does not support the arbitrary discarding of aliquots. There is some argument for recording data on the first aspirate separately, but even this is very doubtful, as the cells are few in number and frequently of poor viability. We believe that all the aspirates should be amalgamated into a single collection for assessment.

14. If a person being considered for BAL is a smoker or has an infection then this is liable to be (overwhelmingly) what the cellular results of the procedure will reflect.

15. A good "wedge" of the bronchoscope into the airway is crucial. If not obtained, a characteristic proximal airway wash results, which yields low numbers of cells with low viability and a high percentage of epithelial cells. This has some implications for medication: if the subject is uncomfortable and coughing the estab-

lishment/maintenance of a "wedge" will be more difficult. The inclusion of atropine and a sedative in the premed and adequate lignocaine (plus time to allow the medication to work) may help to make the patient more comfortable and help to avoid this problem.

16. Reduced suction should be used during the aspiration of BAL. This may help return by decreasing dynamic airway closure and trapping of fluid and should reduce the incidence of red cell contamination.

17. Filtration and washing of BAL cells affects subsequent total and differential cell counts. Unfortunately, the fact that BAL total cell counts have been performed at different stages in the processing of the sample *(39)* and that BAL differentials have been performed in ways that systematically lead to biased results *(40)*, means that it can be very hard to compare results between centers. This applies to even the most basic of cellular indices.

18. The centrifugation of cells followed by resuspension in fresh media (or "washing" of BAL cells as sometimes termed) leads to a well-documented loss of up to a third of cells *(41)*. In addition, filtration of the BAL aspirate is a common practice, in order to remove mucus. In some circumstances this is necessary (e.g., running a BAL sample for automated analysis/cell sorting, but this is rarely the case for obtaining a straight forward total and differential cell count). Further, filtration is frequently performed using variable layers of gauze *(42)* whose thickness and presumably absorption characteristics vary *(43)*. The use of complex organic materials such as cotton in such procedures may risk an effect on cell function. It is therefore unfortunate that detail regarding BAL filtration is frequently not specified. We evaluated the effect of a standardized filtration process with a 200-μm stainless steel mesh on the BAL total and differential cell count in 21 subjects undergoing BAL *(44)*. We found a mean 23% reduction in BAL total cell count. The BAL differentials indicated that this could be accounted for by a predominant removal of alveolar macrophages. Some centers, where the detail has been reported, perform a total and differential cell count on a BAL aspirate that has been both filtered and washed, indicating that this is one possible explanation for the wide range of data relating to BAL indices in the literature. Because processing, such as filtration and "washing" effects BAL parameters so markedly the protocol in this chapter advocates a total and differential cell count performed on a raw, unprocessed aspirate. If this is found to be technically impossible in more than a minority of cases, our experience would again tend to indicate a possible dysfunction within the vital interface between a technically competent clinical bronchoscopist and the laboratory.

19. The cytospin is the most widely used method for generating a differential cell count from BAL. However, other techniques for determining BAL differentials have been successfully reported. Results using the millipore filter method *(45)*, cell smear *(46)*, and glass cover technique *(47)* are practicable and provide robust data, although they are technically more difficult. These alternatives to the cytospin method suffer the drawback that they are technically demanding and time consuming (particularly the millipore method), and can require the

use of modified staining protocols *(45)*. Comparison of such alternative methods with cytospins have indicated that the latter may lead to a selective and variable loss of cells, and particularly of lymphocytes, probably into the cytospin filter *(47)*.

20. It is important to recognize the limitations of cytospins and to take steps to minimize these. We have extensively studied different BAL counting methods. As part of this work we analyzed BAL samples from 21 subjects with cell differentials prepared using variable cytospin spin speeds (28.23g and 81.57g) and durations (1, 2, and 10 min) *(48)*. These conditions were chosen since they represent the range quoted in the literature. We found that the lymphocyte percentage from cytospins made at 81.57g for 2 min were not significantly different from those gained from glass cover preparations, with a slightly lower general result for the cytospin (mean lymphocyte counts 23%, mean difference between glass cover and cytospin methods 3 ± 2%). In contrast, the mean difference at 28.23g was up to 10% lower using cytospins, which was statistically significant. It is obviously important to urge that appropriate spin speeds and times for cytospin preparation are used. Unfortunately, many centers continue to use and publish spin speeds which are consistent with an appreciable and statistically significant underestimate of lymphocyte percentages, particularly in patients with high true lymphocyte counts *(48)*.

21. Fixation and staining protocols for differential cell counts require standardization *(49)*, but fortunately this seems to be less variable with most groups using the method quoted in this chapter, or a similar protocol *(4)*.

22. Red blood cells are always present in BAL samples, although contamination is usually minor (*see* **Fig. 1b**). Substantial erythrocyte contamination that would interfere with subsequent counting is usually secondary to overt bleeding and should be infrequent. However, when this occurs erythrocytes should be removed using appropriate proprietary lysing reagents: e.g., incubate 1 mL of cells with 1-mL Ortho-mune lysing solution for 10 min at room temperature. Cells are then washed and resuspended in PBS. Such a procedure is a "fix" to the problem, and will inevitably lead to cell loss, and an effect on the total and differential cell counts.

23. The question of how to best express BAL results has remained a hotly debated point for the last 15 years. This is a fundamental question for BAL researchers, and its importance has led the ERS BAL task force to work on publishing a consensus guideline document *(12)*.

24. As outlined above (*see* **Note 13**), there remains doubt about the anatomical location of the area sampled by BAL. The assumption is made that regardless of the balance of sampling between airway and alveoli, the fluid that is sampled is essentially that termed the ELF. The majority of the fluid in the aspirate is assumed to be restricted to that portion of the infusate that has "washed out" or lavaged ELF. Unfortunately, a number of studies have indicated that this basic assumption is simplistic, and probably misleading. The situation is exacerbated by the common practice of trying to "calculate" ELF volume, usually by proportionality by comparing the concentration of urea in BAL and plasma *(50)*. The assumption is that

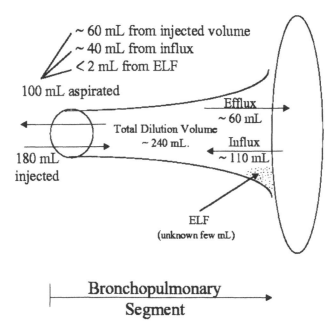

Fig. 5. Complex fluid movement during "typical" BAL-schematic representation.

urea is equilibrated between plasma and ELF and so the dilution of urea in the BAL aspirate compared to plasma gives the ELF dilution. This model does not allow for any possible movement of urea and/or water from the blood to airway during BAL. However, and rather unfortunately for the BAL literature, it has been convincingly demonstrated that movement of urea and water does occur during BAL, so the concept of being able to accurately calculate ELF in BAL fluid is discredited. Despite this, the urea method continues to be used, with increasingly complex means being suggested for trying to calculate it *(51)*.

Using radioisotope markers, we have shown that the fluid dynamics during BAL are complex (*see* **Fig. 5**). Of the 180-mL injected, ~60mL effluxes from the bronchopulmonary segment into the interstitium or vasculature. But at the same time, approx 110 mL is drawn into the available dilution volume, presumably mainly from the circulation, owing to the high aspiration pressure. If, in a typical case, 100 mL is finally aspirated up the bronchoscope, then approx 40 mL of that fluid will have come directly from the interstitium or blood compartment *(52)*. In a study using inulin as a dilution marker of BAL, very similar figures were obtained for net dilution of BAL fluid *(53)*. The fact that the net dilution factor in both asthmatics and normal controls was very similar in this study was at least reassuring for asthma researchers, and would indicate that the fundamental nature of the samples was similar between asthmatic subjects and normal controls.

25. Urea cannot be used as a marker of dilution of ELF because it moves into the lung segment with the large influx of water, as would be expected by the physical process

of "solvent drag" *(54)*, and also by diffusion along the concentration gradient between plasma and BAL fluid in the lung *(55)*. Albumin or other proteins cannot be used because we do not know their physiological concentration in ELF, although it is likely to be a fraction of that in plasma, and it also varies with disease state and therapy *(56,57)*. Hence, this chapter would commend the current position of the ERS BAL task force, that solute and cellular BAL data should be given as "per mL of BAL return" *(12)*, as long as the volume of BAL used and the volume of return are comparable *(58)*. Ideally, preliminary studies in any new disease state being studied should also be undertaken to ascertain that the net dilution of BAL by the balance of efflux/influx of fluid is also comparable to any controls being used *(54)*. Potentially misleading data has been reported in asthma studies where such confounding factors have not been allowed for i.e., different BAL volumes and returns in the disease group compared to the controls *(59)* with inevitable differences in dilution of the solute of interest, giving apparent but possibly artefactual increases in concentrations in the disease state in this example. Within individual studies, very large alterations from normal in the ratio of one solute to another in different groups are most convincing of a real pathological abnormality *(60)*.

Acknowledgments

The work carried out in the Department of Respiratory Medicine is supported by:The National Health and Medical Research Council of Australia, The Alfred Hospital Research Committee, The Alfred Hospital Whole Time Medical Specialists, and Glaxo Wellcome.

References

1. Prakash, U. B. S. (1997) Gustav Killian Centenary: The celebration of a century of progress in bronchoscopy. *Journal of Bronchology* **4**, 1–2.
2. Jackson, C. (1928) Bronchoscopy; past, present and future. *N. Engl. J. Med..* **199**, 759–763.
3. Ikeda, S. (1970) Flexible bronchofiberscope. *Ann. Otol. Rhinol Laryngol.* **79**, 916–919.
4. Task Group Report. (1989) Technical recommendations and guidelines for bronchoalveolar lavage (BAL). *Eur. Respir. J.* **2**, 561–585.
5. Woodcock, A.C., Boe, J., and Cordier, J. F. (Eds.) (1998) Investigative measures for airway inflammation. *Eur. Respir. Rev.* **64**, 1065–1132.
6. The BAL Cooperative Group Steering Committee. (1990) Bronchoalveolar lavage constituents in healthy individuals, idiopathic pulmonary fibrosis and selected comparison groups. *Am. Rev. Respir. Dis.* **141**, S169–201.
7. Kotsimbos, T. and Walters, E. H. (1995) Bronchoscopy, Lavage, Needle and Other Biopsies, in *Medicine International* (Muers, M. and Hopkin, J., eds.), **23**, 250–256.
8. Ramirez, R. J., Schultz, R. B., and Dutton, R.E. (1963) Pulmonary alveolar proteinosis. A new technique and rationale for treatment. *Arch. Intern. Med.* **112**, 419–431.
9. Wilt, J. L. and Banks, D. E. (1995) Reactions to inorganic dusts, in *Immunology and management of interstitial lung diseases* (Walters, E. H. and du Bois, R. M., eds.), Chapman and Hall, London, p 199–222.

10. Baughman, R. P. (1998) Diagnosis of lower respiratory tract infections: what we have and what would be nice. *Chest* **113,** 219S–223S.

11. de Gracia, J., Bravo, C., Miravitlles, M., Tallada, N., Orriols, R., Bellmunt, J., Vendrell, M., and Morell, F. (1993) Diagnostic value of bronchoalveolar lavage in peripheral lung cancer. *Am. Rev. Respir. Dis.* **147,** 649–652.

12. Haslam, P. L. and Baughman, eds. (1999)Report of the European Respiratory Society Task Force: Guidelines for measurement of cellular componants and recommendations for standardization of bronchoalveolar lavage (BAL), *European Respiratory Review*, **9,** 66.

13. Keimowitz, R. I. (1964) Immunoglobulins in normal human tracheobronchial washings. A qualitative and quantitative study. *J. Lab. Clin. Med.*, **63,** 54–59.

14. Laviolette, M. (1985) Lymphocyte fluctuation in bronchoalveolar lavage fluid in normal volunteers. *Thorax*, **40,** 651–656.

15. Ramirez, R. J., Kieffer, R. F., and Ball, W.C. (1965) Bronchopulmonary lavage in man. *Ann. Intern. Med.* **63,** 819–828.

16. Kelly, C. A., Ward, C., Stenton, S. C., Bird, A. G., Hendrick, D. J., and Walters, E. H. (1988) Number and activity of inflammatory cells in bronchoalveolar lavage fluid in asthma and their relation to airway responsiveness. *Thorax*, **43,** 684–692.

17. Davidson, A. C., Barbosa, I., Kooner, J. S., Hamblin, A. S., Stokes, T. C., Bateman, N.T., and Gray, B. (1986) The influence of topical anesthetic agent at bronchoalveolar lavage upon cellular yield and identification and upon macrophage function. *Br. J. Dis. Chest* **80,** 385–390.

18. Djuaknovic, R., Dahl, R., Jarjour, N., and Aalbers, R. (1988) Safety of biopsies and bronchoalveolar lavage. *Eur. Respir. J.* **11,** 39s–41s, Suppl.

19. O'Day, R., Chalmers, D.R.C., Williams, K.M., and Campbell, T.J. (1998) The death of a healthy volunteer in a human research project: implications for Australian clinical research. *M.J.A.* **168,** 449–451.

20. Booth, H., Richmond, I., Ward, C., Gardiner, P. V., Harkawat, R., and Walters, E.H. (1995) Effect of high dose inhaled fluticasone propionate on airway inflammation in asthma. *Am. J. Respir. Crit. Care Med.* **152,** 45–52.

21. Ward, C., Snell, G. I., Orsida, B., Zheng, L., Williams, T. J., and Walters, E. H. (1997) Airway versus transbronchial biopsy and BAL in lung transplant recipients: different but complementary. *Eur. Respir. J.* **10,** 2876–2880.

22. Richmond, I., Booth, H., Ward, C., and Walters, E. H. (1995) Intrasubject variability in airway inflammation in biopsies in mild to moderate stable asthma. *Am. J. Respir. Crit. Care Med.* **153,** 899–903.

23. Ward, C., Gardiner, P. V., Booth, H., and Walters, E. H. (1995) Intrasubject variability in airway inflammation sampled by bronchoalveolar lavage in clinically stable mild to moderate asthmatics. *Eur. Respir. J.* **8,** 1866–1871.

24. Gardiner, P. V., Ward, C., Booth, H., Allison, A., Hendrick, D. J., and Walters, E. H. (1994) Effect of eight weeks treatment with salmeterol on bronchoalveolar lavage inflammatory indices in asthmatics. *Am. J. Respir. Crit. Care Med.* **150,** 1006–1011.

25. Eschenbacker, W. L., and Gravelyn, T. R. (1987) A technique for isolated airway segment lavage. *Chest* **92,** 105–109.

26. Humphreys, H., Winter, R., Baker, M., and Smith, C. (1997) Comparison of bronchoalveolar lavage and catheter lavage to confirm ventilator-associated lower respiratory tract infection. *J. Med. Microbiol.* **45,** 226–231.
27. National Institutes of Health. (1991) Workshop summary and guidelines–investigative use of bronchoscopy, lavage and bronchial biopsies in asthma and other airway diseases. *J. Allergy Clin. Immunol.* **88,** 808–814.
28. van Vyve, T., Chanez, P., Bousquet, J., Lacoste, J., Michael, F., and Godard, P. (1992) Safety of bronchoalveolar lavage and bronchial biopsies in patients with asthma of variable severity. *Am. Rev. Respir. Dis.* **146,** 116–121.
29. Chetta, A., Foresi, A., Bertorelli, G., Pesci, A., and Olivieri, D. (1992) Lung function and bronchial responsiveness after bronchoalveolar lavage and bronchial biopsy performed without premedication in stable asthmatic subjects. *Chest* **101,** 1563–1568.
30. Djukanovic, R., Wilson, R. W., Lai, C. K. W., Holgate, S. T., and Howarth, P. H. (1991) The safety aspects of fiberoptic bronchoscopy, bronchoalveolar lavage and endobronchial biopsy in asthma. *Am. Rev. Respir. Dis.* **143,** 772–777.
31. Duddridge, M., Kelly, C. A., Ward, C., Hendrick, D. J., and Walters, E. H. (1990) The reversible effect of lignocaine on the stimulated metabolic activity of bronchoalveolar lavage cells. *Eur. Respir. J.* **3,** 1166–1172.
32. Kelly, C., Hendrick, D., and Walters, H. (1988) The effect of bronchoalveolar lavage on bronchial responsiveness in patients with airflow obstruction. *Chest* **93,** 325–328.
33. Kirby, J. G., O'Byrne, P. M., and Hargreave, F. E. (1987) Bronchoalveolar lavage does not alter airway responsiveness in asthmatic subjects. *Am. Rev. Respir. Dis.* **135,** 554–556.
34. Gianiorio, P., Bonavia, M., Crimi, E., et al. (1991) Bronchial responsiveness is not increased by bronchoalveolar and bronchial lavage performed after allergen challenge. *Am. Rev. Respir. Dis.* **143,** 105–108.
35. Dohn, M. N. and Baughman, R. P. (1985) Effect of changing instilled volume for bronchoalveolar lavage in patients with interstitial lung disease. *Am. Rev. Respir. Dis.* **132,** 390–392.
36. Davis, G. S., Giancola, M. S., Constanza, M. C., and Low, R. B. (1982) Analyses of sequential bronchoalveolar lavage samples from healthy human volunteers. *Am. Rev. Respir. Dis.* **126,** 611–616.
37. Kelly, C. A., Kotre, J. C., Ward, C., Hendrick, D. J., and Walters, E. H. (1987) Anatomical distribution of fluid at bronchoalveolar lavage. *Thorax* **42,** 625–629.
38. Duddridge, M., Kelly, C. A., Fenwick, J., Hendrick, D. J., and Walters, E. H. (1988) Assessment of mixing between sequential aliquots during bronchoalveolar lavage. *Thorax* **43,** 822–823.
39. Klech, H. and Pohl, W. (1989) Technical recommendations and guidelines for bronchoalveolar lavage. European working party report. *Eur. Respir. J.* **2,** 561–585.
40. Gardiner, P. V., Ward, C., Allison, A., Hendrick, D.J., and Walters, E. H. (1991) An evaluation of methods for quantification of cells recovered by bronchoalveolar lavage (BAL). *Am. Rev. Respir. Dis.* **143,** A666.

41. Mordelet-Dambrine, M., Arnoux, A., and Stanislas-Leguern, G. (1984) Process- ing of lung lavage fluid causes variability in bronchoalveolar cell count. *Am. Rev. Respir. Dis.* **130,** 305–306.
42. Hoidal, J. R., White, J. G., and Repine, J. E. (1979) Impairment of human alveolar macrophage oxygen consumption, and superoxide anion production by local anesthetics used in bronchoscopy. *Chest* **75,** 243–246.
43. Danielle, R. P., Dauber, J. H., and Altose, M. D. (1977) Lymphocyte studies in asymptomatic cigarette smokers–a comparison between lung and peripheral blood. *Am. Rev. Respir. Dis.* **116,** 997–1005.
44. Kelly, C. A., Ward, C., Bird, A. G., Hendrick, D. J., and Walters, E. H. (1989) The effect of filtration on cell counts in bronchoalveolar lavage fluid. *Respir. Med.* **83,** 107–110.
45. Saltini, C., Hance, A. J., Ferrans, V. J., Basset, F., Bitterman, P. B., and Crystal, R. G. (1984) Accurate quantification of cells recovered by bronchoalveolar lav- age. *Am. Rev. Respir. Dis.* **130,** 650–658.
46. Thompson, A. B., Teschler, H., Wang, Y. M., Konietzko, N., and Costabel, U. (1996) Preperation of bronchoalveolar lavage fluid with microscope slide smears. *Eur. Respir. J.* **9,** 603–608.
47. Laviolette, M., Carreau, M., and Colombe, R. (1988) Bronchoalveolar lavage cell differential on microscope glass cover. A simple and accurate technique. *Am. Rev. Respir. Dis.* **138,** 451–457.
48. Booth, H., Ward, C., Gardiner, P. V., and Walters, E. H. (1993) Bronchoalveolar lavage cell counting: alterations in cytocentrifugation technique reduce lymphocte loss. *Eur.Resp.J.* **6,** S436.
49. Moumouni, H., Garaud, P., Diot, P., Lemarie, E., and Anthonioz, P. (1994) Quan- tification of cell loss during Bronchoalveolar lavage fluid processing: effects of fixation and staining methods. *Am. J. Respir. Crit. Care Med.* **149,** 636–640.
50. Rennard, S. I., Basset, G., Lecossier, D., O'Donnell, K. M., Martin, P. G., and Crystal, R. G. (1986) Estimation of the volume of epithelial lining fluid recovered by lavage using urea as a marker of dilution. *J. Appl. Physiol.* **60,** 532–538.
51. von Weichert, P., Joseph, K., MÅller, B., and Franck, W.M. (1993) Bronchoalveolar lavage. Quantitation of intraalveolar fluid? *Am. Rev. Respir. Dis.* **147,** 148–152.
52. Kelly, C. A., Fenwick, J. D., Corris, P. A., Fleetwood, A., Hendrick, D. J., and Walters, E.H. (1988) Fluid dynamics during bronchoalveolar lavage. *Am. Rev. Respir. Dis.* **138,** 81–84.
53. Restrick, L. J., Sampson, A. P., Piper, P. J., Costello, J. F. (1995) Inulin as a marker of dilution of bronchoalveolar lavage in asthmatics and normal subjects. *Am. J. Respir. Crit. Care Med.* **151,** 1211–1217.
54. Ward, C., Duddridge, M., Fenwick, J., et al. (1992) The origin of water and urea sampled at bronchoalveolar lavage in asthmatics and control subjects. *Am. Rev. Respir. Dis.* **146,** 444–447.
55. Merrill, W., O'Hearn, E., Rankin, J., Naegel, G., Matthay, R. A., and Reynolds, H. Y. (1982) Kinetic analysis of respiratory tract proteins recovered during a sequential lavage protocol. *Am. Rev. Respir. Dis.* **126,** 617–620.

56. Ward, C., Fenwick, J., Weddle, A., Booth, H. and Walters, E.H. (1997) Albumin is not suitable as a marker of Bronchoalveolar lavage (BAL) dilution in interstitial lung disease (ILD). *Eur. Respir. J.* **10**, 2029–2033.

57. Ward, C., Duddridge, M., Fenwick, J., Williams, S., Gardiner, P. V., Hendrick, D. J., and Walters, E. H. (1993) An evaluation of albumin as a reference marker for bronchoalveolar lavage fluid in asthmatic and control subjects. *Thorax* **48,** 518–522.

58. Walters, E. H., and Gardiner, P. V. (1991) Bronchoalveolar lavage as a research tool. *Thorax* **46,** 613–618.

59. Wardlaw, A.J., Hay, H., Cromwell, O., Collins, J.R., and Kay, A.B. (1989) Leukotrienes, LTC4 and LTB4 , in bronchoalveolar lavage in bronchial asthma and other respiratory disease. *J. Allergy Clin. Immunol.* **84,** 19–26.

60. Wardlaw, S. J., Dunnette, S., Gleich, G. J., Collins, J. R., and Kay, A. B. (1988) Eosinophils and mast cells in bronchoalveolar lavage in subjects with mild asthma: relationship to bronchial hyperreactivity. *Am. Rev. Respir. Dis.* **137,** 62–69.

4

Nasal Secretions and Exudations

Collection and Approaches to Analysis

Lennart Greiff, Morgan Andersson, and Carl G.A. Persson

1. Introduction

Nasal and bronchoalveolar lavage techniques, as well as sputum induction-techniques, are frequently used for sampling of airway mucosal surface liquids, together with their contents of cell products, plasma proteins, glandular secretions and cells. These techniques continue to provide new information on the nature and pharmacology of airway inflammation in rhinitis and asthma. The relative ease and safety by which nasal lavage techniques can be employed, their repeatability, and the possibility for control of important factors, make it advantageous to use the nose in clinical studies of airway disease mechanisms. The nasal airway thus offers the attractive possibility of exploring gross as well as molecular events directly in the complex, but relevant, disease biosystem. A patient-orientated *in* vivo focus is also needed, we think, for original discovery of important airway disease mechanisms. This need seems increasingly urgent since many central airway in vivo events have been incompletely researched and since concepts built on data from reductive test systems, such as cell culture and mouse models, may not always translate well into human in vivo events *(1,2)*. Additionally, the nasal studies are important because they may provide insights into the biology, physiology, and pharmacology of human mucosal mechanisms, also of other parts of the respiratory tract, notably the difficult-to-reach bronchial mucosa *(3)*.

Solutes on the mucosal surface frequently reflect on-going processes in the airway mucosal tissue, an important site of airway disease mechanisms. By contrast, luminal inflammatory cells may generally reflect a *post-festum* con-

From: *Methods in Molecular Medicine, vol. 56:*
Human Airway Inflammation: Sampling Techniques and Analytical Protocols
Edited by: D. F. Rogers and L. E. Donnelly © Humana Press Inc., Totowa, NJ

dition. It thus appears logical to view luminal entry of granulocytes as an important part of the resolution phase of an exacerbation of airway disease rather than being involved in driving the disease *(4)*. Further, after entry into the lumen, cell phenotypes may change significantly from those relevant to the actual airway disease process *(4)*.

This chapter deals with nasal lavage procedures in adults and children including the controlled exposure of the nasal mucosa to different agents and tracers. The focus is on sampling of nasal mucosal surface liquids for the analysis of solutes. Tentative experimental means by which airway (nasal and bronchial) mucosal surface liquids may be enriched with sub-epithelial inflammatory cell products are also discussed. Methods involved in the analysis of important molecules contained in the nasal samples are not detailed.

2. Materials

All reagents were from Sigma Chemical Co. unless stated otherwise.

1. Isotonic saline for nasal lavage (at room temperature when administered).
2. Histamine.
3. Hypertonic saline or buffered solutions for specific studies (at room temperature when administered).
4. Filter paper disks for nonlavage sampling methods.
5. Elution buffer: 0.1 M TRIS buffer, pH 7.4, 0.01% sodium azide, 0.002% Tween, 0.3% human serum albumin.
6. ^{51}Cr-ethylenediaminotetraacetic acid (EDTA).
7. Desmopressin.

3. Methods
3.1. Nasal Lavage in Adults

It is desirable that nasal lavage techniques should be well-controlled (*see* **Note 1**) and reproducible with regard to the following points:

1. Distribution of the lavage fluid.
2. Mucosal surface area in contact with the lavage fluid.
3. Duration of mucosal exposure to the lavage fluid.
4. When a nasal lavage technique is used for the controlled exposure of the nasal mucosa to active agents and/or probes, concentrations of agents and tracers in contact with a defined airway mucosal surface area should be reasonably well controlled and assessable.
5. The techniques should be noninjurious.
6. Recovery of lavage fluids should be quantitative.
7. Employment of the techniques should be repeatable without undue effects on nasal mucosal physiology.

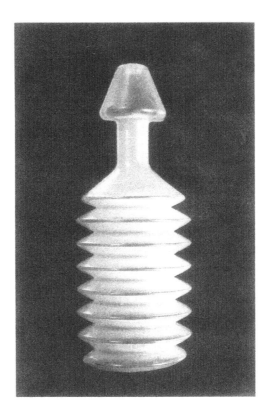

Fig. 1. A nasal pool-device. (From Ref. 18, with permission.)

To try and meet the above requirements, we have introduced a "nasal pool-technique" *(5)*, which is the focus of the present chapter. Several other nasal lavage techniques are in use, including the "head-back lavage" *(6)* and different spray methods *(7)*. Although less compliant with the above requirements than the nasal pool-technique and depending of the type of investigation each of these other lavage techniques have individual merits.

3.1.1. The Nasal Pool Device

The nasal pool-device is a compressible plastic container equipped with a nasal adapter (*see* **Fig. 1**). Unfortunately, this particular device is not available commercially. However, adjusted for fluid-tight contact with the nasal orifice a syringe may be used in accord with the present technique *(8)*.

1. The adapter is inserted into one of the nostrils.
2. The seated subject leans forward in a 60°C flexed neck position and compresses the container. Any fluid escaping an overfilled nasal cavity will not be swallowed but pass into and disappear through the other nasal passage.

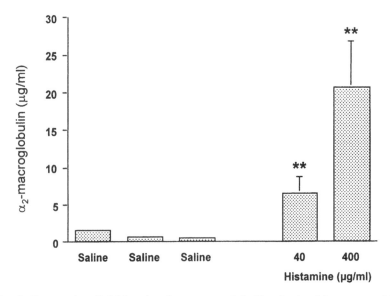

Fig. 2. Decreasing fluid levels of α_2-macroglobulin obtained by repeated isotonic saline lavages (left-side columns). Subsequently, exudation of α_2-macroglobulin evoked by different concentrations of histamine is determined by the use of the nasal pool-technique for concomitant nasal mucosal exposure and lavage (right-side columns). Repeated isotonic saline lavages are thus used to remove surface material and to create an experimental low-level "baseline" from which changes (e.g., after challenge) can be determined accurately. [**]$p<0.01$ compared with third saline control.

3. The nasal pool-fluid is instilled by the subjects themselves into one of the nasal cavities. Equally, each participating subject keeps the nasal cavity filled with fluid by keeping the device compressed.

By these means nasal pool-fluid is maintained in contact with a large and reasonably well-defined area of the mucosal surface for an extended period of time. When the pressure on the device is released, the fluid returns almost quantitatively into the container. Using X-ray visualization of radiodense nasal lavage fluid, we have demonstrated the distribution of the nasal pool instillate from the nostril to the posterior aspect of the nasal septum (5). The recovery of lavage fluid (saline) (in the nonblown nose) was quantitative (92 ± 3%). Gamma camera detection over the facial and gut areas 15 min after administration and subsequent recovery of ^{51}Cr-EDTA indicated that displacement of the lavage fluid to the sinuses or the gut occurred rarely.

Repeated instillations of saline produced stable and low albumin concentrations in recovered nasal pool-fluids, reflecting the noninjurious nature of the technique. Indeed, the gentleness of the nasal pool-lavage may make it less useful alone in studies where particularly sticky material on the mucosal surface shall be sampled. In these instances the pool-sampling may be acutely followed by sampling of the additional material that is retrieved by a forceful blowing of the nose.

To eliminate indices of interest that may have accumulated on the airway surface for unknown periods of time repeated saline lavages are carried out first, prior to study of challenge agents. Thus, stable low-level "baseline" conditions are created and responses to different challenges are detected with optimal sensitivity/accuracy (*see* **Fig. 2**).

3.1.2. Histamine (and Other Mediator) Challenge

Histamine challenge-induced plasma exudation responses have been evaluated to characterize the use of the nasal pool technique for concomitant challenge and lavage *(5)* (*see* **Note 3**). Different concentrations of histamine have thus been present in the lavage fluid. During the few minutes of keeping the nasal cavity filled with such test fluids it may be assumed that the introduced histamine concentrations practically equated those present in the biophase close to the mucosal surface. Consistent concentration response to histamine was also obtained (*see* **Fig. 2**). The coefficient of variation for three repeated individual measurements was 13% for a moderate dose of histamine (40 µg/mL) and 12% for a high dose of histamine (400 µg/mL). Hence, the reproducibility of histamine-induced exudation of plasma was considered acceptable, and we conclude that the nasal-pool-technique permits concomitant provocation and lavage of a large and defined area of the nasal mucosal surface for extended and variable periods of time.

It is anticipated that other inflammatory mediators, that similar to histamine evoke acute microvascular-epithelial exudation of bulk plasma, will be equally suited for studies of nasal exudative responses and responsiveness. The technique of mixing agents in the nasal pool-fluid can also be used with advantage for detailed studies of potency and other properties of pharmacological antagonists. Indeed, concentration-response relationships may thus be explored in vivo in the human airway mucosa in organ bath-like conditions *(9)*. The latter kind of challenge and lavage scheme is preferably carried out with incremental concentrations of the active agent and such a test series may preferably be ended with a few additional saline lavages to avoid any continued exposure to drugs.

Depending on the type of challenge different analytes may appear in nasal mucosal surface liquids at different time points after challenge, for example plasma proteins and secretions within minutes *(5,10)* and eosinophil cationic protein (ECP) within hours *(11)*. Timing of the challenge and lavage scheme with allergen and other causative insults is thus more complex than with simple acutely effective exudative or secretory agents. Generally, the inter-individual variability of nasal mucosal output of cell products, plasma proteins, and glandular secretions must also be considered. Thus, intra-individual observations may be desired as opposed to nonpaired comparisons.

3.1.3. Absorption Permeability Measurements

The nasal pool-technique has the extra merit that the lavage fluid may contain tracer molecules allowing well-controlled determination of the absorption permeability of the nasal mucosa *(12)*. Suitable absorption tracers (e.g., ^{51}Cr-EDTA and desmopressin) have thus been added to the nasal pool-fluid. By the subsequent nasal pool-procedure selected concentrations of these tracers are kept in contact with a large and reasonably well-controlled (absorption) area of the mucosal surface. Importantly, the duration of the absorption process is controlled by the time the fluid is kept in the nasal cavity and by abortion of absorption through removal of any remaining amount of tracer on the mucosal surface by repeated irrigations with isotonic saline. By keeping the absorption-area, the absorption-time, and the tracer concentration controlled, important prerequisites for proper absorption measurements are met. With this technique we have examined the mucosal absorption permeability during disease conditions as well as effects on the mucosal absorption permeability by concomitant challenges *(12)*.

3.2. Nasal Lavage in Children

Different techniques have been used to obtain nasal mucosal liquids in children:

1. Absorption by filter paper *(13)*.
2. Suction by catheters *(14)*.
3. Saline lavage using syringes *(15)*.
4. Instillations in the "lateral decubitus position" *(16)*.
5. Administration of saline with nasal metered dose inhalers followed by collection of nasal "drippings" *(17)*.

However, collectively these techniques exhibit inadequacies regarding baseline data and reproducibility already in their application in adults (*see* **Note 2**). Also, the characteristics in children of these methods have been little described. Where recovery of the nasal lavage fluids has been reported it has been 50% at best *(17)*, where a metered dose inhaler was used to administer 7-mL saline to children aged 7–12 y. The previously employed techniques where the devices are generally handled by the investigator may also have limitations owing to some infringement upon the integrity of the child.

It was of interest to learn that the nasal pool-technique could be used for challenge and lavage of the nasal mucosa in children (7–11 yr-old) *(18)*. After a single demonstration of the technique and without any practical training, these children managed to carry out lavages as well as concomitant histamine challenges and lavages. None of the children reported any degree of discomfort (as assessed by a written summary). In the above-mentioned study in children *(18)*, the recovery of four 1-min saline lavages was $85 \pm 2\%$, $92 \pm 3\%$, $90 \pm 2\%$, and $89 \pm 2\%$. The mean of the intra-individual coefficients of variation was 9%. Histamine-induced exudation of plasma (α_2-macroglobulin) was employed. The recovery of nasal lavage fluids after the concomitant histamine-challenge and lavage in these children was $92 \pm 2\%$, $85 \pm 2\%$, and $89 \pm 2\%$ for isotonic saline, histamine (40 µg/mL), and histamine (400 µg/mL), respectively. Thus, the recovery of the nasal lavage fluid (in the nonblown nose) was quantitative, almost as in studies involving adults.

Taken together our so far limited experiences suggest that the nasal-pool-technique may be an important tool in studies of the pathophysiology and pharmacology of the nasal airway mucosa in children. As an additional asset of the nasal pool-technique, and potentially of special value for this age group, the challenge and lavage procedures can be performed by subjects themselves after minimal training. Whether the "nasal pool" technique can be employed in young preschool children remains to be examined.

3.3. "Lamina Propria" Lavage

The graded airway plasma exudation response is relatively specific to inflammation and may reflect the intensity of inflammatory disease processes *(19)*. It is induced by histamine-type mediators including leukotrienes and bradykinins, but not by simple secretagogues such as methacholine or neural irritants (both capsaicin and nicotine cause pain and secretion in the nose without inducing plasma exudation). The basic physiologic nature of the plasma exudation process is confirmed by the fact that microvascular-epithelial exudation of bulk plasma can occur in human airways without injury and without affecting the ability of the mucosa to absorb surface solutes. Since extravasation, distribution in the extracellular spaces of the mucosa, and para-epithelial luminal entry of plasma occur by mechanisms that allow almost nonsieved flux of macromolecules, the whole plasma exudation process may be best measured by determination of large plasma proteins, notably α_2-macroglobulin, in the airway surface liquids. An additional aspect on the plasma exudation process relates to the possibility that plasma proteins, during their passage through interstitial spaces of the airway mucosa, may bind and move important cell products to the mucosal surface.

In experimental studies, we have thus observed that histamine challenge-induced plasma exudation responses may "transport" cellularly released subepithelial molecules including cytokines and eosinophil granule proteins into the airway lumen *(20,21)*. The luminal appearance of inflammatory cell indices may thus occur secondary to the extensive lamina propria distribution and

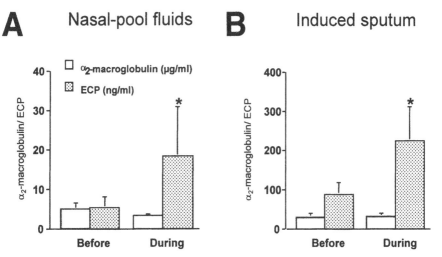

Fig. 3. (**A**) Levels of ECP and α_2-macroglobulin in nasal pool-fluids obtained in children with allergic rhinitis after concomitant histamine (40 µg/mL) challenge and lavage, before and during the pollen season. The levels of α_2-macroglobulin reflect histamine-induced plasma exudation (baseline data not shown). This response to histamine was unaffected by the seasonal allergen exposure. However, the histamine-induced exudation of plasma (α_2-macroglobulin) was associated with an increase in nasal mucosal output of ECP into the pollen season compared with before the season. (From Ref. 20, with permission.) (**B**) Levels of ECP and α_2-macroglobulin in induced sputum obtained after histamine challenge, before and during the pollen season, in patients with allergic rhinitis. The levels of α_2-macroglobulin reflect histamine-induced plasma exudation (baseline data not shown) and this response to histamine was unaffected by the seasonal allergen exposure. Histamine produced an increase in bronchial mucosal output of ECP into the pollen season compared with before the season. Nasal as well as bronchial histamine-challenges thus increase airway mucosal outputs of ECP selectively during the pollen season. These observations suggest the possibility that plasma exudation responses evoked by the challenges moves "free" ECP from the subepithelial compartment into the airway lumen. *$p < 0.05$ compared with before pollen season.(From Ref. 21, with permission. *BMJ Publishing Group* Copyright 1999, *33–36, 54*).

epithelial passage of extravasated bulk plasma that occur within minutes after topical mucosal challenge with histamine. Plasma proteins, especially α_2-macroglobulin, have been demonstrated to bind mediators such as ECP *(22)* as well as many cytokines *(23)*. Hence, we have hypothesized that an "induced exudation" method may be used to bring important mucosal indices of airway inflammation to appear in the nasal mucosal surface liquids.

In a study involving children with allergic rhinitis, we carried out isotonic saline and histamine lavages before and during a pollen season *(20)*. Exclusively during the active allergic disease period the histamine challenge-induced exudation of plasma (α_2-macroglobulin) acutely increased the lavage fluid levels of ECP (*see* **Fig. 3a**). Thus, after repeated nasal lavages with isotonic saline, creating baseline conditions, the histamine-induced plasma exudation response was associated with a six-fold increase in nasal lavage fluid levels of ECP. There is no known mechanism by which histamine could have increased luminal ECP by direct effects on the airway eosinophils. Hence, we interpret these data as an indirect effect involving a histamine-induced "lamina propria lavage" producing luminal entry of subepithelial cell products along with the luminal entry of plasma-derived binding proteins.

Using induced sputum in healthy subjects we have recently demonstrated that histamine challenges, in similarity to our findings in the nose, produce acute luminal entry of α_2-macroglobulin *(24)*. As mentioned above, plasma contains many binding proteins that bind inflammatory cell products. Bronchial luminal entry of extravasated plasma may thus enrich sputum with molecules that otherwise would have remained in the extracellular matrix of the epithelium and the lamina propria. This may be a particularly important consideration for studies of the lower airways since baseline conditions cannot be established in the bronchi by repeated rinsing with saline before challenge and sampling. Indeed, by combining induced exudation with subsequent induced sputum, the sputum samples exhibited increased levels of ECP in patients who have no history of asthma but who suffer from seasonal allergic rhinitis (*see* **Fig. 3b**) *(21)*. It is of a particular note that the increased sputum levels of ECP were evident only after the induced bronchial exudation of plasma. These data may thus suggest that a degree of eosinophilic inflammation with increased baseline release of granule proteins into the mucosal tissue occurs in the bronchi of these patients.

We have also examined effects of the topical hypertonic saline, which is used for sputum induction, on mucosal levels of plasma proteins in the human nasal airway in the absence and presence of histamine *(25)*. Isotonic saline and hypertonic saline (18–36 mg/mL), with and without histamine (400 µg/mL), were administered onto the nasal mucosa using the "nasal-pool" technique. The lavage fluid levels of α_2-macroglobulin were measured as an index of mucosal exudation (luminal entry) of plasma. Briefly, hypertonic saline did not affect the baseline levels of α_2-macroglobulin, but it increased the histamine-induced mucosal exudation (luminal entry) of plasma ($p < 0.05$). Whether hypertonic saline may augment on-going plasma exudation responses, and whether this is a potential drawback for the use of this challenge (e.g., for inducing sputum) remains to be clarified. It is possible that in the bronchial "dual induction" method related previously (induced exudation followed by induced sputum) a useful interaction between the mediator and the hypertonic exposures may have occurred regarding the efficiency of getting plasma exudation-enriched sputum samples.

Results obtained in nasal as well as bronchial airways thus support the possibility that histamine-induced plasma exudation may constitute a "lamina-propria-lavage" in part rinsing the airway mucosal tissue of its free solutes. Exudative challenges in combination with airway lavages and other surface sampling techniques may thus be important experimental tools whereby events occurring within the airway mucosal tissues may be monitored more directly than at baseline lavage only. It is inferred from the present hypothesis that information regarding on-going plasma exudation processes in the airways may be of general importance for proper interpretation of the determined levels of several indices in different airway samples.

3.4. Filter Paper Disks

A longstanding technique to sample airway mucosal "surface" liquids is by the application of absorbing disks of filter paper *(26)* (*see* **Note 4**). In experimental studies involving guinea-pig tracheal airways it was demonstrated that such absorbing disks actually drag subepithelial fluid and solutes, including macromolecules, into the airway lumen *(27)*. Accordingly, filter paper disks may not qualify for selective sampling of airway mucosal surface liquids. On the other hand, the fact that filter paper disks collect a combination of mucosal surface and epithelial/subepithelial liquids and molecules may also be used with distinct experimental advantage (compare the discussion above on "lamina propria lavage"). Furthermore, the sampled fluids are not diluted by this technique which has experimental advantages for determination of indices that are present in the nasal mucosa at low concentrations *(26)*.

1. Cut filter paper disks to suitable sizes.
2. Weigh disks.
3. Place disks in contact with the nasal mucosa for a selected period of time.
4. Reweigh disks (to allow calculation of recovered volume).
5. Disks may be dried at room temperature and frozen awaiting elution.
6. Elute solutes using the elution buffer.
7. Shake overnight at 4°C, and centrifuged at 400g for 15 min.
8. Store eluate at −70°C awaiting analysis.

Using filter paper disks, we have recently demonstrated that single dose allergen challenge produces a nonsymptomatic and nonexudative, late-phase mucosal output of inflammatory cytokines 3–9 h after challenge *(28)*. These cytokines are not readily detectable in similar challenge experiments where unconcentrated nasal lavage fluids have been sampled and analyzed. Finally, filter paper disks have been successfully used for strictly local challenges (e.g., prior to its application the filter paper could have been allowed to absorb a defined dose of allergen) in combination with the local sampling of mucosal fluids and their content of inflammatory indices *(29)*.

3.5. Approaches to Analysis

Only general aspects on handling of samples are briefly reviewed here. In studies designed to examine soluble factors of airway inflammation (inflammatory cell products, plasma proteins, and glandular secretions) it may be important to remove cells that release mediators in the test tube. This is routinely accomplished by centrifugation ($105g$, 10 min, 4°C) and sampling of supernatants. These may need preparation before being frozen for later analysis. In order to improve stability of analytes such as bradykinins, it may be necessary to add EDTA (0.2 mol/L) to the obtained lavage samples (one part EDTA per four parts lavage fluid).

The nasal lavage fluids may contain mucous portions to a variable degree, and this may be a problem. The sample may be homogenized either by mucolytic substances (e.g., dithiotreitol) or by ultrasonication. Our experience with induced sputum samples suggests that the employment of mucolytic substances may greatly affect sample levels of common indices including ECP. Unfortunately, too little is known at present about the distribution of different analytes between the sol and gel phases of airway surface samples.

4. Notes

1. The most critical issue regarding nasal lavage procedures, in general, may be the recovery of nasal lavage fluids and the overall reproducibility and variability of the technique employed. It is essential that these characteristics are checked for and reported.

2. One important option with nasal lavage procedures is the use of repeated saline lavages for the creation of an experimental "baseline" condition where any disturbing mucosal surface material has been removed. This procedure may be vital to the success of studying effects of challenges and similar interventions.

3. Histamine challenges may be employed to produce transient plasma exudation responses that could move "free" molecules from the lamina propria and epithelium into the airway lumen to be picked up by the lavage fluid. Theoretically, this measure would improve the yield of inflammatory mediators and cytokines and improve the possibility that airway surface sample data directly reflect processes occurring in the diseased mucosal tissue. However, it must be underscored that this is a newly introduced hypothesis/technique and continued validation of its employment and further development are warranted.

4. When analytes are present in nasal mucosal surface liquids in very low concentrations, filter papers may be employed to retrieve these solutes in a nondiluted sample. The caveat with absorbing disk techniques is that they do not merely sample surface liquids but they drag subepithelial fluid and solutes into the sample.

References

1. Persson, C. G. A. (1996) *In vivo veritas:* the continuing importance of discoveries in complex biosystems. *Thorax.* **51,** 441–443.
2. Persson, C. G. A. (1999) Clinical research, or classical research? *Nature Med.* **5,** 714–715.
3. Persson, C. G. A, Svensson, C., Greiff, L., Andersson, M., Wollmer, P., Alkner, U., and Erjefält, I. (1992) The use of the nose to study the inflammatory response in the respiratory tract. *Thorax* **47,** 993–1000.
4. Erjefält, J.S. and Persson, C. G. A. New aspects on degranulation and fates of airway mucosal eosinophils. *Am. J. Resp. Crit. Care. Med.* In press.
5. Greiff, L., Pipkorn, U., Alkner, U., and Persson, C. G. A. (1990) The "Nasal Pool-device" applies controlled concentrations of solutes on human nasal airway mucosa and samples its surface exudations/secretions. *Clin. Exp. Allergy.* **20,** 253–259.
6. Naclerio, R.M., Meier, H.L., Kagey-Sobotka, A., Adkinson, Jr., N.F., Meyers, D.A., Norman, P.S., and Lichtenstein, L.M. (1983) Mediator release after nasal airway challenge with allergen. *Am. Rev. Respir. Dis.* **128,** 597–602.
7. Mygind, N. and Versterhauge, S. (1978) Aerosol distribution in the nose. *Rhinology* **16,** 131–136.
8. Wihl, J.A., Baumgarten, C. R., and Petersson, G. (1995) Contralateral differences among biomarkers determined by a modified nasal lavage technique after unilateral allergen challenge. *Allergy* **50,** 3308–3315.
9. Svensson, C., Andersson, M., Greiff, L., Alkner, U., and Persson, C.G.A. (1995) Exudative hyperresponsiveness of the airway microcirculation in seasonal allergic rhinitis. *Clin. Exp. Allergy* **25,** 942–950.
10. Greiff, L., Erjefält, I., Wollmer, P., Andersson, M., Pipkorn, U., Alkner, U., and Persson, C.G.A. (1993) Effects of nicotine on the human nasal airway mucosa. *Thorax.* **48,** 651–655.
11. Bisgaard, H., Grønborg, H., Mygind, N., Dahl, R., Lindqvist, N., and Venge, P. (1990) Allergen-induced increase of eosinophil cationic protein in nasal lavage fluid: effect of the glucocorticoid budesonide. *J. Allergy. Clin. Immunol.* **85,** 891–895.
12. Greiff, L., Lundin, S., Svensson, C., Andersson, M., Wollmer, P., and Persson, C.G.A. (1997) Reduced airway absorption in seasonal allergic rhinitis. *Am. J. Respir. Crit. Care. Med.* **156,** 783–786.
13. Onda, T., Nagakura, T., Uekusa, T., Masaki, T., and Iikura, Y. (1990) Drug effects on antigen-induced release of high molecular weight neutrophil chemotactic activity and histamine in nasal secretion from children with allergic rhinitis. *Allergy. Proc.* **11,** 235–240.
14. Sigurs, N., Bjarnason, R., and Sigurbergsson, F. (1994) Eosinophil cationic protein in nasal secretion and in serum and myeloperoxidase in serum in respiratory syncytial virus bronchitis: relation to asthma and atopy. *Acta. Pediatr.* **83,** 1151–1155.
15. Wang, D., Clement, P., and Lauwers, S. (1994) Comparison of bacterial culture results in bronchoalveolar lavage and nasal lavage fluid in children with pulmonary infection. *Int. J. Ped. Otorhinolaryngol.* **28,** 149–155.

16. Noah, T. L., Henderson, F. W., Wortman, I. A., Devlin, R. B., Handy, J., Koren, H. S., and Becker, S. (1995) Nasal cytokine production in viral acute upper respiratory infection of childhood. *J. Inf. Dis.* **171**, 584–592.
17. Noah, T. L., Henderson, F. W., Henry, M. M., Peden, D. B., and Devlin, R. B. (1995) Nasal lavage cytokines in normal, allergic, and asthmatic school-age children. *Am. J. Respir. Crit. Care. Med.* **152**, 1290–1296.
18. Greiff, L., Meyer, P., Svensson, C., Persson, C. G. A., and Andersson, M. (1997) The "Nasal Pool"-device for challenge and lavage of the nasal mucosa in children: Histamine-induced plasma exudation responses. *Pediatr. Allergy. Immunol.* **8**, 137–142.
19. Persson, C. G. A., Erjefält, J. S., Greiff, L., Andersson, M., Erjefält, I., Godfrey, R. W., et al. (1998) Plasma-derived proteins in airway defence, disease and repair of epiethelial injury. *Eur. Respir. J.* **11**, 958–970.
20. Meyer, P., Persson, C.G.A., Andersson, M., Wollmer, P., Linden, M., Svensson, C., and Greiff, L. (1999) α_2-Macroglobulin and eosinophil cationic protein in the allergic airway mucosa in seasonal allergic rhinitis. *Eur. Respir. J.* **13**, 633–637.
21. Greiff, L., Andersson, M., Svensson, C., Linden, M., Wollmer, P., and Persson, C. G. A. (1999) Demonstration of bronchial eosinophil activity in seasonal allergic rhinitis by induced plasma exudation combined with induced sputum. *Thorax.* **54**, 33–36.
22. Peterson, C. G. and Venge, P. (1987) Interaction and complex-formation between the eosinophil cationic protein and α_2-macroglobulin. *Biochem. J.* **245**, 781–787.
23. James, K. (1990) Interactions between cytokines and α_2-macroglobulin. *Immunol. Today.* **11**, 163–166.
24. Haldorsdottir, H., Greiff, L., Wollmer, P., Andersson, M., Svensson, C., and Persson, C. G. A. (1997) Effect of inhaled histamine, methacholine, and capsaicin on sputum levels of a_2-macroglobulin. *Thorax.* **52**, 964–968.
25. Greiff, L., Wollmer, P., Svensson, C., Andersson, M., Alkner, U., and Persson, C. G. A. (1994) Effects of hypertonic saline on mucosal exudation of plasma in human airways. *Allergy. Clin. Immunol. News.* Suppl. **2**, 76.
26. Sim, T. C., Grant, J. A., Kimberly, A., Hilsmeier, H., Fukuda, Y., and Alam, R. (1994) Proinflammatory cytokines in nasal secretions of allergic subjects after antigen challenge. *Am. J. Respir. Crit. Care. Med.* **149**, 339–344.
27. Erjefält, I. and Persson, C. G. A. (1990) On the use of absorbing disks to sample mucosal surface liquids. *Clin. Exp. Allergy.* **20**, 193–197.
28. Linden, M., Svensson, C., Andersson, E., Andersson, M., Greiff, L., and Persson, C. G. A. (1999) Acute effects of topical budesonide on nasal mucosal GM-CSF and IL-5 after allergen challernge in allergic rhintis *J. Allergy. Clin. Immunol.* **103**, S250.
29. Wagenmann, M., Baroody, F. M., Kagey-Sobotka, A., Lichtenstein, L. M., and Naclerio, R. M. (1994) The effect of terfenadine on unilateral challenge with allergen. *J. Allergy. Clin. Immunol.* **93**, 594–605.

II

SAMPLE COLLECTION

NONINVASIVE TECHNIQUES

5

Induced Sputum

Selection Method

Margaret M. Kelly, Ann Efthimiadis, and Frederick E. Hargreave

1. Introduction

Sputum consists of a mixture of mucus, inflammatory and epithelial cells, and cellular degradation products from the lower respiratory tract. In normal subjects, the inflammatory cells are mainly neutrophils and macrophages, with small numbers of lymphocytes, eosinophils, mast cells, and basophils. When expectorated the sputum is commonly contaminated with a variable amount of saliva, which has abundant squamous epithelial cells, and sometimes with secretions from the nasopharynx. These can be reduced by blowing the nose, rinsing the mouth, and swallowing water before expectoration. Contamination with saliva can be minimized by selecting the sputum from the expectorate and discarding the remainder. Selection of sputum *(1)* improves between-observer repeatability of differential cell counts *(2,3)* and allows standardization of measurements of total cell counts (expressed per gram of sputum) and fluid-phase mediators (by knowledge of the dilution factor of the processed sample).

The examination of sputum has been hindered by difficulties in obtaining a homogeneous dispersed sample. These have been overcome with the use of an inhalation of saline aerosol to induce sputum *(4)* and with the use of mucolytics to disperse it *(5,6)*. The induction has been demonstrated to be safe in mild asthma *(7,8)* and, with modifications, it is safe in more severe asthma or chronic airflow limitation *(9,10)*.

Once expectorated, the cells in the sputum will degenerate. The speed with which this happens and methods to prevent it have not been investigated. Hence for the moment, it is suggested that the sputum be processed as soon as pos-

From: *Methods in Molecular Medicine, vol. 56:*
Human Airway Inflammation: Sampling Techniques and Analytical Protocols
Edited by: D. F. Rogers and L. E. Donnelly © Humana Press Inc., Totowa, NJ

sible, at least within 2 h, and that it be kept in the fridge at 4°C during any delay. Being viscid, sputum is not homogeneous. The examination of unprocessed smears has the disadvantage of sampling only a circumscribed part of the sputum. In addition, the cells are entrapped in mucus and often overlap which makes them difficult to identify. The introduction of efficient mucolytics to release the entrapped cells, and the use of cytospins to ensure a monolayer of cells *(11)* has made the quantification and characterization of cells reliable *(4)*. In addition, the cells may be removed by centrifugation, and the fluid-phase stored for later analysis. The mucolytic used here is dithiothreitol (DTT) *(12)* which reduces disulphide bonds which crosslink glycoprotein fibers and maintain sputum in its gel form. DTT is an efficient, convenient mucolytic which causes minimal damage to the cells *(13–15)*.

Cell counts and some fluid-phase measurements in selected DTT-processed sputum have been shown to have good reproducibility and validity *(2,4,16,17)*, and a comprehensive set of normal values of cellular indices in healthy subjects has been compiled *(18)*. Using the technique to be described, examination of sputum for cell and inflammatory components is increasingly being recognized as a useful investigative tool *(19–22)*.

2. Materials

2.1. Reagents

1. Dulbecco's phosphate-buffered saline (PBS) (Gibco Diagnostics, Tucson, AZ).
2. Dithiothreitol. (Sputolysin, a mixture of dithiothreitol in phosphate buffer, Calbiochem, La Jolla, CA) (*see* **Note 1**).
3. Trypan blue stain, 0.4% (w/v).
4. Wright's stain (*see* **Note 2**).
5. Toluidine blue.

2.2. Apparatus

1. Polypropylene funnel (top diameter 5.5 cm).
2. Nylon gauze, mesh 48 μM (Sefar Inc., Mississauga, ON, Canada).
3. Cytospin 3 Cytocentrifuge, (Shandon Inc., Pittsburgh, PA).
4. Cytocentrifuge sample chambers, cytoclips, and filter cards (Shandon Inc.).

3. Methods

3.1. Sputum Processing

1. Examination of sputum: the expectorate is tipped into a Petri dish, and examined on a black background. The color and consistency of the sputum is noted, and is described as mucoid if clear or white, purulent if yellow or green, or mucopurulent if in-between. The latter two states usually indicate the presence of numerous neutrophils.

2. Selection of sputum from expectorate: the expectorate is inspected for viscid, dense areas which are often fairly well-circumscribed, and these can be selected using blunt-toothed forceps. It is useful to inspect the overall quality of the sample under an inverted microscope and, if the expectorate is watery and contaminated by a large amount of saliva, selection can be guided by the microscope. Salivary areas are easily recognized under the microscope by the characteristic squamous cells, identified by their sharp borders, single round central nucleus, and voluminous cytoplasm. The smaller, round cells, often in densely crowded groups, are indicative of inflammatory cells from the bronchial airways (*see* **Note 3**). Occasionally columnar epithelial cell groups are seen. Areas of squamous contamination are avoided as far as possible and areas with inflammatory cells present are selected.

3. Select approx 200 mg of sputum. This has been found to be adequate for the purposes of cell counts and allows the collection of ~1 mL of supernatant after processing (*see* **Note 4**). Purulent sputum is often of large volume, in the order of several mL, and not usually contaminated by saliva, making selection easy.

4. Dispersion of sputum: the sputum is placed in a preweighed 15-mL polystyrene tube, and weighed. DTT is freshly prepared by diluting Sputolysin 1:10 with distilled water to give a solution of 6.5 mM DTT in 100 mM phosphate buffer, pH 7.0. Four volumes of DTT are then added to the sputum (4 µL DTT for every 1 mg sputum) (*see* **Note 5**).

5. The mixture is then briefly vortexed (for about 5 s), and placed on a bench rocker at room temperature (*see* **Note 6**) for 15 min.

6. Briefly vortex the mixture again and inspect for nondispersed particles. If these are seen, gentle tituration using a disposal pipet is performed to break up these stubborn clumps (*see* **Note 7**). The dispersed sputum is then passed through a nylon gauze filter (48µ*m* pore-size) lining a funnel into a pre-weighed 15mL polystyrene tube. The filtered cell suspension is then weighed.

3.2. Total Cell-Count and Viability

1. The filtrate is again vortexed briefly, and 10 µL removed and mixed with 10 µL 0.4% trypan blue in an Eppendorf tube (*see* **Note 8**).

2. 10 µL of the mixture is placed into an Improved Neubauer hemocytometer (*see* **Note 9**) and the total numbers of nonsquamous cells, both stained and unstained, are counted. Squamous cells (usually <5% in our hands with this method), can be recognized by their large size and morphology and are ignored. All nonsquamous cells are counted in the chamber (*see* **Notes 10** and **11**).

3. Based on the original sputum weight, the weight of the filtrate and the number of cells per square, the total nonsquamous cells present in the sputum are calculated and expressed as the number per gram or mL of sputum (*see* **Note 12**).

4. The cell viability is performed simultaneously by counting the number of cells staining with trypan blue (*see* **Note 13**).

Table 1
Morphology of Cells Seen on Sputum Cytology

Cell	Diameter (μM)	Nucleus	Cytoplasm
Neutrophil	10–14	multilobed	numerous small granules visible on Wright's stain
Eosinophil	10–17	bilobed	large eosinophilic granules
Macrophage	up to 25	nonsegmented	pale vacuolated cytoplasm with occasional pigmented granules
Monocyte	up to 20	irregular, often notched on one side	pale blue, vacuolated cytoplasm
Basophil	14–16	bilobed, condensed chromatin	large dark-blue granules, often obscure the nucleus, stains metachromatically with toluidine blue
Mast cell	14–16	nonsegmented	ovoid or spindle shaped, stains metachromatically with toluidine blue
Lymphocyte	6–9 (occasionally 9–15)	nonsegmented	blue cytoplasm, usually only a thin rim
Columnar epithelial cell	up to 30	often basal	may be ciliated (up to 6 mm in length); may be in cohesive groups
Squamous epithelial cell	40–60	small, pyknotic	Voluminous cytoplasm

3.3. Preparation of Cytospins

1. A portion of the filtrate is removed, and adjusted to a total cell count of 1×10^6 cells/mL of filtrate if necessary (*see* **Note 14**).
2. 70–80 µL (*see* **Note 15**) of the cell suspension is placed in the sample chamber of the cytocentrifuge, and centrifuged at 23g (*see* **Note 16**) for 6 min (*see* **Notes 17** and **18**).
3. The unstained slides are examined under the microscope by lowering the condenser slightly to increase contrast and allowing the cell outlines to be seen and thereby determining if there is a uniform monolayer with minimal overlap.
4. The slides are air-dried and stained with Wright's stain (*see* **Note 19**) which stains the nuclei blue and the cytoplasm pale pink. Eosinophil granules stain a bright pink, whereas basophil granules stain dark purple. **Table 1** lists the main features to aid recognition of cells encountered in sputum.
5. A differential count is performed on at least 400 nonsquamous cells (*see* **Note 20**).
6. If metachromatic cells (mast cells and basophils) are to be investigated, additional cytospins are fixed with Carnoys fixative (*see* **Note 21**) and stained with toluidine blue, and at least 1500 nonsquamous cells are counted.

Table 2
Normal Values of Sputum Total and Absolute Differential Cell Counts
($\times 10^6$ cells/mL)

	Mean (SD)	Normal range Mean -2SD	Mean +2SD	Median (IQR)	Percentiles 10	90
Total cell count	4.13 (4.81)	-4.6	13.76	2.4 (3.19)	0.67	9.73
Eosinophils	0.01 (0.04)	-0.06	0.09	0.00 (0.01)	0	0.04
Neutrophils	1.96 (3.03)	-4.09	8.02	0.87 (1.96)	0.1	4.86
Macrophages	2.13 (2.03)	-1.93	6.18	1.64 (1.87)	0.3	4.86
Lymphocytes	0.04 (0.07)	-0.1	0.18	0.02 (0.05)	0.01	0.09
Bronchial epithelial cells	0.01 (0.04)	-0.06	0.09	0.01 (0.01)	0	0.03

Table 3
Sputum Differential Cell Counts (%)

	Mean (SD)	Normal range Mean -2SD	Mean +2SD	Median (IQR)	Percentiles 10	90
Eosinophils	0.4 (0.9)	-1.4	2.2	0.0 (0.3)	0	1.1
Neutrophils	37.5 (20.1)	-2.7	77.7	36.7 (29.5)	11	64.4
Macrophages	58.8 (21.0)	16.8	100.8	60.8 (28.9)	33	86.1
Lymphocytes	1.0 (1.1)	-1.2	3.2	0.5 (1.8)	0.01	2.6
Metachromatic cells	0.0 (0.0)	-0.1	0.1	0.0 (0.0)	0	0
Bronchial epithelial cells	1.6 (3.9)	-6.2	9.4	0.3 (1.3)	0	4.4

3.4. Interpretation of Cell Counts and Differentials

Normal values for the total and differential cell counts (when sputum is processed by the method described) are given in **Tables 2** and **3**. The accuracy of the counts can be reduced by low cell viability (<40%), excessive cell degeneration or excessive squamous contamination. Apoptotic eosinophils, which may be increased after corticosteroid therapy, have a condensed, unilobed nucleus *(23)*. However, the characteristic eosinophilic granules are usually still evident, making identification possible. Immature macrophages or monocytes may be difficult to distinguish from large lymphocytes *(24)*. The presence of macrophages indicates that the sample is from the lower respiratory tract. Ciliated columnar epithelium can be derived from the bronchial or nasal mucosa.

The total cell count increases in uncontrolled asthma *(4,9)*, smokers *(4,10,25)*, and particularly in viral and bacterial infections *(20)*. The proportion of neutrophils is increased in asthma *(4)*, smokers bronchitis with or without chronic airflow limitation *(10,25,26)* and in infections *(20,27)*. In smokers with chronic airflow limitation, the proportion of neutrophils correlates inversely with the degree of airflow limitation *(17,28,29)*. Few eosinophils are present in healthy subjects (<2%). An increase in sputum eosinophils can be observed in asthma, chronic cough without asthma (when asthma is defined as variable airflow limitation) *(30,31)* and in some patients with chronic airflow limitation *(10,32)*.

3.5. Immunoassay and Histochemical Analysis of Supernatant

The sputum cell suspension is centrifuged at $290g \times 4$ min, and the supernatant removed. It can then be stored at $-70°C$ for future measurements of soluble mediators (*see* **Note 22**). Numerous cytokines and inflammatory mediators can be measured in sputum supernatant *(4,6,25,33–42)*:

1. Cytokines: e.g., interleukin (IL)-1β, 5, 6, and 10, tumour necrosis factor (TNF)α, transforming growth factor (TGF)β.
2. Cytokine receptors: e.g., IL-1 receptor antagonist (IL-1ra) and type II TNF soluble receptor (sTNFRII).
3. Chemokines: e.g., eotaxin, IL-8, regulation on activation normal T-cell expressed and secreted chemokine (RANTES).
4. Eosinophil proteins: e.g., eosinophil cationic protein (ECP), eosinophil peroxidase (EPO).
5. Neutrophil products: e.g., myeloperoxidase (MPO), human neutrophil lipocalin (HNL).
6. Markers of vascular leakage: e.g., albumin, fibrinogen, α2-macroglobulin.
7. Eicosanoids: leukotrienes and prostaglandins.
8. Proteases: e.g., elastase, cathepsin G, matrix metalloproteinase-9, tryptase.
9. Protease-inhibitors: e.g., α1-antitrypsin.
10. Soluble products of nitric oxide.
11. Miscellaneous: e.g., substance P, endothelin-1, and vascular cell adhesion molecule-1 (VCAM-1).

The use of DTT has not been shown to interfere with the measurement of ECP, total IL-8, IL-5, tryptase, or IgA *(43,44)*. The addition of protease-inhibitors to sputum prior to processing appears to increase IL-5 levels *(45)*.

3.6. Further Applications

3.6.1. Special Stains

Sputum has shown clinical application in diagnosis of oropharyngeal reflux (and possible microaspiration), using the oil-red O stain which stains lipid within macrophages *(46)*. Hemosiderin-laden macrophages can be identified with Perls' stain, and can be used as a discriminatory test for left ventricular dysfunction when other causes of pulmonary hemorrhage are excluded *(21)*. The full description of these stains is beyond the scope of this chapter, and readers should refer to the references.

3.6.2. Immunocytochemistry

Cytospins should be fixed soon after preparation. The choice of fixative depends on the antigen to be detected, but 50:50 acetone:methanol, 4% paraformaldehyde, and periodate-lysine-paraformaldehyde *(47)* are fixatives commonly used. Once fixed, the slides should be dried overnight and can then be stored at −70°C indefinitely after being wrapped tightly in metal foil. Various cellular markers have been detected in sputum cells using immunocytochemistry *(25,48–51)*. DTT has been shown to effect the expression of some markers on cells, and appropriate controls for each marker should be performed *(52)*.

3.6.3. Polymerase Chain Reaction

This technique has been applied to sputum cells to detect cytokine mRNA (IL-1α, IL-2, IL-6, IL-8, RANTES, TNF-α, IFN-α, IFN-γ) *(53)*, as well as DNA from numerous infectious agents *(54,55)*. The reader is referred to the references for more information.

3.6.4. In Situ *Hybridization*

Cytospins can be prepared in Rnase-free conditions and the prepared cytospins used for *in situ* hybridization *(56)*.

3.6.5. Transmission Electron Microscopy

Electron microscopy can be performed on the cell pellet. This should be fixed in 2% glutaraldehyde in 0.1 *M* cacodylate buffer at 4°C for 2 h taking care not to agitate or break up the pellet. Once fixed, it can be processed in a manner similar to a small biopsy, and ultrathin sections cut *(57)*.

3.6.6. Flow Cytometry

Using flow cytometry, various surface markers have been detected on sputum cells *(50,58–61)*.

4. Notes

1. According to the manufacturer, DTT is stable for 2–3 yr at room temperature. The DTT can be aspirated through the rubber bung at the top of the container,

using a 1-mL syringe to prevent air entering into the vial. Once in use, it should be stored at 4°C and used within 1 or 2 wk.

2. Other stains suitable for air-dried slides may be used, such as May-Grunwald-Giemsa or the Diff-Quik stain. It is recommended that the same stain should be used regularly, to ensure uniformity. It is important that the various stains are made up freshly so as to keep the staining reliable. Wright's stain has been demonstrated to be more effective at identifying basophils *(24)* than the Diff-Quik stain. Chromotrope 2R *(62)* is a bright red stain for eosinophil granules, and may be preferred if only eosinophils are being counted.

3. Nasal secretions can be a source of contamination, and can be difficult to exclude on microscopy. This can usually be recognized by the operator doing the induction, and can be minimized by instructing the patient to blow his or her nose and not sniff back before expectoration. A similar procedure should be followed when collecting spontaneous sputum.

4. With increasing volumes of sputum processed, there is a decrease in the proportion of cells recovered after processing owing to difficulties with dispersion and also during filtration where blockage of the filter occurs. However, if numerous fluid-phase measurements or several cytospins are required, it may be necessary to process a larger volume of sputum.

5. For practical purposes, it is assumed that the specific gravity of sputum is 1, and therefore 1 g sputum is considered to have a volume of 1 mL. The specific gravity is usually slightly less, 0.8–0.9, although in purulent sputum it may be more.

6. Some investigators incubate the sputum-DTT mixture at 37°C, although there is no evidence that dispersal is more effective than at room temperature *(43)*.

7. It is extremely important to completely disperse the sample since failure to do this results in the loss of cells on the filter with resultant reduction in the total cell counts as well as difficulties with staining. Some investigators employ a shaking water bath to break up the clumps, but a direct comparison has not been performed with a bench-rocker.

8. The trypan blue sputum mixture should be allowed to stand for 3–5 min to allow equilibration. Nonviable cells are unable to exclude dye from their cytoplasm, and consequently take up the blue stain. Cells that still have a functioning cell membrane do not take up dye and are not stained. Extended intervals of equilibration should be avoided, since trypan blue is toxic to cells.

9. The heavy glass cover slip recommended for use with the hemocytometer should be used (and not the cover slips used for slides) to ensure an accurate volume of fluid floods the chamber. The chamber should be filled by capillary action without forcing the suspension into it. It should not be over- or underfilled.

10. Each chamber of the hemocytometer consists of nine large squares subdivided into several smaller ones. Nonsquamous cells in all nine squares are usually counted, but if the specimen is very cellular (as in purulent samples), less squares may be counted. At least 200–300 cells are counted in total.

11. To ensure that the same cell is not counted twice, count cells touching the top and left line of the perimeter of each square and avoid counting cells touching the bottom and right perimeter.

12. Each large square (9 in total), with cover slip in place, represents a total volume of 0.1 mm^3 or 10^{-4} cm^3 (the square has an area of 1 mm^2 and is 0.1 mm deep from coverglass down to chamber). Since 1 cm^3 is equivalent to approx 1 mL, each large square has a volume of 10^{-4} mL (or 0.1 μL).
    The formula used to calculate the number of cells in the filtrate/mL is:

$$\text{Cells/mL} = \text{No. of cells} \times \text{dilution factor}$$

No. of large squares counted × volume of each square (mL)

Dilution factor = dilution of sputum in trypan blue (= 2 in this method).
Since the volume of each square is 10^{-4} mL, the formula can then be given as

$$\text{Cells/mL} = \frac{\text{No. of cells} \times 2 \times 10^{4}}{[\text{No. of large squares counted}]}$$

Total cells in the filtrate = cells/mL x volume of filtrate (mL)
(The volume of filtrate in mL is assumed to be equal to the weight in grams)
    Assuming total cells in filtrate is equal to total cells in sputum, then:
Total cells/mL of sputum = total cells in filtrate/sputum wt. (g)
This may also be expressed per sputum volume in mL, since 1 g sputum is ~1mL:
Example: sputum weight is 0.2 g, filtrate weighs 1.8 g (approx 1.8mL), average number of cells counted per square is 50, then the filtrate contains $50 \times 2 \times 10^4$ cells/mL:

Total cells in filtrate $= 50 \times 2 \times 10^4 \times 1.8$

Total cells/mL sputum $= 50 \times 2 \times 10^4 \times 1.8/0.2$

$= 1.5 \times 10^6$ cells/mL sputum (or 1.5×10^6 cells/g sputum).

13. Calculation of cell viability: if the total number of cells counted in all squares is 250, and the number staining with trypan blue is 50, then the % of viable cells is
$$= (250 - 50/250) \times 100$$
$$= 80\%.$$
14. Since the cell count/mL of the filtrate has been measured, the dilution factor required can be calculated. PBS is used to dilute the suspension.
15. Shandon (the manufacturers of the cytocentrifuge used) recommend that the samples chambers be loaded with 100–500 μL, but we have found lesser volumes to be suitable.
16. This speed has been found to produce minimal distortion of cells. However, slow speeds (23 g as opposed to 90 g) to may result in greater loss of small cells such as lymphocytes *(11,63)*.
17. Filter cards are placed between the sample chamber and slide, held in place by cytoclips. These are used to ensure a tight fit and to absorb excess fluid after the cells have been deposited on the slide. White, absorbent filters are generally used,

but for samples with very low cell counts ($<2 \times 10^6$/mL) brown, less absorbent filters may be used.

18. The sample chambers should be loaded after they have been assembled and inserted into the sealed head. The sample should not be forcibly injected into the chamber, neither should the specimen be allowed to run down the sides of the chamber. Rather, the sample should be directly deposited into the bottom of the chamber.

19. Wright's stain is used routinely in many hematology laboratories, hence it is often easily available. Like May-Grunwald-Giemsa and Diff-Quik stains, it is used for air-dried slides, which are then fixed briefly in methanol before staining. There is greater distortion of cell morphology with air-drying than if the cells are immediately fixed, but this is within acceptable limits for cell differentials.

20. The use of cytocentrifuge preparations does result in a disproportionate loss of small cells, especially lymphocytes, so this should be borne in mind *(11,63)*.

21. Carnoys fixative contains methanol, chloroform, and glacial acetic acid.

22. If numerous cytospins are required for extra histochemical stains or immunocytochemistry, and supernatant is also required for measurement of mediators, the supernatant can be removed first, and the cell pellet resuspended to approx 1×10^6 cells/mL in PBS. This suspension may then be used to prepare numerous cytospins without wastage of supernatant.

References

1. Pizzichini, E., Pizzichini, M. M. M., Efthimiadis, A., Hargreave, F. E., and Dolovich, J. (1996) Measurement of inflammatory indices in induced sputum:effects of selection of sputum to minimize salivary contamination. *Eur. Respir. J.* **9,** 1174–1180.

2. Ward, R., Woltmann, G., Wardlaw, A. J., and Pavord, I. D. (1998) Between-observer repeatability of sputum differential cell counts. Influence of cell viability and squamous cell contamination. *Clin. Exp. Allergy* **29,** 248–252.

3. Spanevello, A., Beghe, B., Bianchi, A., Migliori, G. B., Ambrosetti, M., Neri, M., and Ind, P. W. (1998) Comparison of two methods of processing induced sputum: selected versus entire sputum. *Am. J.Respir. Crit. Care Med.* **157**, 665–668.

4. Pizzichini, E., Pizzichini, M. M. M., Efthimiadis, A., Evans, S., Morris, M. M., Squillace, D., et al. (1996) Indices of airway inflammation in induced sputum: reproducibility and validity of cell and fluid-phase measurements. *Am. J. Respir. Crit. Care Med.* **154**, 308–317.

5. Popov, T., Gottschalk, R., Kolendowicz, R., Dolovich, J., Powers, P., and Hargreave, F. E. (1994) The evaluation of a cell dispersion method of sputum examination. *Clin . Exp. Allergy* **24,** 778–783.

6. Pizzichini, M. M. M., Popov, T., Efthimiadis, A., Hussack, P., Evans, S., Pizzichini, E., et al. (1996) Spontaneous and induced sputum to measure indices of airway inflammation in asthma. *Am. J. Respir. Crit. Care Med.* **154,** 866–869.

7. Wong, H. H. and Fahy, J. V. (1997) Safety of one method of sputum induction in asthmatic subjects. *Am. J. Respir. Crit. Care Med.* **156,** 299–303.

8. de la Fuente, P. T., Romagnoli, M., Godard, P., Bousquet, J., and Chanez, P. (1998) Safety of inducing sputum in patients with asthma of varying severity. *Am. J. Respir .Crit. Care Med.* **157,** 1127–1130.

9. Pizzichini, M. M. M., Pizzichini, E., Clelland, L., Efthimiadis, A., Mahony, J., Dolovich, J., and Hargreave, F.E. (1997) Sputum in severe exacerbations of asthma. Kinetics of inflammatory indices after prednisone treatment. *Am. J. Respir. Crit. Care Med.* **155,** 1501–1508.

10. Pizzichini, E., Pizzichini, M. M. M., Gibson, P., Parameswaran, K., Gleich, G. J., Berman, L., Dolovich, J., and Hargreave, F.E. (1998) Sputum eosinophilia predicts benefit from prednisone in smokers with chronic obstructive bronchitis. *Am. J. Respir. Crit. Care Med.* **158,** 1511–1517.

11. Fleury-Feith, J., Escudier, E., Pocholle, M. J., Carre, C., and Bernaudin, J. F. (1987) The effects of cytocentrifugation on differential cell counts in samples obtained by bronchoalveolar lavage. *Acta Cytologica.* **31,** 606–610.

12. Cleland, W.W. (1964) Dithiothreitol, a new protective reagent for SH groups. *Biochemistry* **3,** 480–482.

13. Wooten, O. J. and Dulfano, M. J. (1978) Improved homogenization techniques for sputum cytology counts. *Ann.Allergy* **41,** 150–154.

14. Hirsch, S. R., Zastrow, J. E., and Kory, R. C. (1969) Sputum liquefying agents: A comparative in vitro evaluation. *J. Lab. Clin. Med.* **74,** 346–353.

15. Tockman, M. S., Qiao, Y., Li, L., Zhao, G., Sharma, R., Cavenaugh, L. L., and Erozan, Y. S. (1995) Safe separation of sputum cells from mucoid glycoprotein. *Acta Cytologica.* **39,** 1128–1136.

16. Spanevello, A., Migliori, G. B., Sharara, A., Ballardini, L., Bridge, P., Pisati, P., et al. (1997) Induced sputum to assess airway inflammation: a study of reproducibility. *Clin. Exp. Allergy* **27,** 1138–1144.

17. Peleman, R. A., Rytila, P. H., Kips, J. C., Joos, G. F., and Pauwels, R. A. (1999) The cellular composition of induced sputum in chronic obstructive pulmonary disease. *Eur. Respir J* **13,** 839–843.

18. Belda, J., Leigh, R., Parameswaran, K., O'Byrne, P. M., Sears, M. R., and Hargreave, F. E. (2000) Induced sputum cell counts in healthy adults. *Am. J. Respir.Crit. Care Med.* **161,** 475–478.

19. Hargreave, F. E. (1999) Induced sputum for the investigation of airway inflammation: evidence for its clinical application. *Can. Respir. J.* **6,** 169–174.

20. Parameswaran, K., Pizzichini, M. M. M., Pizzichini, E., Jeffery, P. K., and Hargreave, F. E. (1998) Serial sputum cell counts in the management of chronic airflow limitation. *Eur. Respir. J.* **11,** 1405–1408.

21. Leigh, R., Sharon, R. F., Efthimiadis, A., Hargreave, F. E., and Kitching, A. D. (1999) Diagnosis of left-ventricular dysfunction from induced sputum examination. *Lancet* 833–834.

22. Jayaram, L., Parameswaran, K., Sears, M. R., and Hargreave, F. E. (2000) Induced sputum cell counts: their usefulness in clinical practice. *Eur. Respir. J.* **16,** 150–158.
23. Woolley, K. L., Gibson, P. G., Carty, K., Wilson, A. J., Twaddell, S. H., and Woolley, M. J. (1996) Eosinophil apoptosis and the resolution of airway inflammation in asthma. *Am. J. Respir. Crit. Care Med.* **154,** 237–243.
24. Willcox, M., Kervitsky, A., Watters, L. C., and King, T. E. (1988) Quantification of cells recovered by bronchoalveolar lavage. *Am. Rev. Respir. Dis.* **138,** 74–80.
25. Keatings, V. M. and Barnes, P. J. (1997) Granulocyte activation markers in induced sputum: comparison between chronic obstructive pulmonary disease, asthma, and normal subjects. *Am. J. Respir. Crit. Care Med.* **155,** 449–453.
26. Ronchi, M.C. (1996) Role of sputum differential cell count in detecting airway inflammation in patients with chronic bronchial asthma or COPD. *Thorax* **51,** 1000–1004.
27. Pizzichini, M.M.M., Pizzichini, E., Efthimiadis, A., Chauhan, A.J., Johnston, S.L., Hussack, P., et al. (1998) Asthma and natural colds. Inflammatory indices in induced sputum: a feasibility study. *Am. J. Respir. Crit. Care Med.* **158,** 1178–1184.
28. Gibson, P., Girgis-Gabardo, A., Morris, M. M., Mattoli, S., Kay, J. M., Dolovich, J., et al. (1989) Cellular characteristics of sputum from patients with asthma and chronic bronchitis. *Thorax* **44,** 693–699.
29. Stanescu, D., Sanna, A., Veriter, S., Kostianev, P. G., Calcagni, P. G., Fabbri, M., and Maestrelli, P. (1996) Airways obstruction, chronic expectoration, and rapid decline of FEV_1 in smokers are associated with increased levels of sputum neutrophils. *Thorax* **51,** 267–271.
30. Gibson, P. G., Dolovich, J., Denburg, J. A., Ramsdale, E. H., and Hargreave, F. E. (1989) Chronic cough: eosinophilic bronchitis without asthma. *The Lancet* **1,** 1346–1348.
31. Gibson, P., Hargreave, F. E., Girgis-Gabardo, A., Morris, M. M., Denburg, J.A., and Dolovich, J. (1995) Chronic cough with eosinophilic bronchitis: examination for variable airflow obstruction and response to corticosteroid. *Clin. Exp. Allergy* **25,** 127–132.
32. Balzano, G., Stefanelli, F., Iorio, C., de Felice, A., Melillo, E.M., Martucci, M., and Melillo, G. (1999) Eosinophilic inflammation in stable chronic obstructive pulmonary disease. Relationship with neutrophils and airway function. *Am. J. Respir. Crit. Care Med.* **160,** 1486–1492.
33. Sulakvelidze, I., Inman, M.D., Rerecich, T., and O'Byrne, P. M. (1998) Increases in airway eosinophils and interleukin-5 with minimal bronchoconstriction during repeated low-dose allergen challenge in atopic asthmatics. *Eur. Respir. J.* **11,** 821–827.
34. Buttle, D. J., Burnett, D., and Abrahamson, M. (1990) Levels of neutrophil elastase and cathepsin B activities and cystatins in human sputum: relationship to inflammation. *Scand. J. Clin. Lab. Invest.* **50,** 509–516.
35. Chalmers, G. W., Thomson, L., Macleod, K. J., et al, and Thomson, N. C. (1997) Endothelin-1 levels in induced sputum samples from asthmatic and normal subjects. *Thorax* **52,** 625–627.

36. Salva, P. S., Doyle, N. A., Graham, L., Eigen, H., and Doerschuk, C. M. (1996) TNF-alpha, IL-8, soluble ICAM-1, and neutrophils in sputum of cystic fibrosis patients [see comments]. *Pediatr. Pulmonol.* 11–19.

37. Konno, S., Gonokami, Y., Kurokawa, M., Kawazu, K., Asano, K., Okamoto, K., and Adachi, K. (1996) Cytokine concentrations in sputum of asthmatic patients. *Int. Arch. Allegy. Immunol.* **109,** 73–78.

38. Pavord, I. D., Ward, R., Woltmann, G., Wardlaw, A. J., Sheller, J. R., and Dworski, R. (1999) Induced Sputum Eicosanoid Concentrations in Asthma. *Am. J. Respir. Crit. Care Med.* **160,** 1905–1909.

39. Osika, E., Cavaillon, J. M., Chadelat, K., Boule, M., Fitting, C., Tournier, G., and Clement, A. (1999) Distinct sputum cytokine profiles in cystic fibrosis and other chronic inflammatory airway disease. *Eur. Respir. J.* **14,** 339–346.

40. Culpitt, S. V., Maziak, W., Loukidis, S., Nightingale, J. A., Matthews, J. L., and Barnes, P. J. (1999) Effect of high dose inhaled steroid on cells, cytokines, and proteases in induced sputum in chronic obstructive pulmonary disease. *Am. J. Respir. Crit. Care Med.* **160,** 1635–1639.

41. Fahy, J. V., Liu, J., Wong, H., and Boushey, H. A. (1993) Cellular and biochemical analysis of induced sputum from asthmatic and from healthy subjects. *Am. Rev. Respir. Dis.* **147,** 1126–1131.

42. Keatings, V. M., Collins, P. D., Scott, D. M., and Barnes, P. J. (1996) Differences in IL-8 and TNF-alpha in induced sptum from patients with chronic obstructive pumonary disease or asthma. *Am. J. Respir. Crit. Care Med.* **153,** 530–534.

43. Louis, R., Shute, J., Goldring, K., Perks, B., Lau, L.C., Radermecker, M., and Djukanovic, R. (1999) The effect of processing on inflammatory markers in induced sputum. *Eur. Respir. J.* **13,** 660–667.

44. Kelly, M. M., Evans, S., Leigh, R., Efthimiadis, A., Gleich, G. J., Horsewood, P., and Hargreave, F. E. (1999) Recovery of radiolabelled interleukin-5 (IL-5) from sputum fluid phase differs when estimated by gamma counter or immunoassay. *Am. J. Respir. Crit. Care Med.* **159,** A849.

45. Kelly, M. M., Evans, S., Leigh, R., Efthimiadis, A., Gleich, G. J., Horsewood, P., and Hargreave, F. E. (1999) Assayed levels of interleukin-5 (IL-5) in the fluid phase of induced sputum may be increased by protease-inhibitors. *Eur. Respir. J.* **14,** 166S.

46. Parameswaran, K., Efthimiadis, A., Allen, C. J., and Hargreave, F. E. (1999) Lipid-laden macrophages in induced sputum. *Am. J. Respir. Crit. Care Med.* **159,** A514.

47. McLean, I.W. and Nakane, P.K. (1974) Periodate-lysine-paraformaldehyde fixative. A new fixation for immunoelectron microscopy. *J. Histochem. Cytochem.* **22,** 1077–1083.

48. Girgis-Gabardo, A., Kanai, N., Denburg, J. A., Hargreave, F.E., Jordana, M., and Dolovich, J. (1994) Immunocytochemical detection of granulocyte-macrophage

colony-stimulating factor and eosinophil cationic protein in sputum cells. *J. Allergy Clin. Immunol.* **93,** 945–947.

49. Lensmar, C., Elmberger, G., Sandgren, P., Skold, C. M., and Eklund, A. (1998) Leukocyte counts and macrophage phenotypes in induced sputum and bronchoalveolar lavage fluid from normal subjects. *Eur. Respir. J.* **12,** 595–600.

50. in 't Veen, J. C. C. M., Grootendorst, D. C., Bel, E. H., Smits, H. H., Van der Keur, M., Sterk, P. J., and Hiemstra, P. S. (1998) CD11b and L-selectin expression on eosinophils and neutrophils in blood and induced sputum of patients wtih asthma compared with normal subjects. *Clin. Exp. Allergy* **28,** 606–615.

51. Gauvreau, G. M., Watson, R. M., and O'Byrne, P. M. (1999) Kinetics of allergen-induced airway eosinophilic cytokine production and airway inflammation. *Am. J. Respir. Crit. Care Med.* **160,** 640–647.

52. Qiu, D. and Tan, W. C. (1999) Dithiothreitol has a dose-response effect on cell surface antigen expression. *J. Allergy Clin. Immunol.* **103,** 873–876.

53. Gelder, C. M., Thomas, P. S., Yates, D. H., Adcock, I. M., Morrison, J. F. J., and Barnes, P. J. (1995) Cytokine expression in normal, atopic, and asthmatic subjects using the combination of sputum induction and the polymerase chain reaction. *Thorax* **50,** 1033–1037.

54. Shimomoto, H., Hasegawa, Y., Takagi, N., Ichiyama, S., Takamatsu, J., Saito, H., and Shimokata, K. (1995) Detection of Pneumocystis carinii, Mycobacterium tuberculosis, and cytomegalovirus in human immunodeficiency virus (HIV)-infected patients with hemophilia by polymerase chain reaction of induced sputum samples. *Intern. Med.* **34,** 976–981.

55. Weir, S. C., Fischer, S. H., Stock, F., and Gill, V. J. (1998) Detection of Legionella by PCR in respiratory specimens using a commercially available kit. *Am. J.Clin. Pathol.* **110,** 295–300.

56. Olivenstein, R., Taha, R., Minshall, E. M., and Hamid, Q. (1999) IL-4 and IL-5 mRNA expression in induced sputum of asthmatic subjects:Comparison with bronchial wash. *J. Allergy Clin. Immunol.* **103,** 238–245.

57. Kelly, M. M., Leigh, R., McKenzie, R., Kamada, D., Ramsdale, E. H., and Hargreave, F. E. (2000) Induced sputum examination: diagnosis of pulmonary involvement in Fabry disease. *Thorax,* **55,** 720–721.

58. Louis, R., Shute, J., Biagi, S., Stanciu, L., Marrelli, F., Tenor, H., et al. (1997) Cell infiltration, ICAM-1 expression, and eosinophil chemotactic activity in asthmatic sputum. *Am. J. Respir. Crit. Care Med.* **155,** 466–472.

59. Hansel, T. T., Braunstein , J. B., Walker, C., Blaser, K., Bruijnzeel, P. L. B., Virchow, J. C. J., and Virchow, C. (1991) Sputum eosinophils from asthmatics express ICAM-1 & HLA-DR. *Clin. Exp. Immunol.* **86,** 271–277.

60. Kidney, J. C., Wong, A. G., Efthimiadis, A., Morris, M. M., Sears, M. R., Dolovich, J. and Hargreave, F. E. (1996) Elevated B cells in sputum of asthmatics: close correlation with eosinophils. *Am. J. Respir. Crit. Care Med.* **153,** 540–544.

61. Fireman, E., Greif, J., Schwarz, Y., Man, A., Ganor, E., Ribak, Y., and Lerman, Y. (1999) Assessment of hazardous dust exposure by BAL and induced sputum. *Chest* **115,** 1720–1728.
62. Hakansson, L., Westerlund, D., and Venge, P. (1987) New method for the measurement of eosinophil migration. *J. Leukoc. Biol.* **42,** 689–696.
63. Mordelet-Dambrine, M., Arnoux, A., Stanislas-Leguern, G., Sandron, D., Chretien, J., and Huchon, G. (1984) Processing of lung lavage fluid causes variability in bronchoalveolar cell count. *Am. Rev. Respir. Dis.* **130,** 305–306.

6

Induced Sputum

Whole Sample

Vera M. Keatings and Julia A. Nightingale

1. Introduction

With the introduction of fiberoptic bronchoscopy and the ability to carry out bronchoscopic biopsy and broncho-alveolar lavage (BAL) in patients and control subjects, characterisation of inflammation in airways diseases such as asthma and chronic obstructive respiratory disease (COPD) has been possible. This has allowed emphasis to be placed on the role of inflammation in diseases such as asthma (*1*) and COPD (*2*). Bronchoscopy, being an invasive procedure, carries an associated morbidity (*3,4*). Although bronchoscopy is carried out in patients with moderate or even severe airflow limitation for clinical indications, it is not ethically justified to carry out research bronchoscopies on such patients, as it is essential to pursue research procedures carrying the minimum risk to volunteer subjects. Thus BAL, for the purposes of research in airways diseases, is limited to patients with mild airflow obstruction, thus requiring extrapolation of findings to a more heterogeneous group of patients. As a consequence of its invasive nature, the number of times the procedure can be repeated is limited so that it may be difficult to study the kinetics of the inflammatory response. In addition, it may be difficult to recruit volunteers for studies that necessitate bronchoscopy.

Induced sputum has the advantage that it is simple and safe to perform, acceptable to patients and allows collection of airway lining fluid from control subjects. It is an especially valuable procedure in the study of moderate to severe asthma or COPD in whom invasive research procedures are not ethically viable.

From: *Methods in Molecular Medicine, vol. 56:*
Human Airway Inflammation: Sampling Techniques and Analytical Protocols
Edited by: D. F. Rogers and L. E. Donnelly © Humana Press Inc., Totowa, NJ

Bearing in mind the need to sample subglottic secretions as purely as possible whereas minimizing salivary contamination, different methods have been used in the collection and processing of induced sputum. We reduce salivary contamination during the induction procedure by asking patients to differentiate between sputum and saliva which is discarded into a separate bowl *(5)*.

As it is possible that some airway lining fluid is coughed up in liquid form, not necessarily forming plugs, and that the liquid part of the airway lining fluid may contain a different cellular and protein composition, we choose to process the sputum sample in its entirety. In reducing salivary contamination during the collection, and processing the sputum in this way, the possibility of sampling a misrepresentative part of the sputum is avoided.

2. Materials

2.1. Reagents

1. Dilute 7% hypertonic saline 1:1 with water to give a 3.5% solution.
2. 50-mL centrifuge tubes for the collection of induced sputum samples. (Corning Costar, High Wycombe, UK.)
3. DL-Dithiothreitol (Sigma Chemicals, Poole, UK) is purchased as a powder and dissolved in Hanks Balanced Salt Solution (HBSS) to make a 0.25% (w/v) solution. This solution should be stored at 4°C and discarded after 1 wk.
4. Kimura stain or Trypan Blue for cell counts. Trypan Blue allows simultaneous measurement of cell counts and cell viability.
5. HBSS.
6. Diff-Quik to allow differential cell counting.
7. 2-mL Eppendorf tubes.

2.2. Apparatus

1. For the sputum induction: an ultrasonic nebulizer, such as a DeVilbiss 2000 (DeVilbiss Co., Heston, Middlesex).
2. For preparation of cytospin slides: a cytospin (Shandon, Runcorn, Cheshire) and glass slides.
3. A hemocytometer for determining cell counts.
4. Standard benchtop centrifuge.
5. Standard microscope for the determination of total and differential cell counts.

3. Methods

3.1. Sputum Induction Procedure

1. Record FEV_1 at baseline and 10 min after inhalation of salbutamol 200 µg via a metered dose inhaler using a spacer device (*see* **Notes 1** and **2**).
2. Fully explain the procedure to the patient, indicating that the aim of the procedure is to obtain secretions originating in the chest, with as little salivary contamination as possible (*see* **Note 3**). Also explain that the inhalation of saline

may give a dry or irritating feeling in the throat but that this will pass as the induction proceeds. The subject should be advised that if he/she experiences any chest tightness or wheeze during the procedure, the investigator should be informed.

3. Ensure subject mouthwashes thoroughly with water.
4. The subject inhales 3.5% saline at room temperature, nebulized via an ultrasonic nebulizer (De Vilbiss 2000, De Vilbiss, Middlesex, UK) with output set at 4.5 mL/min (*see* **Note 4**).
5. At any time during the procedure, if the subject experiences excessive salivation, he/she should discard saliva into a bowl.
6. If at any time, the FEV_1 falls by 20% or more, the procedure should be stopped and salbutamol 2.5 mg given by nebulizer.
7. Record FEV_1 at 3-minintervals and immediately following this, the subject is encouraged to cough deeply. Sputum is collected into a polypropylene pot and saliva is discarded into a separate bowl (*see* **Note 5**).
8. The sputum induction should continue for a fixed period, usually 15–20 min (*see* **Note 6**).
9. The sputum sample should be kept at 4°C for not more than 2 h prior to further processing.

3.2. Sputum Processing

The whole sputum sample is processed.

1. Sputum is homogenized by the addition of 0.25% dithiothreitol (DTT). The volume of DTT added is a fixed multiple (6 times) of the weight of the sputum sample. The sample is then vortexed at room temperature.
2. Centrifuge at 300g for 10 min.
3. Separate the supernatant and freeze at -70°C until further analysis (*see* **Note 7**).
4. Resuspend the cell pellet in 1mL HBSS.
5. Total cell counts are determined on a hemocytometer slide using Kimura stain or Trypan Blue stain and slides are prepared using a cytospin (Shandon, Runcorn, Cheshire), and then stained with DiffQuik stain. 300 nonsquamous cells are counted on each of the two slides for each sputum sample. Differential cell counts are expressed as a percentage of lower airway cells, that is, excluding squamous epithelial cells. Squamous cells should be counted and reported separately to provide internal quality control of sampling. Samples are considered adequate for analysis if there is <50% squamous cell contamination.

3.3. Sputum Supernatant Assays

Sputum supernatant samples have been assayed for a number of different cytokines or inflammatory markers, including interleukin (IL)-8 *(6)*, TNFα *(6)*, granulocyte macrophage-colony stimulating factor (GM-CSF) *(7)*, neutrophil and eosinophil myeloperoxidases (MPO and EPO) *(8)*, human neutrophil lipocalin (HNL) *(8)* and eosinophil cationic protein (ECP) *(8)*. Assays are performed as they would be for cell culture supernatants except that the effect of DTT on the assay must be established, since DTT can interfere with a number of assays (*see* **Note 8**). All standard curves should be run with the appropriate concentration of DTT in the standards. All sputum supernatants must have the same concentration of DTT to be comparable.

4. Notes

1. All sputum inductions within a particular study are carried out at the same time of day, generally between 9AM and 2PM, particularly if the study involves asthmatic subjects.
2. Prior to sputum induction, all subjects inhale salbutamol 200 μg via MDI. This is because hypertonic saline is known to be a potent stimulus to bronchospasm. For uniformity, this is also given to the control subjects although hypertonic saline is not a bronchoconstrictive agent in normal subjects.
3. Subjects are asked to differentiate between sputum originating from the airways, and saliva from the buccal cavity. We have found that during sputum induction, subjects are able to distinguish between saliva and subglottic secretions and that after a little education and instruction can, in the majority of cases, produce an adequate sample of sputum. Subjects should be discouraged from clearing their throat during the sputum induction, instead being encouraged to cough deeply. Inhalation of hypertonic saline can cause hypersalivation. If saliva and sputum are not separated during the sputum induction, large volumes (>20 mL) of sample are produced resulting in unquantifiable dilution of sputum with saliva *(9)*.
4. The De Vilbiss nebulizer has an output control knob which is not marked with output parameters. It is necessary to calibrate the output knob in advance of the procedure. Unpublished observations suggest that a higher nebulizer output leads to better quality induced sputum samples. However, there are no published data comparing the effects of different nebulizer outputs. A good success rate has been found using nebulizer outputs as low as 0.9 mL/min, but this was using a different induction protocol with sequential 5-min inhalations of 3–5% saline *(10)*.
5. It will be noted that it is easier to induce sputum from patients with airways diseases than from control subjects. The reasons for this are twofold. Patients are more likely to produce sputum spontaneously and to recognise sputum as distinct from saliva and may have more airway lining fluid present initially. Care should be taken to ensure that control subjects who do not normally produce sputum can distinguish between saliva and sputum. Many individuals find the act of coughing sputum an embarrassing one and should be encouraged to cough deeply and given privacy where deemed necessary. These measures are essential to the production of an adequate sputum sample.
6. The composition of sputum samples changes during the course of the sputum induction procedure, with higher differential neutrophil and lower differential macrophage counts in early compared with later samples *(11)*. The reason for these changes in composition with time is not clear, but may reflect sampling from progressively lower levels within the airway during the induction proce-

dure. In view of this, the duration of sputum induction should be standardized within studies. Bias might be introduced in studies where sputum induction is continued for different times in different groups, or in those studies where sputum induction is halted once sufficient sputum has been collected.

7. Sputum supernatants retained for future analysis (of cytokines and so on) should be stored as aliquots (in 2 mL Eppendorf tubes) in order to prevent repeated freezethawing as this may decrease the levels of cytokines detected.

8. DTT is known to interfere with a number of assays. Therefore, it must be established that DTT does not interfere with the assay or that any changes with DTT are linear. This is checked by running standard curves with and without DTT to determine the linearity of the standard curve. In addition, it is important to validate the assay by spiking raw sputum with a known concentration of the mediator in question to determine its recoverability following the processing technique. In all assays, standard curves should be run with the same concentration of DTT as that in the sputum supernatant samples. This requires that all sputum supernatants have the same fixed final concentration of DTT.

9. Repeated sputum induction within a short time can lead to an increase in differential neutrophil counts in subsequent samples taken within a 24-h period *(12,13)*.

References

1. Barnes, P. J. (1989) New concepts in the pathogenesis of bronchial hyperresponsiveness and asthma. *J. Allergy Clin. Immunol.* **83,** 1013–1026.
2. Martin, T. R., Raghu, G., Maunder, R. J., and Springmeyer, S. C. (1985) The effects of chronic bronchitis and chronic airflow obstruction on lung cell populations recovered by bronchoalveolar lavage. *Am. Rev. Respir. Dis.* **132,** 254–160.
3. Kirby, J. G., O'Byrne, P. M., and Hargreave, F. E. (1987) Bronchoalveolar lavage does not alter airway hyperesponsiveness in asthmatic subjects. *Am. Rev. Respir. Dis.* **135,** 554–556.
4. Van Vyve, T., Chanez, P., Bousquet, J., Lacoste, J.-Y., Michel, F.-B., and Godard, P. (1992) Safety of bronchoalveolar lavage and bronchial biopsies in patients with asthma of variable severity. *Am. Rev. Respir. Dis.* **146,** 116–121.
5. Gershman, N. H., Wong, H. H., Liu, J. T., Mahlmeister, M. J., and Fahy, J. V. (1996) Comparison of two methods of collecting induced sputum in asthmatic subjects. *Eur. Respir. J.* **9,** 2448–2453.
6. Keatings, V. M., Collins, P. D., Scott, D. M., and Barnes, P. J. (1996) Differences in interleukin-8 and tumor necrosis factor-alpha in induced sputum from patients with chronic obstructive pulmonary disease or asthma. *Am. J. Respir. Crit. Care Med.* **153,** 530–534.
7. Nightingale, J. A., Rogers, D. F., Hart, L. A., Kharitonov, S. A., Chung, K. F., and Barnes, P. J. (1998) Effect of inhaled endotoxin on induced sputum in normal, atopic, and atopic asthmatic subjects. *Thorax* **53,** 563–571.
8. Keatings, V. M.,Barnes, P. J. (1997) Granulocyte activation markers in induced sputum: comparison between chronic obstructive pulmonary disease, asthma, and normal subjects. *Am. J. Respir. Crit. Care Med.* **155,** 449–453.

9. Fahy, J. V., Liu, J., Wong, H., and Boushey, H. A. (1993) Cellular and biochemical analysis of induced sputum from asthmatic and from healthy subjects. *Am. Rev. Respir. Dis.* **147,** 1126–1131.

10. Hunter, C. J., Ward, R., Woltmann, G., Wardlaw, A. J., and Pavord, I. D. (1999) The safety and success rate of sputum induction using a low output ultrasonic nebulizer. *Respir. Med.* **93,** 345–348.

11. Holz, O., Jörres, R. A., Koschyk, S., Speckin, P., Welker, L., and Magnussen, H. (1998) Changes in sputum composition during sputum induction in healthy and asthmatic subjects. *Clin. Exp. Allergy* **28,** 284–292.

12. Nightingale, J. A., Rogers, D. F., and Barnes, P. J. (1998) The effect of repeated sputum induction on cell counts in normal volunteers. *Thorax* **53,** 87–90.

13. Holz, O., Richter, K., Jörres, R. A., Speckin, P., Mücke, M., and Magnussen, H. (1998) Changes in sputum composition between two inductions performed on consecutive days. *Thorax* **53,** 83–86.

7

Measurement of Exhaled Nitric Oxide and Carbon Monoxide

Sergei A. Kharitonov

1. Introduction

Nitric oxide (NO) can be detected in the exhaled air and the concentration of exhaled NO is increased in patients with airway inflammation such as asthma and bronchiectasis. This suggests that exhaled NO may provide a noninvasive means of monitoring inflammation in the respiratory tract.

The "inflammatory origin" *(1–5)* of elevated levels of exhaled NO in asthma *(4,6)*, its high responsiveness to corticosteroids *(7,8)*, and accumulating evidence of its association with asthma severity *(9–11)* makes exhaled NO an effective and practical marker to monitor the effect of corticosteroid treatment in asthma. Dose-dependent reduction in exhaled NO has been recently reported in mild asthmatics treated with low doses of budesonide *(12)*.

Recently, elevated levels of exhaled carbon monoxide (CO), by-product of hemoglobin cleavage by heme oxygenase, have been detected in atopic asthma *(13–16)* and allergic rhinitis *(17)*, patients with cystic fibrosis *(18,19)*.

Here, the detailed methods for exhaled NO and CO measurements are described, which are in accordance with the European Respiratory Society *(20)* and American Thoracic Society *(21)* recommendations.

2. Materials

2.1. System Design and Terminology

Equipment in clinical use varies widely in complexity, but the basic principles are the same. All systems based on the chemical reaction between the O_3 and the NO (chemiluminescence). A photomultiplier measures the light intensity emitted, and the quantity of light is proportional to the NO concentration.

From: *Methods in Molecular Medicine, vol. 56:*
Human Airway Inflammation: Sampling Techniques and Analytical Protocols
Edited by: D. F. Rogers and L. E. Donnelly © Humana Press Inc., Totowa, NJ

Exhaled CO measurements are made by electrochemical sensor and the amount of electrical current generated during the reaction between the sensor and CO is proportional to the CO concentration.

2.1.1. Online Measurement

Measurements of eNO or eCO during an exhalation. NO and CO output represents the rate, that is the amount of NO, CO exhaled per unit time. NO is calculated from the product of NO concentration in nanoliters per liter and expiratory flow rate in liters per minute, corrected to BTPS. CO is expressed as a concentration in parts per million (ppm).

2.1.2. Offline NO and CO Measurements

eNO and eCO measured in a reservoir in which expired air was collected. Exhalation flow should be added as a subscript, for example, $eNO_{0.35}$, with the flow rate in liters per second.

2.1.3. Nasal NO

Concentration of nasal NO, is the rate of nasal NO exhaled and should be represented as nasal V_{NO}, or expressed in parts per billion (ppb).

2.2. Equipment Requirements

Minimum standards for equipment include (*see* **Note 1**):

1. Analyzers should be equipped with disposable mouthpieces connected to the sampling tubing with an internal restrictor to allow the exhalation with mild resistance (1.0 ± 0.2 mm Hg), in order to close the soft palate and separate nasal and oral cavities, and to prevent nasal NO contamination.
2. Chemiluminescence analyzer has to be calibrated daily using a certified concentration of NO in nitrogen (50–400 ppb), and certified 5% CO_2 (BOC, Special Gases, Surrey Research Park, Guildford, UK). The CO analyzer has to be calibrated once a week using 500 ppm CO calibration gas and miniFlo Valve and Flow indicator (Bedfont Scientific Ltd, Kent, UK).

2.3. Equipment Quality Control

2.3.1. Each Day

1. Leak testing (loose connections).
2. Changing filters (after 5–8 measurements).
3. Staff (standard subject, e.g., healthy nonsmoking technician performing NO/CO measurements) should be tested to assure overall stability of the system. When sufficient data on a standard individual are obtained, laboratories may choose to establish their own outliner criteria to serve as indicators of potential problems with their NO/CO analyzer.
4. Calibration using a certified concentration of NO in nitrogen (preferentially <100 ppb for exhaled NO measurements and 400–800 ppb for nasal NO measurements).

2.3.2. Each Week

Calibration using a certified concentration of CO_2 and CO.

Records of equipment checks and standard subject tests should be dated, signed, and kept in a laboratory log book.

2.3.3. Infection Control

The major goal of infection control is to prevent the transmission of infection to patients and staff during NO/CO measurements. Infection may be transmitted by two modes (*see* **Note 2**):

1. Direct contact: through direct contact with potential pathogens, there is the potential for transmisssion of upper respiratory tract infection (URTI), enteric infections, and blood-borne infections. Although infection with hepatitis and HIV are unlikely via saliva, the possibility exists when there is hemoptysis, open sores on the oral mucosa, or bleeding gums. The most likely surfaces for contact are mouthpieces and the immediately proximal surfaces of valves or tubing.
2. Indirect contact: contaminated aerosol droplets have the potential for transmitting tuberculosis, various viral infections, and possibly opportunistic infections and nosocomial pneumonia to susceptible patients. Mouthpieces and proximal valves and tubing are likely candidates for contamination by aerosols.

2.4. Factors Influencing Exhaled NO Values

A variety of factors affect the accurate measurement of exhaled NO (*see* **Note 3**).

2.5. Factors Influencing Exhaled CO Values

A variety of factors affect the accurate measurement of exhaled CO (*see* **Note 4**).

3. Methods

3.1. On-Line NO/CO Measurements

1. The conditions that may affect exhaled, nasal NO and exhaled CO production should be avoided or registered and used for the data interpretation (*see* **Notes 3** and **4**).
2. Seated position could be recommended as a standard position.
3. Before beginning the test, the maneuvers should be demonstrated and the subject carefully instructed.
4. Inspiratory maneuver: the exhalation NO/CO maneuver begins with exhalation to residual volume (RV) followed by rapid inhalation to total lung capacity (TLC). Inspiratory time in healthy subjects averages 1.5 to 2 s. In patients with moderate to severe airflow obstruction, i.e., the ratio of forced expiratory volume in 1 s (FEV_1) to vital capacity (VC) <0.5, inspiratory times average about 2 s, with 95% less than 4 s. The increase in inspiration time might lead to exhaled NO/CO alterations.

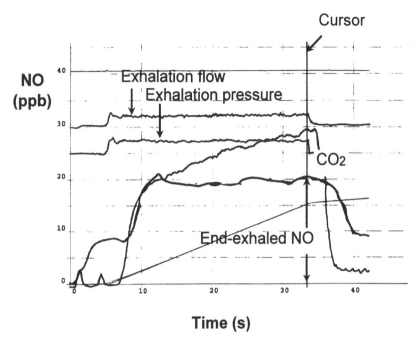

Time (s)

Fig. 1. Schematic illustration of end-exhaled NO/CO measurement for the single slow exhalation against a resistance.

5. The inspiration should be rapid (no longer than 2.5 s in healthy subjects and 4 s in patients with moderate to severe airway obstruction).

6. Inspiratory air or gas mixture: no relationship has been found between ambient and exhaled NO levels, whether breathing ambient or NO-free air. However, notwithstanding which technique is employed, ambient NO at the time of each test should be recorded.

7. Ambient CO should be recorded as close as possible to the time of the measurements and subtracted from the exhaled CO levels.

8. Exhalation procedure: after inspiration, the subject should exhale without hesitation or interruption. For the end-exhaled NO measurements subjects were exhaling slowly from TLC over 15–25 s with exhalation flow 0.05 L/s and with minimal exhalation pressure between 5 and 20 cm H_2O. Created backpressure is sufficient to keep soft palate closed, so that nasal cavities are partitioned from the remainder of the respiratory tract preventing the contamination of exhaled air with nasal NO. There is no need to use this resistance to measure exhaled CO, as there is no nasal CO production.

9. The mean value of the last 100 NO measurements, acquired with 0.04 s interval, was taken from the point corresponding to the plateau of end-exhaled CO_2 reading (5–6% CO_2), and representing the lower respiratory tract sample (*see* **Fig. 1**). Exhaled CO levels should be taken at the same time point, as NO.

10. Nasal NO measurements: nasal NO should be measured with a probe inserted into one of the nares, whereas the subject breathheld, i.e., with no active exhala-

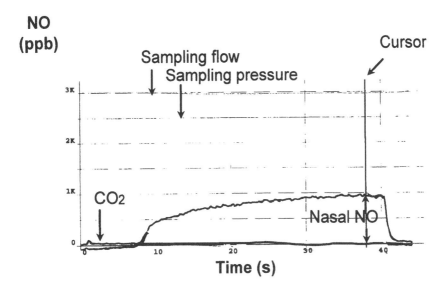

Fig. 2. Schematic illustration of nasal NO measurement for the direct sampling from nasal cavities.

tion. The probe generated flow between the two chambers given that they are in communication with each other. The velopharynx closure allowed analysis of the local NO concentration with free flow of ambient air from one nostril to the other and subsequent direction into analyzer. For all maneuvers the CO_2 levels in the sampled gas should also be monitored. The absence of CO_2 traces on a plot confirms a velopharynx closure (*see* **Fig. 2**).

11. Interval between tests: it is generally recognised that 2–3 breaths should eliminate any excess of NO accumulated during 20–30 s of exhalation. It is reasonable to expect that 2-min interval between tests may be sufficient in some patients with severe maldistribution of ventilation, and 1-min interval is sufficient in normal subjects.

12. Subjects should be asked to refrain from smoking for 24 h before the test. The time of the last cigarette smoked should be recorded. Subjects should avoid alcohol for at least 4 h before testing. Women should be asked about their menstrual cycle and contraception means. The demonstration that URTIs are associated with a high level of exhaled NO indicates that caution should be applied when interpreting elevated values of exhaled NO and it is important to exclude measurements made at the time of an URTI.

3.2. Off-Line NO/CO Measurements

1. A collecting device *(22)* with a fixed flow restriction (mouthpiece diameter = 2.7 cm, restriction diameter = 5 mm to create pressure in the mouth up to 10 cm H_2O and to close the soft palate) should be used to collect the exhaled air.

2. An indication of exhalation flow will be achieved by a mouthpiece pressure gauge calibrated for flow to provide visual guidance for the subjects to maintain a constant flow rate.
3. A three-way valve open to the atmosphere during the first part of the maneuver was used to discard the first portion of exhaled air contaminated with ambient and nasal NO. The time needed to wash out the dead space (t) was estimated to be 1–2 s (t = dead space volume/exhalation flow where dead space was calculated as weight (lb) + age in years, and exhalation flow was 10–11 L/min).
4. Silica gel should be used to prevent the condensation of vapor in the reservoir (the collapsible reservoir, David S. Smith Liquid Packaging, type 5LMA 115).

3.3. On-Line Measurements in Children

1. Online measurements in children 12 yr or older use the same technique recommended for adults.
2. Patients less than 12 yr old: an expiratory flow rate of 50 mL/s, and at least a 2-s plateau duration should be achieved and exhalation has to be maintained for at least 4 s. Repeated exhalations are performed until three NO/CO plateau values agree at the 10% level or two agree at the 5% level.
3. 30-s interval between tests, to allow patients to rest. The mean NO/CO values are then recorded. For children unable to sustain a steady expiration flow, forced vital capacity off-line collection may be ideal.

3.4. Off-Line Measurements in Children

1. Same procedure as for the off-line NO/CO collection and measurements in adults.
2. In children unable to cooperate: tidal expirate for NO/CO measurements is collected over 2 min in the same reservoir.

4. Notes

1. EQUIPMENT SPECIFICATIONS

Measurement unit	ppb or ppm
Accuracy	±1% full range
Lower detectable limit	<1 ppb (NO) and < 1 ppm (CO)
Response time	<500 ms (NO) and < 3 s (CO)
Lag time	5–10 s including the delay between application of
the NO/	CO gas and the rise time to 95% of the final response. To be reported by the investigator.
Signal/noise ratio	>2
Drift	<1% of full scale per 24 h
Reproducibility	Better than 1 ppb (eNO), or 0.1 ppm (nasal NO), or 1 ppm (CO)
Measurement ranges	0.1–5000 ppb and 0.5–500 ppm
Pressure/flow sensors to measure expiration flow, pressure, and exhaled volume in real-time	Flow measurement range 0.5–30 L/min; pressure measurement range 0.5–10 mm Hg

CO$_2$ analyzer (desirable, but not obligatory option)	Range 0–10% CO$_2$, accuracy $\pm$ 0.1%, response time 200 ms to 90% of full scale
Bio-feedback display unit designed to provide a visual guidance for a subject to maintain the pressure and exhalation flow within the certain range, improving test repeatability and enhancing patient cooperation	Exhalation flow rate 5–6 L/min; exhalation pressure 1$\pm$0.2 mm Hg

2. Contamination can be limited by:
   a. Gloves must be worn when handling potentially contaminated equipment if there are any open cuts or sores on technicians' hands. Hand washing must always be performed between patients.
   b. To avoid cross-contamination, reusable mouthpieces, breathing tubes should be disinfected or sterilized regularly. Mouthpieces, nose clips, and any other equipment coming into direct contact with mucosal surfaces should be disinfected or sterilized after each use.
   c. Special precautions must be taken when testing patients with hemoptysis, open sores on the oral mucosa, or bleeding gums. Tubing must be decontaminated before reuse, and internal device surfaces must be decontaminated with accepted disinfectants for blood-transmissible agents.
   d. Extra precautions may be undertaken for patients with known transmissible infectious diseases: testing patients at the end of the day to allow time for disassembly and disinfecting.
   e. In settings where it is not possible to routinely dismantle the tubing, in-line filters may be effective in preventing equipment contamination. If an in-line filter is used, the measuring system must meet the minimal recommendations listed above for system accuracy, flow resistance and equipment must be calibrated with a filter installed.

3. Processes and factors affecting exhaled and nasal NO

Increased NO	Decreased NO
Technical factors, exhalation or sampling techniques, breathing pattern	
Low exhalation or sampling flow rate	High exhalation or sampling flow rate
Breath-holding	Spirometric maneuvers (transiently)
NO modulators, drugs	
Inhaled,IV, or ingested L-arginine	Inhaled, oral, or IV given NOS inhibitors (for example, L-NNMA, L-NAME, aminoguanidine)
	Inhaled or oral glucocorticosteroids
	β_2-agonists (for less than 1 h)
	Leukotrienes antagonists
Physiological, pathophysiological conditions and habits	
	Menstruation

Allergen challenge (late response)
Inhaled LPS in normal subjects

Smoking
Acute ethanol ingestion
Diseases
Asthma   COPD
Allergic rhinitis   Systemic sclerosis with pulmonary
                                                  hypertension
Upper respiratory tract infections
Bronchiectasis and lower respiratory
tract infections   Kartagener's syndrome
                                                  Primary cillia diskynesia
Ulcerative colitis   Cystic fibrosis

4. Processes and factors affecting exhaled CO
   Increased CO   Decreased CO
          Physiological, pathophysiological conditions and habits
   Allergen challenge (early and late response)
   Smoking
                          Diseases
   Asthma
   Allergic rhinitis
   Upper respiratory tract infections
   Bronchiectasis and lower respiratory tract infections
   Cystic fibrosis

References

1. Hamid, Q., Springall, D. R., Riveros-Moreno, V., et al. (1993) Induction of nitric oxide synthase in asthma. *Lancet* **342,** 1510–1513.

2. Saleh, D., Ernst, P., Lim, S., Barnes, P. J., and Giaid, A. (1998) Increased formation of the potent oxidant peroxynitrite in the airways of asthmatic patients is associated with induction of nitric oxide synthase: effect of inhaled glucocorticoid. *FASEB J* **12,** 929–937.

3. Barnes, P. J. and Liew, F .Y. (1995) Nitric oxide and asthmatic inflammation. *Immunology Today* **16,** 128–130.

4. Kharitonov, S. A., Yates, D. H., Robbins, R. A., Logan-Sinclair, R., Shinebourne, E. A., and Barnes, P. J. (1994) Increased nitric oxide in exhaled air of asthmatic patients. *Lancet* **343,** 133–135.

5. Marshall, H. E. and Stamler, J. S. (1999) Exhaled Nitric Oxide (NO), NO Synthase Activity, and Regulation of Nuclear Factor (NF)-kappaB. *Am. J. Respir. Cell. Mol. Biol.* **21,** 296–297.

6. Alving, K., Weitzberg, E., and Lundberg, J. M. (1993) Increased amount of nitric oxide in exhaled air of asthmatics. *Eur. Respir. J.* **6,** 1368–1370.

7. Kharitonov, S. A., Yates, D. H., Chung, K. F., and Barnes, P. J. (1996) Changes in the dose of inhaled steroid affect exhaled nitric oxide levels in asthmatic patients. *Eur Respir J* **9,** 196–201.

8. Kharitonov, S. A., Yates, D. H., and Barnes, P. J. (1996) Inhaled glucocorticoids decrease nitric oxide in exhaled air of asthmatic patients. *Am. J. Respir. Crit. Care Med.* **153,** 454–457.

9. Stirling, R. G., Kharitonov, S. A., Campbell, D., Robinson, D., Durham, S. R., Chung, K. F., and Barnes, P. J. (1998) Exhaled NO is elevated in difficult asthma and correlates with symptoms and disease severity despite treatment with oral and inhaled corticosteroids. *Thorax* **53,** 1030–1034.

10. Lanz, M. J., Leung, D. Y., McCormick, D. R., Harbeck, R., Szefler, S. J., and White, C. W. (1997) Comparison of exhaled nitric oxide, serum eosinophilic cationic protein, and soluble interleukin-2 receptor in exacerbations of pediatric asthma. *Pediatr. Pulmonol.* **24,** 305–311.

11. Lanz, M. J., Leung, D. Y., and White, C. W. (1999) Comparison of exhaled nitric oxide to spirometry during emergency treatment of asthma exacerbations with glucocorticosteroids in children. *Ann. Allergy Asthma Immunol.* **82,** 161–164.

12. Jatakanon, A., Kharitonov, S. A., Lim, S., and Barnes, P. J. (1999) Effect of differing doses of inhaled budesonide on markers of airway inflammation in patients with mild asthma. *Thorax* **54(2),** 108–114.

13. Zayasu, K., Sekizawa, K., Okinaga, S., Yamaya, M., and Sasaki, H. (1997) Increased carbon monoxide in exhaled air of asthmatic patients. *Am. J. Respir. Crit. Care Med.* **156,** 1140–1143.

14. Horvath, I., Donnelly, L. E., Kiss, A., Paredi, P., Kharitonov, S. A., and Barnes, P. J. (1998) Elevated levels of exhaled carbon monoxide are associated with an increased expression of heme oxygenase-1 in airway macrophages in asthma: a new marker of oxidative stress. *Thorax* **53,** 668–672.

15. Yamaya, M., Sekizawa, K., Ishizuka, S., Monma, M., Mizuta, K., and Sasaki, H. (1998) Increased carbon monoxide in exhaled air of subjects with upper respiratory tract infections. *Am. J. Respir. Crit. Care Med.* **158,** 311–314.

16. Uasuf, C.G., Jatakanon, A., James, A., Kharitonov, S.A., Wilson, N.M., and Barnes, P.J. (1999) Exhaled carbon monoxide in childhood asthma. *J. Pediatr.* **135,** 569–574.

17. Monma, M., Yamaya, M., Sekizawa, K., et al. (1999) Increased carbon monoxide in exhaled air of patients with seasonal allergic rhinitis. *Clin. Exp. Allergy* **29,** 1537–1541.

18. Paredi, P., Shah, P. L., Montuschi, P., Sullivan, P., Hodson, M. E., Kharitonov, S. A., and Barnes, P. J. (1999) Increased carbon monoxide in exhaled air of cystic fibrosis patients. *Thorax* **54,** 917–920.

19. Antuni, J. D., Kharitonov, S.A., Hughes, D., Hodson, M. E., and Barnes, P. J. (2000) Increase in exhaled carbon monoxide during exacerbations of cystic fibrosis. *Thorax* **55(2),** 138–142.

20. Kharitonov, S. A., Alving, K., and Barnes, P. J. (1997) Exhaled and nasal nitric oxide measurements: recommendations. *Eur. Respir. J.* **10,** 1683–1693.

21. Anonymous Recommendations for Standardized Procedures for the Online and Offline Measurement of Exhaled Lower Respiratory Nitric Oxide and Nasal Nitric

Oxide in Adults and Children. (1999) *Am. J. Respir. Crit. Care Med.* **160**, 2104–2117.

22. Paredi, P., Loukides, S., Ward, S., Cramer, D., Spiver, M., Kharitonov, S. A., and Barnes, P. J. (1998) Exhalation flow and pressure-controlled reservoir collection of exhaled nitric oxide for remote and delayed analysis. *Thorax* **53,** 775–779.

8

Measurement of Exhaled Hydrocarbons

Paolo Paredi, Sergei A. Kharitonov, and Peter J. Barnes

1. Introduction

Oxidative stress is implicated in the pathogenesis and progression of asthma *(1,2)*, chronic obstructive respiratory disease (COPD) *(3)*, and cystic fibrosis *(4)*. Reactive oxygen species (ROS) are unstable compounds with unpaired electrons, capable of initiating oxidation. Several of the inflammatory cells which participate in the inflammatory response, such as macrophages, neutrophils, and eosinophils release increased amounts of ROS *(1,5)* exceeding the already reduced tissue antioxidant defences of asthmatic and COPD patients *(2)*.

One mechanism by which oxidants may cause lung injury is through lipid peroxidation. ROS, such as superoxide anion ($O_2^{.}$), and hydrogen peroxide (H_2O_2) released by activated immune and inflammatory cells can induce the lipid peroxidation of polyunsaturated membrane fatty acids *(6)*, impair membrane function and inactivate membrane-bound receptors and enzymes, increase tissue permeability *(7)*, and therefore promote airflow limitation.

Volatile hydrocarbons are products of lipid peroxidation and their measurement in the exhaled breath has been proposed as a means to assess lipid peroxidation in vivo *(8)* (*see* **Fig. 1**) *(6,9)*. Ethane derived from n-3 polyunsaturated fatty acids (i.e., linolenic acid), and 1-pentane, derived from n-6 fatty acids (i.e., linolenic and arachidonic acids), are noninvasive markers of lipid peroxidation. These alkanes are produced by β-scission of the lipoalkoxyl radical to produce the alkyl radical followed by hydrogen abstraction to produce ethane or 1-pentane. Although only a small fraction of the lipid peroxides actually produces ethane or 1-pentane, the production of these alkanes reflects the extent of lipid peroxidation and, thereby, the in vivo oxidative stress. In this group of exhaled gases, ethane has received more attention because of its easier

From: *Methods in Molecular Medicine, vol. 56:*
Human Airway Inflammation: Sampling Techniques and Analytical Protocols
Edited by: D. F. Rogers and L. E. Donnelly © Humana Press Inc., Totowa, NJ

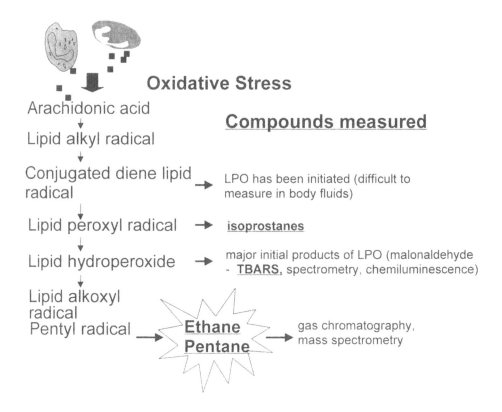

Fig. 1. Markers of the lipid peroxidation of arachidonic acid in biological fluids and exhaled breath. *LPO: lipid peroxidation, TBARS: thiobarbituric acid reactive substances.*

and faster chromatographic measurement compared to other hydrocarbons *(10–12)*. The exhaled air of human subjects was first analyzed for the presence of hydrocarbons in the 1960s *(13)*. Since then, the research in this area has progressed slowly because of technical and practical problems, such as the contamination of ambient hydrocarbons and the need to concentrate exhaled air because of the low concentrations of these volatile compounds.

Two approaches have been used to deal with the problem of ambient air. Some researchers employ washout periods to clear the lungs for 4 or 5 min *(14,15)*, alternatively, the problem of ambient contamination is neglected *(16)* or dealt with correcting for the actual background concentrations *(11,17)*.

The concentration of the sample of exhaled breath has also been addressed in two different ways. In some studies, exhaled breath was concentrated in cartridges containing adsorbing resins (adsorption/desorption method), in other studies, breath was concentrated at low temperatures in a gas sampling loop (the cryofocusing technique).

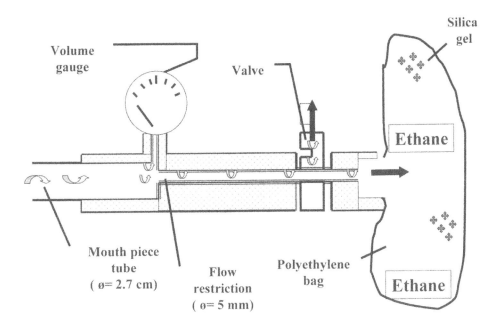

Fig. 2. Schematic diagram of the portable equipment for collection of exhaled ethane. The arrows indicate the direction of the air flow. The three-way valve is in the closed position for reservoir collection of exhaled breath.

We modified a previously developed technique for single breath analysis of exhaled hydrocarbons *(10)* where the sample does not require concentration and the collection is not preceded by washout with hydrocarbon-free air. Exhaled breath is collected at constant exhalation flow and pressure into a reservoir and later analyzed by gas chromatography for the content of hydrocarbons. The levels of ambient ethane are subtracted from exhaled breath concentrations to reduce ambient contamination.

Like other authors *(12)*, we favor ethane over pentane as a measure of lipid peroxidation because of the more rapid metabolism of pentane by animals and man *(18)*. In addition, mass spectroscopic analysis of human exhalate has demonstrated the presence of significant amounts of isoprene, which may be mistaken for pentane during gas chromatographic analysis rendering pentane quantification complex *(11)*.

The measurement of exhaled ethane is simple and noninvasive, it can be repeated and may be applied to children and to patients with severe disease. Measurement of exhaled ethane may provide a means of detecting and monitoring cytokine-mediated inflammation and oxidant stress in the airways and of assessing the efficacy of treatment.

2. Materials

2.1. Apparatus

2.1.1. Portable Device for Exhaled Air Collection

The collecting device (*see* **Fig. 2**) consists of:

1. A fixed flow restriction (mouthpiece diameter = 2.7 cm, restriction diameter = 5 mm) introduced to increase pressure in the mouth up to 10 cm H_2O which is effective in closing the soft palate *(19,20)* and isolating the nasopharynx.
2. An indication of exhalation flow achieved by a mouthpiece pressure gage calibrated for flow to provide visual guidance for the subjects to maintain a constant flow rate.
3. A three-way valve open to the atmosphere during the first part of the maneuver used to discard the first portion of exhaled air contaminated with ambient and nasal ethane.
4. Silica gel used to prevent the condensation of vapor *(21)* in the reservoir.
5. A collapsible reservoir (David S. Smith Liquid Packaging, type 5LMA 115) with an inner polyethylene layer which does not affect ethane levels.

2.1.2. Gas Chromatographic Analysis

1. Gas chromatograph model Philips PU 4500.
2. Signal output to Shimadzu CR6A integrator.
3. Column Poropak Q 1.5m × 4 mm.
4. Calibration gas mixture 50 parts per million (ppm) methane and 50 ppm ethane (Phase Separation, Deeside, Clwyd).
5. Hamilton gas tight Microliter syringe (10 µL).
6. Connect a TH three-way stopcock.

3. Methods

3.1. Exhaled Breath Collection

1. Exhaled ethane is collected into a collapsible reservoir during a single exhalation from total lung capacity to residual volume at a constant flow (10–11 L/min) over 20–30 s (*see* **Notes 1** and **2**) against a mild resistance (*see* **Note 3** and **Fig. 2**). The exhaled breath collecting device should be connected to the reservoir only after ambient air has been removed from the reservoir using a vacuum pump. The inhalation to total lung capacity should be continuous without pauses. A breath-hold can increase the concentration of exhaled ethane. During exhalation, the lips should be tight around the mouthpiece avoiding air leaks.
2. During exhalation, the air coming from the dead space, contaminated with nasal and ambient ethane is discarded in the atmosphere by a three-way valve. The time needed to wash out the dead space (t) is estimated to be 1–2 s (t = dead space volume/exhalation flow where dead space is calculated as weight (lb) + age in years, and exhalation flow was 10–11 L/min) *(22)*.
3. Once the exhalation maneuver is finished and the patient has reached residual volume the three-way valve should be promptly closed to avoid ambient con-

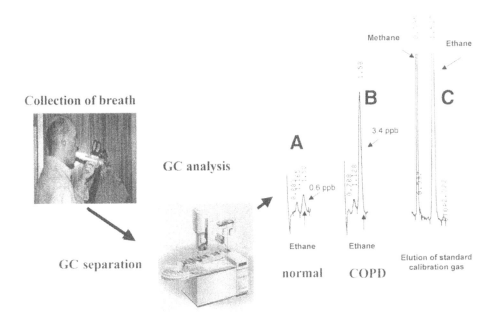

Fig. 3. Single breath collection of exhaled breath and gas chromatograph separation of ethane. Exhaled ethane tracings of a normal subject (**Panel A**) and a patient with chronic obstructive pulmonary disease (**Panel B**) (COPD). **Panel C** shows the elution profile of the calibration gas mixture of methane and ethane. The retention times (1.58 min for ethane) are indicated at the top of each peak.

tamination of the collected air or reflux out of the reservoir.

4. Once the exhaled air is collected, the reservoir is immediately sealed and the sample should be kept at room temperature and analyzed for ethane content within 48 h (*see* **Notes 4** and **5**)

5. The collapsible reservoir is equipped with a rigid plastic ring which should be pressed on a flat surface when the collecting device is removed preventing ambient air contamination. The reservoir should be sealed immediately (*see* **Note 4**).

6. Two samples of exhaled breath and one of ambient should be collected for each patient. The mean of the two samples (with a variability lower than 3%) should be recorded.

3.2. Gas Chromatographic Analysis

1. The column is conditioned overnight at 200°C. After reducing the operating temperature and lighting the detector flame the chromatograph is left to equilibrate for 30 min or until a stable baseline is obtained. Calibration is obtained by external standard method using 1 mL of 50 ppm ethane calibration gas mixture.

2. The oven (column) temperature is set at 60°C, injector temperature at 140°C, and detector temperature at 160°C. The carrier gas is nitrogen at a flow rate of 40 mL/min.

3. A sample (e.g., 2 μL) of the collected expired air is injected into the gas chromatograph using a gas tight Hamilton syringe (*see* **Notes 6** and **7**). 30–40 min should be allowed between each measurement to allow wash out of residual contaminating hydrocarbons in the gas chromatograph column.

With these settings, the retention time for ethane is 1.5 min (*see* **Fig. 3**). The levels of ambient ethane are subtracted from exhaled breath concentrations to reduce ambient contamination.

The reproducibility of this method was proved by the Bland and Altman test *(23)*. The coefficient of variation (standard deviation/mean value × 100) of exhaled ethane levels measured during two successive collections at 5-min intervals (single session variability) was 5.4%, while between sessions variability, (1 d interval) was 6.2%.

3.3. Factors Influencing Exhaled Ethane Levels

3.3.1. Age

Even though there may be increased systemic lipid peroxidation with aging, there is no significant difference in excretion of both ethane and pentane between healthy children and adults *(24)*.

3.3.2. Fasting and Type of Diet

Both type and amount of polyunsaturated fatty acids in the diet may influence hydrocarbon release *(25,26)*, especially in laboratory animals. However, there seems to be no acute effect of ingested lipids on hydrocarbon exhalation in man. A single standard breakfast containing 12.9 g and 0.4 g of linoleic and linolenic acid did not change the concentration of ethane in exhaled air compared to fasting *(27)*.

3.3.3. Antioxidant Nutrients

Vitamin E alone, unlike the combination of vitamins C, E, and β carotene, fails to reduce exhaled ethane in cigarette smokers *(12)*. Therefore, every subject should be asked if taking vitamin supplement.

3.3.4. Drugs

Studies on the physiological effects of drugs on hydrocarbon excretion in man are scarce. Blockers of hepatic cytochrome P-450 monooxygenases, by decreasing the metabolism of hydrocarbons, induce a nonspecific increase of pentane and, to a lesser extent, of ethane excretion. Conversely, phenobarbital, which induces P-450 leads to a decrease in hydrocarbon release in rats.

The β-adrenergic receptor blocking agent, propranolol, was shown to decrease both basal and exercise induced excretion of pentane in human volunteers, but the mechanism of this effect remains unclear *(28)*.

Steroid treatment is associated with lower levels of exhaled ethane in asthma *(29)*, COPD *(30)*, and cystic fibrosis *(31)*. Steroids, in fact, by reducing inflammation, attenuating the release of oxidants by inflammatory cells *(32)*, and suppressing proinflammatory cytokine production *(33)* may reduce lipid peroxidation as shown in previous studies *(34–36)*.

3.3.5. Cigarette Smoking

There is increased lipid peroxidation in the lungs of smokers compared to control subjects as assessed by the content of malonaldeyde in lung parenchyma and of exhaled ethane and pentane. The treatment with vitamins E, C, and beta-carotene effectively reduce the levels of exhaled hydrocarbons *(12)*. Therefore also smoking habits should be investigated when measuring exhaled hydrocarbons.

4. Notes

1. Exhaled ethane is markedly flow-dependent, and there is a significant reduction in ethane concentrations when the exhalation flow rate is increased. The probable reason for the reduction in ethane concentration with increased expiratory flow is that the same amount of ethane will be dispersed in a different exhaled volume. Thus, with a higher exhalation flow, ethane will be diluted in a greater volume and, hence, a lower ethane concentration will be detected. The exhalation flow should be kept steady at 10–11 L/min for as long as possible (*see* **Subheading 3.1., step 1**). Some dummy tests should be undertaken in order for the patients to familiarize themselves with the technique. There is no apparent influence of exhaled volume on ethane levels, provided dead space volume is discarded.
2. The portable collecting device should be equipped with a bio-feedback oral pressure and/or exhalation flow display, designed to provide visual guidance for the subject to maintain the pressure and/or exhalation flow within the desired range, thus improving the repeatability and enhancing patient cooperation (*see* **Subheading 3.1., step 1**)
3. It is important to separate the nasal passages from the remainder of the respiratory tract during exhalation to prevent contamination of exhaled ethane with nasal and ambient ethane. This is achieved by adding a resistance to the exhalation apparatus which generates mouth pressure and the closure of the soft palate separating the nasal cavities from the nasopharynx (*see* **Subheading 2.1., step 1**). Also for this reason it is important for the patient to keep a constant exhalation flow, and therefore mouth pressure, during the collection of exhaled breath.
4. The collecting device should be detached very carefully from the reservoir to avoid ambient contamination.
5. Ethane concentration was equally stable in 5 polyethylene and 5 Tedlar reservoirs for 48 h after collection (% increase: 3±1% and 5±2% for the polyethylene and Tedlar reservoirs, respectively).

6. 2 μL of exhaled breath are injected into the gas chromatograph. The most critical point for ambient contamination of the sample of exhaled breath is the withdrawal of air from the reservoir and the subsequent injection into the gas chromatograph.

7. A gas tight Hamilton syringe equipped with a three-way stopcock should be used. This allows to seal the syringe once the desired volume of air is withdrawn from the reservoir and to reopen it only when the needle is inserted in the gas chromatograph analyzer minimizing contamination with ambient air (*see* **Subheading 3.2., step 3**).

8. Ethane can be produced by bacteria, therefore it is important to use each reservoir only once to reduce bacteria contamination.

9. Age, diet, antioxidant nutrients, drugs, cigarette and smoking habits should be investigated in every subject before measuring exhaled ethane (*see* **Subheading 3.3.**).

References

1. Barnes, P. J. Reactive oxygen species and airway inflammation. (1990) *Free Radic. Biol. Med.* **9,** 235–243.

2. Rahman, I., Morrison, D., Donaldson, K., and MacNee, W. (1996) Systemic oxidative stress in asthma, COPD, and smokers. *Am. J. Respir. Crit. Care Med.* **154,** 1055–1060.

3. Repine, J. E., Bast, A., Lankhorst, I. (1997) Oxidative stress in chronic obstructive pulmonary disease. Oxidative Stress Study Group. *Am. J. Respir. Crit. Care Med.* **156,** 341–357.

4. Brown, R. K., Wyatt, H., Price, J. F., and Kelly, F. J. (1996) Pulmonary dysfunction in cystic fibrosis is associated with oxidative stress. *Eur. Respir. J.* **9,** 334–339.

5. Jarjour, N. N. and Calhoun, W. J. (1994) Enhanced production of oxygen radicals in asthma. *J. Lab. Clin. Med.* **123,** 131–136.

6. Kneepkens, C. M., Lepage, G., and Roy, C. C. (1994) The potential of the hydrocarbon breath test as a measure of lipid peroxidation. *Free Radic. Biol. Med.* **17,** 127–160.

7. Morrison, D., Rahman, I., Lannan, S., and MacNee, W. (1999) Epithelial permeability, inflammation, and oxidant stress in the air spaces of smokers. *Am. J. Respir. Crit. Care Med.* **159,** 473 479.

8. Habib, M. P., Clements, N. C., and Garewal, H. S. (1995) Cigarette smoking and ethane exhalation in humans. *Am. J. Respir. Crit. Care Med.* **151,** 1368–1372.

9. Kazui, M., Andreoni, K. A., Norris, E. J., Klein, A. S., Burdick, J. F., Beattie, C., et al. (1992) Breath ethane: a specific indicator of free-radical-mediated lipid peroxidation following reperfusion of the ischemic liver. *Free Radic. Biol. Med.* **13,** 509–515.

10. Zarling, E.J. and Clapper, M. (1987) Technique for gas-chromatographic measurement of volatile alkanes from single-breath samples. *Clin. Chem.* **33,** 140–141.

11. Kohlmuller, D. and Kochen, W. (1993) Is n-pentane really an index of lipid peroxidation in humans and animals? A methodological reevaluation. *Anal. Biochem.* **210,** 268–276.

12. Habib, M. P., Tank, L. J., Lane, L. C., and Garewal, H. S. (1999) Effect of vitamin E on exhaled ethane in cigarette smokers. *Chest.* Mar. **115,** 684–690.

13. Aulik IV. (1966) Gas chromatographic analysis of exhaled air and acetylene mixture. *Biull. Eksp. Biol. Med.* **62,** 115–117.

14. Lemoyne, M., Van Gossum, A., Kurian, R., Ostro, M., Axler, J., and Jeejeebhoy, K. N. (1987) Breath pentane analysis as an index of lipid peroxidation: a functional test of vitamin E status. *Am. J. Clin. Nutr.* **46,** 267–272.

15. Refat, M., Moore, T. J., Kazui, M., Risby, T. H., Perman, J. A., and Schwarz, K. B. (1991) Utility of breath ethane as a noninvasive biomarker of vitamin E status in children. *Pediatr. Res.* **30,** 396–403.

16. Toshniwal, P. K. and Zarling, E. J. (1992) Evidence for increased lipid peroxidation in multiple sclerosis. *Neurochem. Res.* **17,** 205–207.

17. Moscarella, S., Laffi, G., Buzzelli, G., Mazzanti, R., Caramelli, L., and Gentilini, P. (1984) Expired hydrocarbons in patients with chronic liver disease. *Hepatogastroenterology.* **31,** 60–63.

18. Jeejeebhoy KN. (1991) In vivo breath alkane as an index of lipid peroxidation. *Free Radic. Biol. Med.* **10,** 191–193.

19. Kharitonov, S. A., Chung, K. F., Evans, D., O'connor, B. J., and Barnes, P. J. (1996) Increased exhaled nitric oxide in asthma is mainly derived from the lower respiratory tract. *Am. J. Respir. Crit. Care Med.* **153,** 1773–1780.

20. Kharitonov, S. A. and Barnes, P. J. (1997) Nasal contribution to exhaled nitric oxide during exhalation against resistance or during breath holding. *Thorax* **52,** 540–544.

21. Sato, K., Sakamaki, T., Sumino, H., Sakamoto, H., Hoshino, J., Masuda, H., et al. (1996) Rate of nitric oxide release in the lung and factors influencing the concentration of exhaled nitric oxide. *Am. J. Physiol.* **Jun. 270,** L914–L920

22. Cotes, J. E. (1994) Lung function. In Assessment and application in medicine. Fifth Ed., *Blackwell Scientific Publications,* **Chapter 10,** p 3100.

23. Bland, J. M. and Altman, D. G. (1986) Statistical methods for assessing agreement between two methods of clinical measurement. *Lancet* **1,** 307–310.

24. Kneepkens, C. M., Ferriera, C., Lepage, G., and Roy, C. (1992) Hydrocarbon breath test in cystic fibrosis. evidence for increased lipid peroxidation. *Pediatr. Gastroenterol. Nutr.* **14,** 344

25. Kivits, G. A., Ganguli–Swarttouw, M. A., and Christ, E. J. (1981) The composition of alkanes in exhaled air of rats as a result of lipid peroxidation in vivo. Effects of dietary fatty acids, vitamin E and selenium. *Biochim. Biophys. Acta.* **665,** 559–570.

26. Dillard, C. J., Sagai, M., and Tappel, A. L. (1980) Respiratory pentane: a measure of in vivo lipid peroxidation applied to rats fed diets varying in polyunsaturated fats, vitamin E, and selenium and exposed to nitrogen dioxide. *Toxicol. Lett.* **6,** 251–256.

27. Zarling, E. J., Mobarhan, S., Bowen, P., and Sugerman, S. (1992) Oral diet does not alter pulmonary pentane or ethane excretion in healthy subjects. *J. Am. Coll. Nutr.* **11,** 349–352.

28. Pincemail, J., Camus, G., Roesgen, A., Dreezen, E., Bertrand, Y., Lismonde, M., et al. (1990) Exercise induces pentane production and neutrophil activation in humans. Effect of propranolol. *Eur. J. Appl. Physiol.* **61,** 319–322.

29. Paredi, P., Leak, D., Ward, S., Cramer, D., Kharitonov, S. A., and Barnes, P. J. (1999) Increased ethane in exhaled air of asthmatic patients. *Am. J. Respir. Crit. Care Med.* **159,** A97

30. Paredi, P., Ward, S., Cramer, D., Kharitonov, S. A., and Barnes, P. J. (1999) Exhaled ethane is increased in COPD and correlates with airway obstruction. *Am. J. Respir. Crit. Care Med.* **159,** A475.

31. Paredi, P., Kharitonov, S. A., and Barnes, P. J. (1999) Exhaled ethane is elevated in cystic fibrosis and correlates with carbon monoxide levels and airway obstruction. *Am. J. Respir. Crit. Care Med.* **161,** 1247–1251.

32. Marumo, T., Schini-Kerth, V. B., Brandes, R. P., and Busse, R. (1998) Glucocorticoids inhibit superoxide anion production and p22 phox mRNA expression in human aortic smooth muscle cells. *Hypertension* **32,** 1083–1088.

33. Inoue, H., Aizawa, H., Fukuyama, S., Takata, S., Matsumoto, K., Shigyo, M., Koto, H., and Hara, N. (1999) Effect of inhaled glucocorticoid on the cellular profile and cytokine levels in induced sputum from asthmatic patients. *Lung* **177,** 53–62.

34. Braughler, J. M. (1985) Lipid peroxidation-induced inhibition of gamma-aminobutyric acid uptake in rat brain synaptosomes: protection by glucocorticoids. *J. Neurochem.* **44,** 1282–1288.

35. Kouno, T., Egashira, T., Takayama, F., Kudo, Y., and Yamanaka, Y. (1994) Effect of methylprednisolone on plasma lipid peroxidation induced by lipopolysaccharide. *Jpn. J. Pharmacol.* **64,** 163–169.

36. Chiara, O., Giomarelli, P. P., Borrelli, E., Casini, A., Segala, M., and Grossi, A. (1991) Inhibition by methylprednisolone of leukocyte-induced pulmonary damage. *Crit. Care Med.* **19,** 260–265.

9

Breath Condensate as a Vehicle for Collection of Inflammatory Mediators, Especially Hydrogen Peroxide

Johan C. de Jongste, Rijn Jöbsis, and H. Rolien Raatgeep

1. Introduction

Exhaled air is saturated with water at 37°C, and cooling causes condensation of this water vapor. Breath condensate can be analyzed for the presence of inflammatory mediators and other putative markers of inflammation, among which are hydrogen peroxide (H_2O_2), leukotrienes (LT), prostanoids, thiobarbituric acid reactive products (TBARs), and metabolites of nitric oxide (NO), including nitrites and nitrates. The methodology for these measurements has not been standardized. There is very little, if any, direct evidence that concentrations of substances detected in breath condensate actually reflect their concentration at the level of the intrapulmonary airways. However, studies that have correlated breath condensate findings to the presence and severity of lower airway disease suggest that this might be the case.

Inflammatory cells and pulmonary macrophages produce H_2O_2. Increased H_2O_2 levels have been found in the breath condensate of adult cigarette smokers *(1)*, adults with asthma *(2)* and in children with unstable *(3)* and stable *(4)* asthma. In addition, increased levels of H_2O_2 have been demonstrated in individuals with common colds and in patients with cystic fibrosis (CF) *(5)*. In adult asthmatic patients, the H_2O_2 concentration in breath condensate correlates with sputum eosinophilia, but not with hyperresponsiveness *(6)*. Exhaled H_2O_2 seems to respond to antibiotic treatment in exacerbations of airway infection in CF *(5)*, and is therefore of potential interest for the monitoring of CF treatment. Despite massive airway inflammation in CF, exhaled H_2O_2 is only marginally elevated or within normal limits *(5,7,8)*. This could be owing to abundant viscous airway secretions, which may be a physical barrier or

From: *Methods in Molecular Medicine, vol. 56:*
Human Airway Inflammation: Sampling Techniques and Analytical Protocols
Edited by: D. F. Rogers and L. E. Donnelly © Humana Press Inc., Totowa, NJ

increase antioxidant activity in the airway lumen. Reference ranges for exhaled H_2O_2 have been published for school-aged children *(9)*.

Other putative markers of airway inflammation have been studied less well. There are few reports on levels of eicosanoids in exhaled air condensate, mainly focusing on chemotactic LTB_4 and the cysteinyl LTs, LTC_4, D_4 and E_4. One group has reported increased levels of LT in asthma *(10)*. A weak point in these studies is that salivary contamination was not ruled out, and may account for the findings. In ventilated adults with respiratory distress syndrome, elevated levels of isoprostanes (prostanoids that may reflect oxidant stress in the airways) have been described in breath condensate *(11)*.

Nitrate and nitrite, oxidation metabolites of NO, may be elevated in breath condensate, even if NO is not elevated in the gas phase, perhaps because of local metabolism in abnormal airways. This has been shown in cystic fibrosis patients *(12)*.

TBARs are oxidation products of lipids that are thought to result from oxidant damage of the airway tissues. The presence of TBARs in condensate of exhaled air has been demonstrated in adults with asthma *(2)*.

Exhaled substances can be identified by 2-D polyacrylamide gel electrophoresis (PAGE) in breath condensate using sensitive protein stains. Characterization is possible on the basis of localization in the electropherogram, or by molecular techniques. In one study *(13)*, patients were instructed to exhale forcefully, and it seems likely that contamination with saliva may explain, in part, the findings. We have been unable to detect meaningful quantities of protein in breath condensate that was not contaminated by saliva, using PAGE and highly sensitive enzyme-linked immunosorbent assay (ELISA) techniques (unpublished results).

We will now concentrate on H_2O_2 in breath condensate, as this is the best studied marker thus far, and some standardization is available. We will describe the condensate collection procedure and method of measurement in detail, and discuss a number of pitfalls. Condensate can be obtained by passing exhaled air through a cold tube, the material of which should be appropriate for the retrieval of the substances under examination (e.g., glass in the case of hydrogen peroxide, teflon for cysteinyl LTs). Various types of glass tubes or vessels have been used *(3,4,6,13)*. Usually, cooling is accomplished by countercurrent circulating ice water in a double-jacketed tube. Alternatively, condensate can be obtained by blowing air through a glass vessel that is placed in liquid nitrogen to capture any water vapor in the exhalate as ice on the walls of the vessel *(13)*. Frozen condensate can be stored until analysis, and its H_2O_2 content remains stable for at least a month *(9)*. The importance of storing and even collecting the condensate in the dark to avoid breakdown of substances of interest has not been evaluated.

2. Materials
2.1. Apparatus

1. Collection device consisting of a siliconized double-jacketed 50-cm long glass tube (as commonly used for distillation). The inner tube can either be straight, or have bulb-shaped outpouches to increase its surface area (e.g., Allihn PH5 BD 502, Pulles en Hanique, Veldhoven, The Netherlands).
2. Silicon rubber mouthpieces of different sizes (e.g., Mijnhart, Bilthoven, The Netherlands).
3. Two-way nonrebreathing valve (Hans Rudolph 1420 series small 2-way NRBV Y-shape, Kansas City, MO).
4. Wide-bore silicone tubing with smooth inner surface (we use ventilator tubing by Siemens, Elema, Sweden).
5. Nose-clip.
6. Vial to collect condensate (we use 50-mL Falcon tubes).
7. Cooling pump (e.g., Frigomix-U, Braun Biotech Int., Melsungen, Germany).
8. Fluorimeter (e.g., Perkin-Elmer model 3000, Perkin Elmer, Norwalk).

2.2. Reagents

Reagents are from Sigma Chemical Co., St. Louis, MO.

1. 60 mM *p*-hydroxyphenylacetic acid in H_2O.
2. 10 mg/mL horseradish peroxidase in H_2O.
3. 30% hydrogen peroxide, stabilized (Perhydrol, Merck), in serial dilutions of 0.01–10 µM. These should be made fresh each time. Stock solutions should be kept cold in dark brown bottles and opened bottles replaced at least monthly.
4. Dichlormethylsilan 2% in chloroform.

3. Methods
3.1. Collection of Exhaled Air Condensate

1. Connect mouthpiece to the nonrebreathing valve in such a way that the inspiration port points downward. This will act as a saliva trap and prevent accumulation of any saliva in the collection device (*see* **Notes 1** and **2**).
2. Connect valve to the glass tube via smooth silicone rubber tubing positioned so that the exhaled air travels upward before it enters the glass tube. This is important to prevent saliva contamination of the condensate.
3. Mount the glass tube at a downslope of approx 45°C, and place a collection vial in ice under the open end. This apparatus, as we use it for children, is shown in **Fig. 1**.
4. Seat the subject next to the apparatus, wearing a nose-clip and breathing quietly through the mouthpiece. Prior to the collection, any exercise should be avoided, and the mouth is rinsed with water. The subject is allowed to take the mouthpiece out for a short moment during the procedure if necessary (e.g., because of saliva accumulation or cough) (*see* **Note 2**).

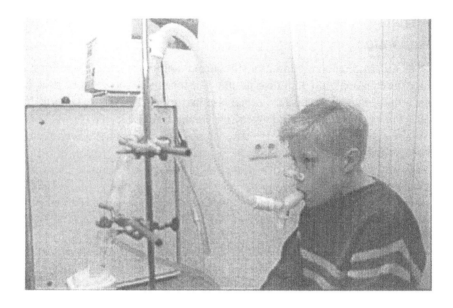

Fig. 1. Apparatus for collection of breath condensate (for details, see text).

5. Encourage the subject to breathe quietly and steadily throughout the procedure, avoiding any cough or forced maneuvers into the tubing. There are data suggesting that expiratory flow rate influences the concentration of peroxide (R. Jorres, Hamburg, personal communication). Hence, hyperventilation should be recognized and corrected whenever it occurs (*see* **Note 3**). Usually, 10–15 min will suffice to obtain 1–2 mL of condensate (*see* **Notes 4** and **5**). The condensate is either stored in a refrigerator at –20°C, or processed directly.

3.2. Measurement of H_2O_2

Peroxide concentrations can be assessed by fluorimetry of the reaction product of peroxide, horseradish peroxidase, and *p*-hydroxyphenyl acetic acid. Concentrations are determined from interpolation of a standard curve of H_2O_2 (*3,4*).

1. Mix 400 µL thawed or fresh condensate, or peroxide standard solution, with 10 µL 60 mM p-hydroxyphenyl acetic acid and 4 µL 10 mg/mL horseradish peroxidase solution, to obtain final concentrations of 1.5 mM and 100 µg/mL, respectively.
2. Vortex at room temperature for a few seconds. This immediately results in a fluorescent product.
3. Measure fluorescence using a fluorimeter at an excitation wavelength of 295 nm and an emission wavelength of 405 nm, using glass cuvets of 0.5 mL. The lower detection limit is aprox 0.01 µM H_2O_2.

4. Notes

1. Avoid contamination of condensate by saliva because it is a rich source of peroxide, mediators, cytokines, and other proteins. Salivary contamination can be checked by determining amylase in the condensates. Amylase is abundant (>30,000 IU/mL) in saliva, whereas only traces are present in lower airway secretions. Any new apparatus should be checked for contamination, and we recommend measuring amylase regularly in all samples of condensate, using routine procedures.

2. A special problem occurring in young children, and occasionally adults, is drooling, which may prevent the valves from functioning properly. Instruction to swallow at intervals, and to remove the mouthpiece to avoid the unpleasant sensation of swallowing against a closed valve is helpful.

3. Hyperventilation is a common problem when subjects breathe through a mouthpiece. This may not only affect the composition of the condensate, but also cause symptoms of dizziness and even fainting. Therefore, we routinely show video programs to distract the patients while condensate is collected, and feel that a video set is an absolute requirement for a successful procedure. Hyperventilation should be corrected whenever it occurs and researchers should be alert to detect it.

4. A limitation to collecting condensate from children is that the amount of condensate necessary for duplicate determination requires about 10–15 min of tidal breathing. This is not feasible for most children younger than ~3 years. Some preschool children will, however, accept mouthpiece and nose-clip while watching television.

5. After 1–2 min, condensate will become visible as drops inside the cold tube. At this time point, it is helpful to tap the glass tube to speed up drainage of condensed water into the collecting vial.

References

1. Nowak, D., Antczak, A., Krol, M., Pietras, T., Shariati, B., Bialasiewicz, P., et al. (1996) Increased content of hydrogen peroxide in the expired breath of cigarette smokers. *Eur. Respir. J.* **9,** 652–657.

2. Antczak, A., Nowak, D., Shariati, B., Król, M., Piasecka, G., and Kurmanowska Z. (1997) Increased hydrogen peroxide and thiobarbituric acid-reactive products in expired breath condensate of asthmatic patients. *Eur. Respir. J.* **10,** 1235–1241.

3. Dohlman, A. W., Black, H. R., and Royall, J. A. (1993) Expired breath hydrogen peroxide is a marker of acute airway inflammation in pediatric patients with asthma. *Am. Rev. Respir. Dis.* **148,** 955–960.

4. Jöbsis, Q., Raatgeep, H. C., Hermans, P. W. M., and De Jongste, J. C. (1997) Hydrogen peroxide in exhaled air is increased in stable asthmatic children. *Eur. Respir. J.* **10,** 519–521.

5. Jöbsis, Q., Raatgeep, H. C., Hermans, P. W. M., and De Jongste, J. C. (2000) Hydrogen peroxide and nitric oxide in ehaled air of children with cystic fibrosis during antibiotic treatment. *Eur. Respir. J.* **16,** 95–100.

6. Horváth, I., Donnelly, L. E., Kiss, A., Kharitonov, S. A., Lim, S., Chang, K. F., and Barnes , P. J. (1998) Combined use of exhaled hydrogen peroxide and nitric oxide in monitoring asthma. *Am. J. Respir. Crit. Care Med.* **158,** 1042–1046.

7. Ho, L. P., Faccenda, J., Innes, J. A., and Greening A. P. (1999). Expired hydrogen peroxide in breath condensate of cystic fibrosis patients. *Eur. Respir. J.* **13,** 103–106.

8. Worlitzch, D., Herberth, G., Ulrich, M., and Döring G. (1998) Catalase, myeloperoxidase, and hydrogen peroxide in cystic fibrosis. *Eur. Respir. J.* **11,** 377–383.

9. Jöbsis, Q., Raatgeep, H. C., Schellekens, S. L., Hop, W. C. J., Hermans, P. W. M., and De Jongste, J. C. (1998) Hydrogen peroxide in exhaled air of healthy children: reference values. *Eur. Respir. J.* **12,** 483–485.

10. Becher, G., Winsel, K., Neubauer, G., and Stresemann E. (1997) Breath condensate as a method of noninvasive assessment of inflammation mediators from the lower airways. *Pneumologie* **51(Suppl. 2)** 456–459.

11. Carpenter, C. T., Price, P. V., and Christman, B. W. (1998) Exhaled breath condensate isoprostanes are elevated in patients with acute lung injury or ARDS. *Chest* **114,** 1653–1659.

12. Ho, L. P., Innes, J. A., and Greening, A. P. (1998) Nitrite levels in breath condensate of CF patients are raised in contrast to exhaled nitric oxide (NO) levels. *Am. J. Respir. Crit. Care Med.* **157,** A125.

13. Scheideler, L., Manke, H. G., Schwulera, U., Inacker, O., and Hammerle, H. (1993) Detection of nonvolatile macromolecules in breath: a possible diagnostic tool? *Am. Rev. Respir. Dis.* **148,** 778–784.

III

Cell Isolation and Culture

10

Airway Epithelial Cells (Primaries vs Cell Lines)

Louise E. Donnelly

1. Introduction

The cells lining the airway consist of epithelial cells, of which there are several types including columnar cells, basal cells, and secretory/goblet cells. It is these cells which are the first lines of defense against airborne inflammatory agents. Initially, it was thought that the epithelium just formed a physical barrier between the lumen and the underlying-cells in the lung. However, epithelial cells themselves do exhibit many anti-inflammatory features and may actively participate in the inflammatory processes in the lung. The development of in vitro cell culture systems of airway epithelia has added to studies into the pathology of airway inflammation.

There are several methods for the culture of human primary epithelial cells *(1–4)*. This chapter will discuss culture of cells from trachea obtained from surgical procedures and from bronchial brushings using a defined cell culture media. The choice of cell culture media has been crucial in the successful culture of human primary epithelial cells. The system routinely used in our laboratory *(5)* is essentially that of Dent et al. 1998 *(6)*. A rich basal media is required and serum supplementation alone is not sufficient for continued proliferation of primary cells. Various growth factors and supplements are added to the media, epidermal growth factor (EGF) is required for proliferation of epithelial cells whereas the addition of hydrocortisone suppresses growth of fibroblasts *(7)* and promotes epithelial differentiation *(8)*. Similarly, retinoic acid also promotes the growth and differentiation of epithelial cells *(9,10)*.

The availability of tissue, requirement of a defined media and the unpredictable growth characteristics of primary epithelial cells has led to many workers using human epithelial cell lines. The most commonly used cell lines are A549 cells and BEAS-2B cells. A549 cells are derived from a human lung carcinoma

From: *Methods in Molecular Medicine, vol. 56:*
Human Airway Inflammation: Sampling Techniques and Analytical Protocols
Edited by: D. F. Rogers and L. E. Donnelly © Humana Press Inc., Totowa, NJ

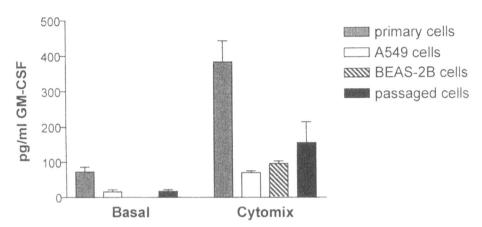

Fig. 1. Release of GM-CSF from epithelial cells following treatment with cytomix. All cells were cultured to confluence in 24-wells plates then cultured for 24 h in serum-free media. Cells were stimulated for 24 h in the presence of 50 ng/mL cytomix and media harvested and GM-CSF levels measured by ELISA. The data are expressed as mean ± SEM, n=34 for primary cells, n=4 for A549 cells, n=4 for BEAS-2B cells, n=7 for passaged cells.

whereas the BEAS-2B cell line is a transformed bronchial epithelial cell. These cells are relatively easy to culture and allow for the completion of numerous and complex experiments. However, it must be remembered that cell lines are only a model of human primary epithelial cells and therefore may differ from primary cells in their response to stimuli. An example of this can be seen in the response of human primary epithelial cells, A549 cells, BEAS-2B cells and passaged human primary epithelial cells to cytomix stimulation (interleukin-1β, tumor necrosis factor-α and interferon-γ). Primary epithelial cells produce significantly higher levels of granulocyte macrophage-colony stimulating factor (GM-CSF) under both basal and stimulated conditions when compared to both A549 cells and BEAS-2B cells and to passaged primary epithelial cells (*see* **Fig. 1**). These data demonstrate the problem of extrapolating data from cell lines to primary epithelial cultures. It is therefore recommended that cell lines should be used to determine mechanistic pathways, which require many cells, and that the definitive experiments should be performed using primary cells as confirmation of the effects in a more relevant model.

2. Materials

All reagents were from Sigma (Dorset, UK) except where noted.

1. Plasticware- *Primaria* flasks, 6-well plates and 24-well plates are obtained from Falcon (Cowley, Oxford, UK). Other tissue culture flasks are obtained from Corning-Costar Ltd. (High Wycombe, Bucks, UK).

2. Coating solution: 1% (v/v) Vitrogen (purified collagen in 0.012 N HCl) (Cohesion, Palo Alto, CA, USA).

3. Ham's F12 Nutrient Media with Glutamax (Gibco BRL, Paisley UK)

4. 7.5% (w/v) $NaHCO_3$.

5. Hydrocortisone 1 mM (0.36 mg/mL): Dissolve 7.2 mg in 2 mL of ethanol; dilute 1:10 in Ham's F12 and store in aliquots at –20°C until required.

6. EGF 5 µg/mL: Dissolve 0.1 mg in 20 mL of Ham's F12 store in aliquots at –20°C until required.

7. Insulin 9.52 mg/mL: Dissolve 100 mg in 10 mL of Ham's F12 + 0.5 mL of 1 M NaOH and store in aliquots at –20°C until required.

8. Retinoic Acid 3 µg/mL: Dissolve 50 mg in 16.67 mL ethanol and dilute 1:100 in ethanol, dilute 1:10 in Ham's F12 then aliquot and store at –20°C until required.

9. Transferrin 0.5 mg/mL: Dissolve 10 mg in 20 mL Ham's F12 and store in aliquots and store at –20°C until required.

10. Triiodothyronine 2 mg/mL: Dissolve 20 mg in 0.5 mL 1 M NaOH and add 9.5 mL Ham's F12, store in aliquots and store at –20°C until required.

11. Antibiotic/antimycotic solution (100X): Penicillin 10000 U/mL, streptomycin 10 mg/mL and amphotericin 25 µg/mL.

12. Anti-PPLO: 100X solution (Gibco-BRL, Paisley UK).

13. Fetal calf serum (FCS).

14. Nuserum IV (Becton Dickinson, Cowley, Oxford UK).

15. Primary cell culture media:
    To 100 mL Ham's F12, add:

Hydrocortisone	100 µL	Final conc. 1 µM
EGF	100 µL	Final conc. 5 ng/mL
Insulin	105 µL	Final conc. 10 µg/mL
Retinoic acid	100 µL	Final conc. 10 nM
Transferrin	100 µL	Final conc. 0.5 µg/mL
Triiodothyronine	100 µL	Final conc. 2 µg/mL
$NaHCO_3$	2 mL	Final conc. 1.5 mg/mL
Antibiotic/antimycotic	1 mL	
Anit-PPLO	1 mL (optional)	
FCS/Nuserum IV 5 mL	Final conc 5% (v/v) (*see* **Note 1**)	

    This medium can be stored at 4°C in the dark for up to one week.

16. Hank's Balanced Salts Solution (HBSS).

17. DNase: 100X solution DNase 1, Dissolve 5 mg in 5mL of HBSS.

18. 100µm mesh cell strainers were obtained from Falcon (Cowley, Oxford, UK).

19. Poly-L-lysine coated glass microscope slides (BDH, Poole, Dorset, UK).

20. 10%(v/v) formalin solution.

21. 1% (w/v) Alcian blue in acetic acid; dissolve 1 g Alcian blue in 3%(v/v) acetic acid and filter through a Whatman No. 1 filter.

22. 0.4% (w/v) basic fuchsin; dissolve 0.4 g basic fuchsin in 100 mL of distilled water and filter through a Whatman No.1 filter paper.

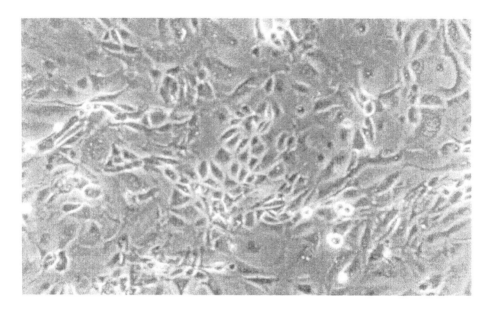

Fig. 2. Culture of human primary epithelial cells. Confluent culture of primary epithelial cells from human tracheal explant.

23. A549 human carcinoma cell line (CCL-185); American Type Culture Collection (ATCC), Rockville, MD.
24. Dulbecco's modified Eagle's media (DMEM).
25. 200 mM glutamine (100X stock solution).
26. A549 cell culture media:
    500 mL DMEM
    50 mL FCS
    5 mL glutamine stock solution
    5 mL antibiotic/antimycotic solution.
    Media should be stored at 4°C and used within 1 wk.
27. Trypsin-EDTA: 10X solution: dilute 1:10 in HBSS before use.
28. Keratinocyte serum-free media complete with supplements 2.5 µg EGF and 25 µg bovine pituitary extract (Gibco-BRL, Paisley, UK).
29. Enzyme-linked immunosorbent assay (ELISA) plates (Greiner Ltd., Gloucester, UK).
30. Coating solution: 0.1 M NaHCO$_3$, pH 8.2. Dissolve 4.2 g of NaHCO$_3$ in 500 mL of distilled water and pH to 8.2.
31. 10X phosphate buffered saline (PBS)/Tween: Dissolve 80 g of NaCl, 11.6 g of Na$_2$HPO$_4$, 2 g KH$_2$PO$_4$, 2 g KCl in 1 L of distilled water and pH to 7.0 then add 5 mL of Tween-20.
32. Blocking solution: 1X PBS/Tween containing 10% (v/v) FCS.
33. Capture antibody: rat antihuman GM-CSF clone BVD2-23B6 (PharMingen International, Becton Dickinson UK Ltd, Cowley, Oxford UK.)

34. Detection antibody: biotinylated rat antihuman GM-CSF clone BVD2-21C11 (PharMingen International. Becton Dickinson UK Ltd, Cowley, Oxford UK).
35. Recombinant human GM-CSF standard (R&D Systems Europe Ltd, Abingdon, Oxfordshire, UK).
36. 0.1 *M* citric acid: dissolve 10.5 g citric acid monohydrate in 500 mL of distilled water.
37. Avidin-peroxidase: dissolve 1 mg in avidin-peroxidase in 1 mL of distilled water and make 25 µL aliquots and store at –20°C until required.
38. ABTS substrate: dissolve 150 mg of 2,2'-azino-*bis*(3-ethylbenzthiazoline-6-sulphonic acid) in 500 mL of 0.1 *M* citric acid, pH to 4.35 with NaOH pellets. Aliquot into 11 mL vials and store at –20°C until required.
39. 30% (v/v) H_2O_2 solution.

3. Methods

3.1. Culture of Human Primary Epithelial Cells from Tracheal Explant

1. Make up cell culture media (*see* **Subheading 2, step 15**).
2. Pieces of trachea are obtained from donor lung from transplant operations (*see* **Note 2**).
3. Pieces of trachea are carefully dissected using a scalpel in a sterile cell culture hood in a Petri dish to remove any connective tissue and smooth muscle (*see* **Note 3**).
4. Pieces of trachea/bronchi are cut into small pieces of approx. 2 mm square and at least three such pieces placed epithelium side down into 6-well plates.
5. 1 mL media is added to each well and the cells are cultured at 37°C in a humidified atmosphere with 95% air, 5% (v/v) CO_2.
6. Media is changed after 1 wk and then three times a week until the cells are 70–80% confluent (*see* **Note 4** and **Fig. 2**).
7. The tracheal pieces are removed and placed into new culture dishes and cultured as above.

3.2. Culture of Human Primary Epithelial Cells from Bronchial Brushings

1. Plates for culture must be coated for at least 1 h with 1% (w/v) collagen at 37°C. 2 mL collagen solution is added to a 25 cm^2 flask. Enough solution should be added to just cover the growth area of a flask or a well. The flask is then incubated at 37°C for at least 1 h prior to use. The collagen solution may be removed and the plasticware rinsed with HBSS prior to use.
2. Brushings are obtained from patients undergoing fiberoptic bronchoscopy according to the method of Kelsen et al (*11*) (*see* **Note 5**).
3. The cell suspension is treated with 50 µg/mL DNase 1 for 20 min at room temperature.
4. The cell suspension is then filtered through a 100 µm mesh into a 50-mL centrifuge tube and washed through the filter with HBSS.

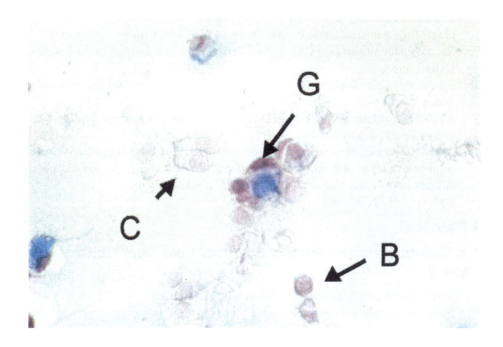

Fig. 3. Cytospin of bronchial brushing epithelial cells. Bronchial brushing cells were fixed onto a poly-L-lysine coated slide and stained with Alcian blue/fuchsin red. Ciliated columnar cells (**C**) and basal cells (**B**) stain pink and secretory/goblet cells (**G**) stain blue.

5. The cell suspension is centrifuged at 300*g* for 10 min and the resultant cell pellet resuspended in 1 mL cell culture media and the cells counted using a standard hemacytometer.
6. Cells are seeded into 24-well plates at a density of 250,000 cells/well. Cells are allowed to attach to the plates for 4 d then fresh media added to the wells and the cells cultured until confluent (*see* **Note 6**).

3.3. Identification of Epithelial Cell Types by Cell Staining

1. Cells are diluted to a density of 10,000 cells/100 µL in HBSS.
2. Cell smears (10,000 cells/slide) are prepared using a Shandon Cytospin 3 centrifuge. 100 µL cell suspension is centrifuged on to a poly-L-lysine coated slide at 40*g* for 6 min.
3. The cells are air-dried onto the slides.
4. The slides are then placed in 10% (v/v) formalin for 10 min to fix the cells onto the slides.
5. The slides are then placed in 1% (w/v) Alcian blue in 3% (v/v) acetic acid for 5 min.

6. The excess stain is then washed off with water.
7. The slides are placed in 0.4% (w/v) basic fuchsin for 1 min.
8. Again excess stain is washed off with water and the slides air-dried.
9. Cells are identified by microscopy (**Fig. 3**). Ciliated cells are identified by the columnar shape and the presence of cilia and red stain, basal cells are round and stain red and secretory cells stain blue within the secretory granules.

3.4. Culture of A549 Epithelial Cells

1. Make up media (*see* **Subheading 2, step 26**).
2. Frozen vials of cells from ATCC should be stored in liquid nitrogen until needed. Cells are then defrosted by placing the vial in a beaker of water heated to 56°C (*see* **Note 7**).
3. As soon as the ice crystals have melted in the vial, the contents are transferred to a 15-mL centrifuge tube containing ice cold media.
4. The cell suspension is centrifuged at 300g for 5 min to pellet the cells.
5. The cell pellet is resuspended into 3 mL of cell culture media prewarmed to 37°C and seeded into a 25 cm^2 flask.
6. Cells are cultured at 37°C in a humidified atmosphere of 95% air, 5% (v/v) CO_2. Cell media must be changed every 2 d until the cells reach confluence.
7. Cells are passaged by removing cell culture media and washing the cells with warm HBSS.
8. Trypsin-ethylenediaminetetraacetic acid (EDTA) solution is added to the flask (approx. 2 mL for a 25 cm^2 flask, 5 mL for a 75 cm^2 flask and 10 mL for a 162 cm^2 flask) and placed in the cell culture incubator for 2–3 min (*see* **Note 8**).
9. As soon as the cells appear rounded under the microscope, the flask is tapped sharply to remove adherent cells from the plastic.
10. An equal volume of media is added to the cell suspension and aspirated into a centrifuge tube to inhibit the action of trypsin.
11. The cell suspension is then centrifuged at 300g for 10 min and the supernatant is aspirated and discarded.
12. The cell pellet is then resuspended in cell culture media and seeded into new flasks (*see* **Note 9**).

3.5. Culture of BEAS-2B Cells

1. Make up media as below: 500-mL Keratinocyte serum-free media; 25 μg bovine pituitary extract; 2.5 μg EGF; 5-mL antibiotic/antimycotic solution. Media should be stored at 4°C and used within 1 wk.
2. All cell culture plastic ware should be coated with 1% (v/v) collagen prior to use (*see* **Subheading 3.2.1.** and **Note 10**).
3. Cells are thawed and cultured essentially as described for A549 cells, with the caveat that these cells are more prone to damage by trypsinization and hence should be passaged at lower split ratios (*see* **Note 9**).

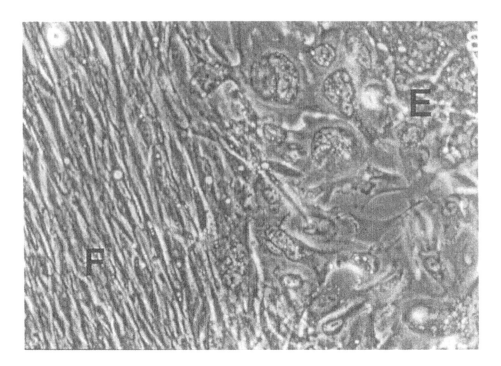

Fig. 4. Coculture of epithelial cells and fibroblasts. Culture of primary epithelial cells (**E**) and contaminating fibroblasts (**F**) from human tracheal explant.

3.6. Granulocyte Macrophage-Colony Stimulating Factor Measurement by ELISA

1. Rat monoclonal capture antibody against GM-CSF is diluted to a concentration of 2 µg/mL in 0.1 *M* NaHCO₃ and 100 µL of this solution is pipeted into a 96-well ELISA plate and incubated overnight at 4°C.
2. The plates are washed five times with 1X PBS/Tween and the plates are pounded onto paper towels to dry.
3. 200-µL blocking solution is then added to each well and the plates incubated for 2 h at room temperature.
4. The plates are then washed 5 times with 1X PBS/Tween as before.
5. Samples and standards are added to the wells and incubated at 4°C overnight (*see* **Note 11**).
6. The plates are washed 5 times and then incubated for 45 min at room temperature with 100 µL/well detection antibody diluted to 2 µg/mL in blocking solution.
7. Plates are then washed 5 times as before.
8. Plates are then incubated for 30 min at room temperature with 100 µL/well of a 1:400 dilution of avidin-peroxidase in blocking solution.
9. Plates are then washed 5 times as before.

10. ABTS substrate solution must be thawed no more than 5 min before use. 11 μL of H_2O_2 is added to the substrate and mixed well. 100 μL substrate solution is added to each well and the plate incubated at room temperature for 10–80 min.

11. The plate is then measured spectrophotometrically at 405 nm and the amount of GM-CSF in each sample calculated from a standard curve.

4. Notes

1. The choice of FCS against Nuserum IV depends on availability. However we have found that Nuserum IV has reduced the level of contamination of fibroblast cells in the cultures and is now used routinely for the culture of primary epithelial cells. Fibroblasts can be easily identified from epithelial cells on the basis of morphology (*see* **Fig. 4**). Epithelial cells form a classical cobblestone monolayer in culture whereas fibroblasts are long thin cells forming a classical tram-track monolayer.

2. It is not always possible to obtain fresh tissue from the operating theater because of various logistical problems that may be out of the control of the experimenter. We have found that if tissue is stored in complete cell culture media at 4°C viable cells may still be cultured from this tissue up to 2 d later.

3. It is important to remove any connective tissue and smooth muscle from the preparation as cells other than epithelial cells may grow out from the explant. This may take time and patience but is an absolute requirement to obtain a pure culture of epithelial cells.

4. The rate of cell proliferation depends on the subject and the quality of tissue. However, for most cultures to reach 70–80% confluence takes approx. 3–4 wk (*see* **Fig. 2.**). We have found that if pieces of tissue are left in the wells for more than 4–5 wk there is a decline in cell proliferation and cells may die. Removal of the tissue and continual feeding of the cells ensures that the cultures survive and approach confluence.

5. This chapter does not go into the details of the bronchoscopy procedures which is described by Kelsen et al. (*11*). However, brushed cells are collected into ice cold media and stored on ice until returned to the cell culture laboratory.

6. Brushed cells may not attach to the plates since many ciliated cells may remain "swimming" in the cell media until their cilia stop beating. This may take up to a week. Therefore cells that have not attached after 4 d may be removed from the wells and plated into fresh wells where they will attach and grow.

7. Ideally, cells should be defrosted from frozen at 1°C/min. However, this is not always possible. Therefore defrosting the vial in warmed water does not give the cells heat shock or allow the defrosted cells to remain in dimethyl sulfoxide (DMSO) which can be toxic to cells.

8. During passaging, cells must be exposed to Trypsin-EDTA for as short a time as possible to prevent damage to the cell surface proteins.

9. We passage cells using a split ratio as the method to determine how many flasks should be used. For A549 cells the split ratio is 1:10 (i.e., one 25 cm^2 flask could be passaged into 10 fresh 25 cm^2 flasks or approximately three 75 cm^2 flasks). BEAS-2B cells require a split ratio of no more than 1:5. If these cells are seeded too thinly, their growth is suppressed.

10. Cell culture plastic ware should be treated for at least 1 h with collagen solution prior to use. It is possible to treat plasticware several days in advance. Not all tissue culture plastic requires such treatment as many companies now produce pretreated plasticware such as Primaria cell culture plastic which can be used without such treatment.

11. GM-CSF standards are diluted in blocking solution with the maximum standard at 2000 pg/mL and doubling dilutions performed with the sensitivity of the assay at 16 pg/mL. Samples may have to be diluted to be within the range of the standard curve.

References

1. Wu, R., Zhao, Y. H., and Chang, M. M. (1997) Growth and differentiation of conducting airway epithelial cells in culture. *Eur. Respir. J.* **10,** 2398–2403.

2. Wu, R., Nolan, E., and Turner, C. (1985) Expression of tracheal differentiated functions in serum-free hormone-supplemented medium. *J. Cell Physiol.* **125,** 167–181.

3. Franklin, W. A., Folkvord, J. M., Varella, G. M., Kennedy, T., Proudfoot, S., and Cook, R. (1996) Expansion of bronchial epithelial cell populations by in vitro culture of explants from dysplastic and histologically normal sites. *Am. J. Respir. Cell Mol. Biol.* **15,** 297–304.

4. Devalia, J. L., Sapsford, R. J., Wells, C. W., Richman, P., and Davies, R. J. (1990) Culture and comparison of human bronchial and nasal epithelial cells in vitro. *Respir. Med.* **84,** 303–312.

5. Donnelly, L. E., Lim, S., Adcock, I. M., Chung, K. F., and Barnes, P. J. (1998) Primary human epithelial cells from both normal and asthmatic patients express iNOS. *Am. J. Respir. Crit. Care Med.* **157,** A769

6. Dent, G., White, S. R., Tenor, H., Bodtke, K., Schudt, C., and Leff, A. R. (1998) Cyclic nucleotide phosphodiesterase in human bronchial epithelial cells: characterization of isoenzymes and functional effects of PDE inhibitors. *Pulm. Pharmacol. Ther.* **11,** 47–56.

7. Vento, R., Torregrossa, M. V., Guiliano, M., Grecomoro, G., and Piccione, F. (1990) Effects of dexamethasone on human synovial fibroblast-like cells, from osteoarthritic joints, in culture. *Life Sci.* **47,** 2199–2205.

8. Darcy, K. M., Shoemaker, S. F., Lee, P. P., Ganis, B. A., and Ip, M. M. (1995) Hydrocortisone and progesterone regulation of the proliferation, morphogenesis, and functional differentiation of normal rat mammary epithelial cells in three dimensional primary culture. *J. Cell Physiol.* **163,** 365–379.

9. Shibagaki, T., Kitamura, H., Inayama, Y., Ogata, T., and Kanisawa, M. (1994) Effects of vitamin A on proliferation of human distal airway epithelial cells in culture. *Virchows Arch.* **424,** 525–531.

10. Niles, R. M., Loewy, B. P., and Brown, K. (1990) The effect of retinoic acid on growth and proto-oncogene expression in hamster tracheal epithelial cells. *Am. J. Respir. Cell Mol. Biol.* **2,** 365–371.

11. Kelsen, S. G., Mardini, I. A., Zhou, S., Benovic, J. L., and Higgins, N. C. (1992) A technique to harvest viable tracheobronchial epithelial cells from living human donors. *Am. J. Respir. Cell Mol. Biol.* **7,** 66–72.

11

Isolation and Culture of Human Alveolar Type II Pneumocytes

Ian R. Witherden and Teresa D. Tetley

1. Introduction

Alveolar type II pneumocytes (alveolar type II cells; TII cells) play an important role in the homeostasis of the alveolar unit. They are the progenitor cells to the type I pneumocyte and are therefore responsible for regeneration of alveolar epithelium following alveolar epithelial cell damage. The type I cell covers over 90% of the alveolar surface, reflecting its capacity to stretch into a flattened cell with very little depth (approx. 0.1 μm), but with a large surface area, to facilitate gas exchange. Nevertheless, the type II cell outnumbers type I cells, estimated to be by 2:1 in rodents. Most of the type II cell lies buried in the interstitium of the alveolus, with only the apical tip of the cell reaching into the airspace, through which another crucial function, provision of alveolar surfactant, occurs. Surfactant synthesis and secretion is a unique feature of type II cells; surfactant consists of a high proportion of phospholipids (approx. 90%) and a small proportion of protein (approx. 10%), which contains surfactant apoprotein (SP), of which four have so far been described, SP-A, SP-B, SP-C, and SP-D *(1,2)*. Surfactant is highly surface active and is essential to prevent alveolar collapse. In addition, surfactant has many other roles, including pulmonary host defense. Compromised surfactant synthesis and function are believed to be a feature of numerous disease states *(1,2)*, including infant respiratory distress syndrome, adult respiratory distress syndrome, alveolar proteinosis, and microbial infection.

To better understand the crucial role of pulmonary surfactant in survival many have studied surfactant metabolism by pure populations of type II cells in vitro. Kikkawa and colleagues *(3)* were the first to describe a method to

From: *Methods in Molecular Medicine, vol. 56:*
Human Airway Inflammation: Sampling Techniques and Analytical Protocols
Edited by: D. F. Rogers and L. E. Donnelly © Humana Press Inc., Totowa, NJ

isolate rat type II cells in 1974. Since then, methods have been modified to provide the optimal isolation and culture conditions for experimental investigation *(4)*. The majority of these have been developed using rodent lung tissue as the source of type II cells *(4)*. The resulting investigations have provided a wealth of information about type II cell function, for example, surfactant – metabolism, important factors in growth and repair of the alveolar epithelium and epithelial transport mechanisms. However, there are some important differences between rodent and human type II cells that make human the best choice for some studies. For example, lysozyme has been located in rat but not human type II cells *(5)* and, although humans express at least two SP-A genes, only one SP-A gene has so far been demonstrated in rats, mice, and rabbits *(1)*. Many investigators have attempted to overcome interspecies differences by using the human pulmonary adenocarcinoma A549 cell line. However, whether these cells are representative of human type II cells is debatable, since they are derived from malignant tissue and do not always exhibit classic type II cell characteristics.

Consequently, a few groups have attempted to develop methods to isolate human alveolar type II cells. Some of these methods result in mixed cell populations, which are useful when specific type II cell characteristics can be dissected out for study *(6,7)*, or when mixed type II and type I cell cultures are required *(8)*. Other methods are cumbersome *(9,10)*.

A previous method *(6)*, developed in our laboratory, that provided a mixed lung cell model, has been modified so that a pure human type II cell monolayer can be studied. This method is highly reproducible, very straightforward, relatively inexpensive, and open to adaptation, for example to construct an air-liquid interface, as previously described for rat type II cells *(11)*. The human cells exhibit characteristic type II cell phenotype—apical microvilli, tight junctions, lamellar bodies containing surfactant and are alkaline phosphatase positive.

2. Materials

2.1. Reagents

1. Low protein hybridoma media (LPHM; Gibco-BRL, Paisley, Scotland). Store at 4°C.
2. Hanks balanced salt solution (HBSS), containing calcium and magnesium (Gibco-BRL). Store at 4°C.
3. Newborn calf serum (NCS: Gibco-BRL): store at –20°C.
4. Trypsin (Sigma Chemical Company, Poole, UK; code T-8003). Store at –20°C.
5. DNase I (Sigma Chemical Company). Store at –20°C.
6. Penicillin/streptomycin (Gibco-BRL; 100-fold concentrate). Store at 37°C.
7. Vitrogen-100, type I collagen (Imperial Laboratories, London, UK). Store at 4°C.
8. 400–500 μm mesh cell strainer (*see* **Note 1**)

9. 40-μm mesh cell strainers (Falcon, Marathon Laboratory Supplies, London, UK).
10. T-75 (75cm²) or T-175 (175 cm²) tissue culture flasks, 96-and/or 24-well tissue culture plates.
11. Naphthol-AS-phosphate (Sigma; code N-5625)
12. Fast red violet (Sigma; code F-3381)
13. Type I collagenase (Sigma; code C0130, from *Clostridium histolyticum*)

2.2. Preparation of Media, Collagen-Coated Plates, and Alkaline Phosphatase Stain

1. Trypsin: Make up 0.25% trypsin in HBSS, filter sterilize (0.2 μm filter, Sartorius Ltd, Epsom, UK or Gelman Sciences, Northampton, UK). Store in aliquots at –20°C.
2. Complete culture medium: 10% NCS in LPHM, 2 mM glutamine, 100-U/mL penicillin and 100-μg/mL streptomycin. Store at 4°C. As glutamine and antibiotics lose potency over time at this temperature (e.g., 2 wk), prepare fresh media at regular intervals.
3. Collagen-coated plates: Dilute Vitrogen-100 to a 1% solution in sterile deionized distilled water. Coat the tissue culture wells, using sterile technique, with either 75 μL (96-well plates) or 300 μL (24-well plates). Leave with lids off, in an operating tissue culture hood, at room temperature, overnight, to dry. The Vitrogen-coated plates can be stored, with lids on, boxed or wrapped, at 4°C for 2 wk.
4. Alkaline phosphatase stain: Dissolve 10 mg naphthol-AS-bisphosphate in 40 μL dimethylsulphoxide. Make up to 10 mL with alkaline phosphatase buffer, 0.625 M MgCl and 0.125M amino methyl propanol in distilled water, pH 8.9. Add 10 mg fast red violet LB salt. Shake the suspension well, leave for 5 minutes at room temperature, then filter (0.2–0.8μm filter; Sartorius or Gelman. Filtering is essential). Make up immediately before use.

3. Methods

3.1. Isolation and Culture of Human Alveolar Type II Cells

Alveolar type II cells can be isolated from normal regions of lung tissue obtained following lobectomy for carcinoma of the lung (*see* **Note 2**). If large pieces of tissue are obtained, we recommend that they are cut into smaller segments of approx. 5 cm³ when inflated with saline (*see* **step 3** below), and processed in parallel to obtain optimal type II cell recovery. Smaller pieces are worth processing as they nevertheless provide sufficient cells for replicate studies using 96-well plates.

1. Wash the tissue with sterile 0.15 M NaCl to remove blood and debris from the surface. Place the tissue into a Petri dish.
2. Perfuse the tissue with 0.15 M saline by inserting the needle (21-gauge) of a 20 mL syringe through one edge and applying gentle pressure to the syringe. Gently massage the tissue to facilitate emptying lavage from the tissue ready for the next instillation.

3. Repeat this procedure at the same site, and then at other sites, until the whole piece of tissue has been perfused and perfusate contains less than 1×10^4 monocytes/mL (this can take up to 500 mL saline). The tissue should appear grey/white in color, as this process removes the red and white blood cells as well as the alveolar phagocytes (*see* **Note 3**). Cut the tissue into pieces approx 5 cm^3.

4. Place the tissue into a fresh Petri dish ready for trypsinization. Instill the trypsin solution (10–15 mL/5 cm^3 piece) into the lung tissue in exactly the same way as the saline lavage, until it overflows into the Petri dish. Instill the fluid into all segments so that all regions of the tissue are fully inflated once. Place the covered Petri dish into a 37°C incubator for 15 min. Any trypsin that has seeped from the tissue into the Petri dish may be aspirated and discarded at this stage if necessary.

5. Instill fresh trypsin solution into the tissue until fully inflated, as before, and incubate for a further 15 min. Repeat the procedure once more to give a total trypsinization period of 45 min. Aspirate and discard excess trypsin solution that has leaked into the Petri dish.

6. Chop the tissue finely into 1–2 mm^3 in the presence of NCS (or fetal calf serum; 10 mL/5 cm^3 piece), to inhibit trypsin activity. Add DNase I (250-µg/mL HBSS; 7 mL/ 5 cm^3 piece) to the suspension to degrade glutinous DNA released from ruptured cells during the mincing process. Shake the minced tissue suspension vigorously by hand for 5 min; this stage is essential and enhances type II cell recovery.

7. Filter the tissue suspension through a large gauge mesh (400–500 µm) then a 40-µm mesh to remove undigested tissue and debris from the enzymatically-released epithelial cells, which pass through the filter.

8. Centrifuge the filtrate, containing mostly single cells, at 300g for 10 min at 12°C. Suspend the cell pellet in 30 mL 50% LPHM and 50% HBSS containing 100 mg/ mL DNase I. Determine the total crude cell number using a hemocytometer (this will be approx. 20×10^6 cells/5 cm^3 piece of tissue). A cytospin of the crude cell preparation may also be prepared for alkaline phosphatase staining (*see* **Note 4**).

9. Plate the resuspended cell suspension into either T-75 or T-175 culture flasks and incubate at 37°C for 1–2 h to enable any contaminating macrophages to adhere (*see* **Note 5**).

10. Remove the media containing the nonadherent, type II cell-enriched cell population and centrifuge at 300g for 10 min at 12°C. Resuspend the cell pellet in 30 mL complete, 10% NCS, culture media and incubate in a T-75 tissue culture flask for 1–2 h at 37°C to allow contaminating fibroblasts to adhere.

11. Remove the nonadherent, type II cell-enriched medium and centrifuge as previously described. Pool the cell pellets from each piece of tissue and resuspend in a known, small volume of complete medium. Count the epithelial cells using a hemocytometer by phase contrast microscopy (*see* **Note 6**). There should be approx. 10×10^6 cells/5 cm piece of tissue. Thus, a piece of tissue, 15 cm × 5 cm × 5 cm, would be expected to yield approx. 30×10^6 cells. Prepare a cytospin for alkaline phosphatase staining if required (*see* **Note 4**).

12. Add complete medium so that there are 1×10^6 epithelial cells/mL and plate onto Vitrogen-coated plates; 0.5–1.0×10^6/well of a 24-well plate and 1.0–1.5×10^5/

Magnification: x10   x40   x10

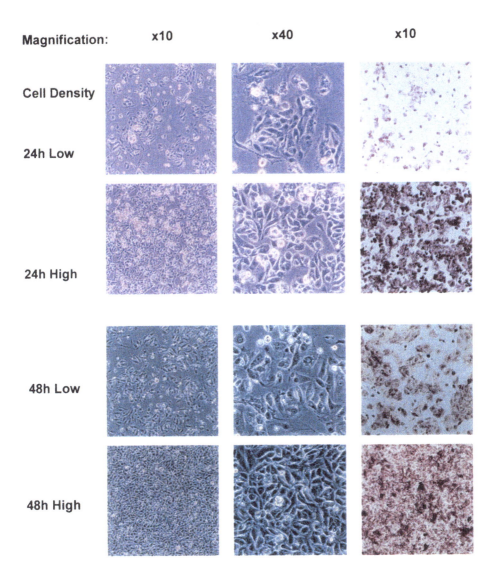

Fig. 1. Light microscopy of human epithelial type II cells seeded at two densities and examined at 24 and 48 h following seeding. The cells are alkaline phosphatase positive and form clusters that increase in size until they merge as a monolayer between 2 and 3 d after seeding, depending on the original cell density.

well of a 96-well plate (make media up to 1 mL/well and 200 μL/well, respectively). Incubate in a humidified atmosphere in 5% CO_2 at 37°C for 24 h.

13. After 24 h (*see* **Note 7**) remove media and nonadherent cells. Do not wash, leave remaining loosely attached cells and apply fresh complete medium.

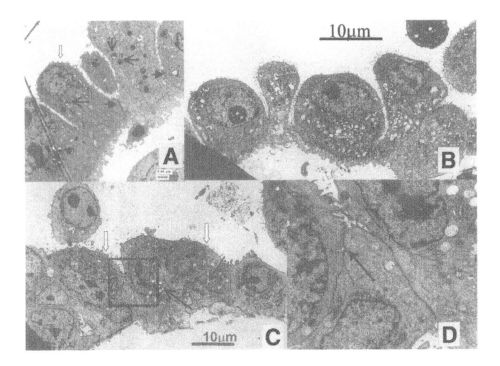

Fig. 2. Electron microscopy of human lung epithelial cells 4 d after seeding. **a** and **b.** Human epithelial type II cells showing cuboidal appearance with apical microvilli (open arrows), lamellar bodies (black arrows, fine tip) and well-formed tight junctions (black arrow, blunt tip) between all the cells (**a**). Low power electron microscopy illustrating a monolayer of connected type II cells (**b**). These cells grow in monolayers. **c** and **d** A549 adenocarcinoma cells showing flattened appearance with disorganized microvilli (open arrows) and sparse, abnormal lamellar bodies (black arrows, fine tip). Note also the multiple cell layers (**c**). High magnification of boxed area from **Fig. 2c** illustrating a rare tight junction (black arrow, blunt tip) (**d**).

14. After another 16–24 h, remove medium and wash off remaining loose cells with HBSS. Apply fresh complete medium. The cells form a confluent monolayer within 3 d of plating.

3.2. Characterization of Human Type II Cells

1. Alkaline phosphatase stain: Cover air-dried (>15 min) cytospin preparations or washed adherent cells with freshly prepared alkaline phosphatase stain and incubate for 20 min at 37°C. Wash with distilled water and examine wet or dry by light microscopy. The intensity of pink stain reflects the amount of alkaline phos-

phatase present (*see* **Note 8**). In this study, the cells were seeded at two densities, 0.5 and 1.0×10^6 cells per well, in 24-well plates. The cells have been stained for alkaline phosphatase 24 and 48 h after seeding and compared with unstained cells, observed at the same stage, by phase contrast light microscopy (*see* **Fig. 1**). Thus, the cells can be seen to be virtually 100% alkaline phosphatase-positive, representing the type II cell purity (*see* **Fig. 1**, last column, and **Fig. 2**). The cells begin as small clusters which increase in size over time, until a monolayer forms, between 2 and 3 d following seeding, depending on seeding density. The cells are ideal to use for experiments on d 3 and 4 after isolation.

2. Electron microscopy: The Vitrogen substrate allows removal of cells as sheets using collagenase. The type II cell monolayers have been incubated with 0.25% collagenase in HBSS until the cells loosened (observe by light microscopy), when they were lifted mechanically using a flat-edged utensil. The cells were pelleted by centrifugation, as previously described, then fixed in 2.5% glutaraldehyde in cacodylate buffer and processed for electron microscopy. The cells are cuboidal in appearance with type II cell characteristics (d 4 after seeding) of numerous surfactant-containing lamellar bodies, apical microvilli, and tight junctions (*see* **Fig. 2a, b**). Electron microscopy confirms the observations by light microscopy, of a virtually 100% type II cell population which grows as a monolayer. An interesting feature is elongated tight junctions which may reflect the type II:type II cell contact rather than type II:type I cell contact that most often occurs in vivo. Electron microscopy of A549 cells, grown for 4 d on Vitrogen, and prepared for electron microscopy in an identical manner, is shown for comparison (*see* **Fig. 2c, d**). Cells often grow in layers at this stage. Note also that lamellar bodies containing lipid inclusions are relatively scarce; where there are lipid inclusions, these are not lamellar bodies. Tight junctions are rare, difficult to visualize and poorly formed. Many cells are flattened, rather than cuboidal, in appearance and the microvilli are irregular.

3. Messenger RNA expression of SPA and SPC: Expression of mRNA for SP-A and SP-C was investigated by harvesting RNA from TII cells (on d 4) and, for comparative purposes, the original, fresh, unprocessed human lung tissue as well as the following lung cell lines: A549 adenocarcinoma, BEAS-2B, NCI-H441, and NCI-H322. Cellular RNA was prepared using commercial kits and then hybridized with random ^{32}P-dCTP primer-labeled cDNA encoding human SP-C (*12*), or SP-A (*13*), or β-actin and exposed to X-ray film for 48 h. Immunolocalization of SP-A and SP-C in human lung tissue suggests that their synthesis is confined to type II cells (*2*). The present study shows that both SP-A and SP-C are expressed strongly in the fresh tissue and in the type II cell monolayers on d 4 (*see* **Fig. 3**). This is also true at d 1 (data not shown). However, expression decreases so that by d 7 in vitro, there is very little SP-A or SP-C (data not shown) and, again, experiments are best carried out on d 3 and 4. Interestingly, there is no expression of either SP-A or SP-C in the A549 adenocarcinoma cell line, which is frequently used as a surrogate for human type II cell studies, although not for surfactant metabolism, reflecting its altered phenotype. None of the other lung

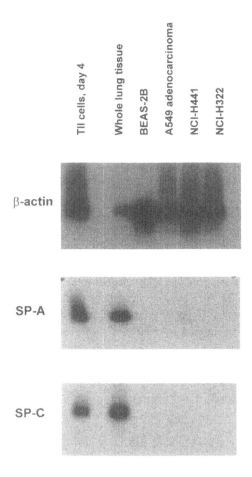

Fig. 3. Messenger RNA expression of surfactant protein (SP)-A and SP-C by human lung tissue and human type II cells 4 d after seeding compared with four human lung epithelial cell lines. Messenger RNA for these proteins was only expressed by fresh human lung tissue and isolated human type II cells.

epithelial cell lines express the surfactant apoproteins (*see* **Fig. 3**).

4. Notes

1. A small stainless steel sieve or tea strainer can be used. It must be oven sterilized.
2. Fresh pieces of tissue can be stored overnight in a sterile flask at 4°C. They can be processed the next day.
3. If necessary, following saline lavage, the tissue can be perfused with LPHM, submerged in LPHM in a sterile, capped container and stored overnight at 4°C. The tissue can be processed the next day.
4. At this point, although epithelial cells will enrich the cell population, it will include airway and tissue macrophages as well as any fibroblasts that may have

been accessed following epithelial stripping, and other contaminating cells. It should nevertheless contain about 50% alkaline phosphatase-positive cells i.e., epithelial, mostly type II, cells *(see* **Note 8**). It is advisable to carry out alkaline phosphatase staining at this stage to evaluate the purity of the crude isolate. This can then be compared with the purity of the final preparation used for seeding.

5. Macrophages adhere readily in a serum-free medium such as LPHM. Inclusion of DNase at this stage facilitates further degradation of free DNA which, if left, can continue to agglutinate, trapping cells and reducing ultimate type II cell recovery.

6. Epithelial cells can be distinguished from contaminating cells as, by phase contrast microscopy, it is possible to adjust the focus so that they have a pink hue. Contaminating macrophages are colorless or contain cigaret smoke particles, whereas other cells are colorless or much smaller than the epithelial cells.

7. At this stage, it will be difficult to see the clusters of adherent type II cells below the nonadherent, mixed cells. Without experience, the isolation may appear by light microscopy to have failed, as any residual contaminating red blood cells, colonies of nonadherent, floating ciliated cells, other cell debris and nonadherent cells mask the successful proliferation of underlying type II cells. Once the media has been changed and cells washed, it is possible to see clusters of proliferating type II cells, which eventually merge to form a monolayer.

8. Alkaline phosphatase has been shown to be a reliable marker of type II cell phenotype both in vitro and in vivo. Loss of alkaline phosphatase-positivity occurs when the cells lose their type II cell phenotype. Staining of fresh cytospin preparations of type II cells and adherent cells for alkaline phosphatase provides insight to the purity and growth characteristics of human type II cells in vitro. Although the crude and final cell preparations may only be 50–80% alkaline phosphatase-positive, many of the nonpositive cells are removed by differential adherence or are nonviable. Use of Vitrogen enhances type II cell adherence and maintenance of phenotype in vitro, so that the monolayers are virtually pure type II cell preparations. It is also possible to use extracellular matrix (ECM) as a substrate (*14*) although our comparative studies (unpublished observations) suggest that human type II cells prefer Vitrogen, whereas rat type II cells grow best on ECM. Use of ECM-prepared plates is more expensive than using Vitrogen.

Acknowledgments

The authors would like to thank Mr. Terry Bull and Ms. Anne Dewar (the Division of Neuroscience and the Division of the National Heart & Lung Institute, Imperial College School of Medicine, London) for carrying out the electron microscopy of human type II epithelial cells and the A549 adenocarcinoma cell line.

References

1. Wright, J. R. (1997) Immunomodulatory functions of Surfactant. *Physiol. Rev.* **77,** 931–962.
2. Mason, R. J., Greene, K., and Voelker D. R. (1998) Surfactant protein A and surfactant protein D in health and disease. *Am. J. Physiol.* **275,** L1–L13.

3. Kikkawa, Y. and Yoneda, K. (1974) The type II epithelial cell of the lung. 1. Method of isolation. *Lab. Invest.* **30,** 76–84.

4. Dobbs, L. G. (1990). Isolation and culture of alveolar type II cells. *Am. J. Physiol.* **258,** L134–L147.

5. Singh, G. Katyal, S. L., Brown, W. E., Collins, D. L. and Mason, R. J. (1988) Pulmonary lysozyme — a secretory protein of type II pneumocytes in the rat. *Am. Rev. Respir. Dis.* **138,** 1261–1267.

6. Bingle, L., Bull, T. B., Fox, B., Guz, A., Richards, R. J., and Tetley, T. D. (1990) Type II pneumocytes in mixed cell culture of human lung: A light and electron microscope study. *Environ. Health Persp.* **85,** 71–80.

7. Alcorn, J. L., Smith, M. E., Smith, J. F., Margraf, L. R., and Mendelson, C. R. (1997) Primary cell culture of human type II pneumocyte: Maintainance of a differentiated phenotype and transfection with recombinant adenoviruses. *Am. J. Respir. Cell Mol. Biol.* **17,** 672–682.

8. Elbert, K. J., Schafer, U. F., Schafers, H. J., Kim, K. J., Lee, V. H. L., and Lehr, C. M. (1999) Monolayers of human alveolar epithelial cells in primary culture for pulmonary absorption and transport studies. *Pharmaceutical Res.* **16,** 601–608.

9. Edelson, J. D., Shannon, J. M., and Mason, R. J. (1989) Effects of two extracellular matrices on morphologic and biochemical properties of human type II cells *in vitro*. *Am. Rev. Respir. Dis.* **140,** 1398–1404.

10. Hoet, P. H. M., Lewis, C. P. L., Demedts, M., and Nemery, B. (1994) Putrescine and paraquat uptake in human lung slices and isolated type II pneumocytes. *Biochem. Pharmacol.* **48,** 517–524.

11. Dobbs, L. G., Pian, M. S., Maglio M., Dumars S., and Allen L. (1997) Maintenance of the differentiated type II cell phenotype by culture with an apical air surface. *Am. J. Physiol.* **273,** L347–L354.

12. Glasser, S. W., Korfhagen, T. R., Wert, S. E., Bruno, M. D., McWilliams, K. M., Vorbroker, D. K., and Whitsett, J. A. (1991). Genetic element from human surfactant protein SP-C gene confers bronchiolar-alveolar cell specificity in transgenic mice. *Am. J. Physiol.* **261,** L349–356.

13. White, R. T., Damm, D., Miller, J., Spratt, K., Schilling, J., Hawgood, S. Benson, B., and Cordell, B. (1985). Isolation and characterization of the human pulmonary surfactant apoprotein gene. *Nature* **317,** 361–363.

14. Bingle, L., Richards, R. J., Fox, B., Masek, L., Guz, A., and Tetley, T. D. (1997) Susceptibility of lung epithelium to neutrophil elastase: Protection by native inhibitors. *Mediators of Inflammation* **6,** 345–354.

12

Pulmonary Artery Endothelial Cells

Joachim Seybold and Norbert Suttorp

1. Introduction

Endothelial cells function as a highly regulated barrier between blood and interstitium. They play a central role in the regulation of vascular permeability by controlling the passage of liquid and nutrients as well as the transit of white blood cells *(1,2)*. The endothelium is involved in the inflammatory response by either secreting cytokines or responding to blood-derived mediators or signals from adjacent cells *(3–6)*. In 1973, Jaffe and coworkers *(7)* first published the culture of endothelial cells isolated from human umbilical veins. Ryan and coworkers *(8)* described, in 1978, the first isolation of pulmonary artery endothelial cells. Porcine endothelial cells have been used to study endothelial permeability in vitro *(2,9,10)* adhesion *(11)*, and blood coagulation *(12)*. Since the regulation of endothelial permeability is critical for pulmonary gas exchange, the close vicinity to airway epithelial cells has drawn attention to interactions between both cell types. Here we describe the isolation and culture of pulmonary artery endothelial cells and outline the in vitro measurement of endothelial permeability.

2. Materials

2.1. Media and Solutions

All cell culture reagents were purchased from Gibco Life Technologies unless otherwise stated. The fetal calf serum, trypsin-ethylenediaminetetraacetic acid (EDTA) and collagenase should be screened (e.g., by use of growth curves) to give optimal results.

From: *Methods in Molecular Medicine, vol. 56:*
Human Airway Inflammation: Sampling Techniques and Analytical Protocols
Edited by: D. F. Rogers and L. E. Donnelly © Humana Press Inc., Totowa, NJ

1. Medium 199 with antibiotics: Medium 199 with Earle´s salt, L-glutamine (2 mM), penicillin (100,000 units/L), streptomycin (100 mg/L), amphotericin B (1 mg/L).
2. Medium 199 with antibiotics and fetal calf serum (FCS) (10% and 20%, v/v): FCS from different suppliers (PAA, Biochroma, Sigma) has to be tested for optimum growth of endothelial cells. Heat inactivation of FCS is not required for porcine endothelial cells. For plating cells on filters, 20% (v/v) FCS is optimal.
3. Hanks balanced salt solution(HBSS) /HEPES (without Ca^{2+} and Mg^{2+}: Ca/Mg free HBSS): 0.4 g/L KCl, 0.06 g/L KH_2PO_4, 8 g/L NaCl, 0.35 g/L $NaHCO_3$, 0.048 g/L Na_2HPO_4, 1 g/L D-Glucose, 6 g/L HEPES, pH 7.4.
4. HBSS/HEPES (with Ca^{2+} and Mg^{2+}: HBSS): 0.185 g/L $CaCl\infty2H_2O$, 0.4 g/L KCl, 0.06 g/L KH_2PO_4, 0.1 g/L $MgCl_2\infty2H_2O$, 0.1 g/L $MgSO_4 \infty7H_2O$, 8 g/L NaCl, 0.35 g/L $NaHCO_3$, 0.048 g/L Na_2HPO_4, 1 g/L D-Glucose, 6 g/L HEPES, pH 7.4.
5. Gelatin, 10X stock solution: 2.5 g gelatin from porcine skin (Sigma) is dissolved in 500 mL distilled water at 60°C. The hot gelatin solution is filtered through a 0.2 μM sterile filter, aliquoted in 50 mL tubes and stored at 4°C. Before plating cells the gelatin is diluted 1:10 in sterile distilled water to obtain a final concentration of 0.5 mg/mL.
6. Trypsin/EDTA: Trypsin [0.5%, approx 5 U/mL (25°C)]/EDTA is supplied in phosphate buffered saline from Boehringer Mannheim. Aliquots (7 mL) are stored at –20°C.
7. Collagenase 0.1% (w/v, Worthington, class II): 1 g/L collagenase is dissolved in HBSS, sterilized by filtration through 0.2 μM sterile filter, stored at –20°C for up to 2 w. Collagenase should be thawed and warmed up to 37°C shortly before use.

2.2. Instruments and Materials

The following instruments have to be sterile:

1. Scalpels.
2. Blunt forceps.
3. Surgical scissors.
4. Surgical clips.
5. Beaker.
6. Thread.
7. Glass pipets or disposable pipets (5 and 10 mL).
8. Pasteur pipets.
9. Gloves.
10. Cell culture flasks (75 cm^2, T75, Nunc).
11. 50 mL tubes (Falcon).
12. 15 mL tubes (Nunc).
13. Sterile filter 0.2 μM (Millipore).
14. Polycarbonate filter membranes (25 mm diameter, pore size 5 μM, polyvinylpyrrolidone (PVP)-free, Nucleopore, Tübingen, Germany) *(see* **Note 1**).
15. Petri dishes (60 × 15 mm), Falcon 1016 (Easy grip).

3. Method

3.1. Isolation of Pulmonary Artery Endothelial Cells

The isolation of endothelial cells is performed under sterile conditions using a laminar flow biosafety hood. All solutions are warmed to 37°C prior to the isolation of the endothelial cells.

1. Resected aortas are transported to the laboratory on ice in a sterile plastic bag.
2. The bottom of each cell culture flask (T75) is covered with 5 mL of the diluted gelatin (0.5 mg/mL). The flasks are kept in the incubator at 37°C for 1 h.
3. Dissect the pulmonary artery from the aorta. Put a piece of thread tightly around the bottom end of the pulmonary artery, close to the pulmonary valve. Wash the lumen three times with 10 mL of HBSS (37°C). Fix three clips on the top (i.e., open) end of the artery and place it in a beaker, in such a way that the lumen of the artery is held open by the weight of the clips hanging down beside the beaker.
4. Fill the artery with warm collagenase and incubate at 37°C for 30 min. Remove the collagenase and massage the artery carefully for 1 min.
5. Rinse the artery thoroughly with 10 mL Medium 199 using a pipetting device and transfer the suspension, which now contains the endothelial cells, into a 15 mL Falcon tube. Rinse and massage the artery again and collect into a new Falcon tube.
6. Centrifuge the Falcon tubes (300g, 10 min) at room temperature, discard the supernatant, resuspend the cells in 10 mL Medium 199 and centrifuge again.
7. Remove supernatant and resuspend cells carefully in 1 mL Medium 199 + 10% (v/v) FCS.
8. Discard the gelatin from the cell culture flasks (step 2), and add 14 mL Medium 199 + 10% (v/v) FCS. Pipet the cell suspension into the medium and incubate at 37°C, 5% (v/v) CO_2. Change the medium every 3 to 4 d. The endothelial cells will reach confluence within 5–7 days (*see* **Note 2**).
9. Passage the monolayers after reaching confluence. Wash twice with Ca/Mg free HBSS and detach the cells with 3.5 mL of Trypsin-EDTA (37°C), add 56 mL of Medium 199 + 10% (v/v) FCS and split the cell suspension in 3-cell culture flasks (T75) which have been treated with gelatin, as described in step 2. Within 2 to 3 d the monolayer will reach confluence with a density of approx 0.6×10^6 cells/cm^2.

3.2. Measurement of Endothelial Permeability

The in vitro system for the measurement of endothelial permeability (**Fig. 1**) allows the quantification of the smallest volumes of liquid passing through a monolayer of endothelial cells grown on polycarbonate filter membranes. The cell-covered membrane is mounted in a modified chemotaxis chamber (**Fig. 1**) and exposed to a hydrostatic pressure of 10 cm H_2O. The water filtration rate determined allows the calculation of the hydraulic conductivity (porosity). The system is accurate enough to measure an increase in filtration vol-

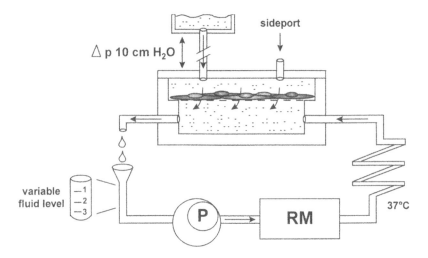

Fig. 1. System for the measurement of endothelial permeability. Pulmonary endothe-lial cells are grown on a polycarbonate filter membrane and are mounted in a modified chemotaxis chamber. Hydrostatic pressure (10 cm H_2O) is applied to the luminal side of the endothelial monolayer. Through the second drill-hole drug(s) of interest can be injected into the compartment. A constant flow (10 mL/min) of HBSS buffer (37°C) through the abluminal side is maintained by the roller pump (P). Variable fluid levels can be measured with the glass capillary on the left side with an accuracy of 10 μL. The volume in the lower compartment is 10 mL, and in the upper compartment is 1 mL. In order to calculate the albumin reflection coefficient (RC), the radioactivity monitor (RM) measures the flux of ^3H_2O and [^{14}C]-albumin added to the upper compartment.

umes as little as 10 μL over 5 min. The albumin reflection coefficient can be calculated by measuring the passage of ^3H_2O and [^{14}C]-albumin through the endothelial monolayer as described below (**Subheading 3.2.1**).

3.2.1. Culture of Endothelial Cells on Polycarbonate Filter Membranes

1. Incubate the polycarbonate filter membranes for 1 h in gelatin solution (0.2%, w/v) and 30 min in glutaraldehyde (3%, v/v) in order to crosslink the gelatin. The membranes are sterilized for 4 h in 70% (v/v) ethanol before thorough washing with sterile Ca/Mg free HBSS. The filter membranes can be kept in sterile Ca/Mg free HBSS at 37°C for up to 3 d.
2. Place the pretreated filter membranes in a fresh Petri dish and allow to dry. Fix the membrane on the Petri dish by carefully touching the edge of the filter at 4 points with a hot needle.
3. Use two cell culture flasks (T75) from the same pulmonary artery which will be enough for 5 filter membranes. Wash twice with Ca/Mg free HBSS and detach the cells with 3.5 mL of Trypsin-EDTA (37°C). Add 6 mL of Medium 199 + 20% (v/v) FCS, transfer the suspension to a 15-mL Falcon tube and centrifuge at 200g for 5

min. Remove the supernatant and resuspend the cells in 2.5 mL of Medium 199 + 20% (v/v) FCS. Place the cell suspension (approx 0.6×10^6 endothelial cells/cm^2) carefully with a pipet on the filter membrane and allow the endothelial cells to attach to the membrane while incubating for 4 h at 37°C and 5% (v/v) CO_2 (*see* **Note 3**).

4. Once the cells adhere to the filter membranes add *carefully* 10 mL of Medium 199 + 20% (v/v) FCS to the Petri dishes and allow the cells to form a confluent monolayer within approx 2 d (*see* **Note 4**).

3.2.2. Experimental Protocol for Measurement of Endothelial Permeability

1. The confluent endothelial monolayer grown on polycarbonate filter membranes is placed in the modified chemotaxis chamber (**Fig. 1**) between rubber gaskets (one on the bottom, two on top of the membrane) (*see* **Notes 5 and 6**). The cells face the upper compartment which is covered by a plexiglass lid. This lid is screwed tightly on the bottom rubber gasket. One hole in the lid is connected to a syringe adjusted to an appropriate height in order to apply 10 cm H_2O hydrostatic pressure. The other hole (usually closed with a rubber plug) allows addition of drugs or removal of samples. The bottom compartment is perfused continuously (10 mL/min), using roller pumps (*see* **Note 7**), with a total volume of 10 mL HBSS. Before applying the hydrostatic pressure, the system should equilibrate for 20 min. The control filter is prepared in the same way on a parallel system (*see* **step 3** below).

2. Apply hydrostatic pressure (10 cm H_2O) which leads within 30 to 60 min to a gradual reduction of the liquid volume filtered through the monolayers from initially 50–150 µL/min to a basal rate of less than 20 µL/min (referred to as sealing) (*see* **Notes 8–10**).

3. Add the drug to be tested to the upper compartment and measure the volume filtered every 5 min. As a negative control, apply the vehicle of the respective drug to the control system, running in parallel.

4. At the end of the experiment a potent permeability-inducing agent is added as a positive control: e.g., staphylococcus α-toxin (10 µg/mL), A 23187 (10^{-7}M) or mellitin (10 µg/mL).

3.2.3. Calculation of Hydraulic Conductivity

The hydraulic conductivity is the result of the filtration rate (µl/min) divided by the area, and the hydrostatic pressure difference. In Subheading 3.2.1, Fig. 1, with an area of 3.46 cm^2 and a hydrostatic pressure difference of 10 cm H_2O, the conversion factor for the calculation of the hydraulic conductivity from the filtration rate is 20.78: e.g., 10 µL/min (0.01 cm^3/min) filtration results in a hydraulic conductivity of 4.82×10^{-6} cm $\times$ s^{-1} $\times$ cm H_2O^{-1}.

3.2.4. Calculation of the Reflection Coefficient for Albumin

The membrane selectivity for albumin [albumin reflection coefficient, RC] is determined by adding 100 nCi ^3H_2O and 100 nCi [^{14}C]-albumin to the upper compartment. To prevent nonspecific absorption of albumin to the walls of the filter system, the buffer was supplemented with 0.25% (w/v) unlabeled albumin. The amount of ^3H_2O and $[^{14}C]$-albumin in the lower compartment is continuously measured (**Fig. 1**) using a radioactivity monitor (Ramona LS-5, Raytest, Heidelberg, Germany) consisting of a flow-through cell, a splitter/mixer, and a personal computer for data calculation. One mL HBSS buffer is removed every 5 min from the lower compartment and mixed with 4 mL Quickszint 212 scintillation fluid. The volume withdrawn by the splitter is continuously substituted by a pump. The resulting dilution of the fluid of the lower compartment has to be considered in the calculation of the albumin reflection coefficient. In addition, 50 μL of fluid from the upper compartment is withdrawn every 5 min, mixed with 10 mL scintillation fluid, and counted in a Packard liquid scintillation analyzer (model 2000 CA, Packard, Frankfurt, Germany).

RC is calculated according to the formula:

$$RC = 1 - (A/B \times D/C)$$

where A is difference in $[^{14}C]$-albumin (in cpm/mL), multiplied by the volume of the lower compartment, between time points x and $x + 5$ minutes,

B is the sum of $[^{14}C]$-albumin (in cpm/mL), in the upper compartment, at time points x and $x + 5$ min, divided by 2,

C is the difference in ^3H_2O (in cpm/mL), multiplied by the volume of the lower compartment, between time points x and $x + 5$ min,

and D is the sum of ^3H_2O (in cpm/mL) in the upper compartment at time points x and $x + 5$ min, divided by 2.

For example, for $A = 300$, there was an increase of 30 cpm/mL $[^{14}C]$-albumin in the lower compartment of the filter system between 10 and 15 min. The volume of the lower system is 10 mL, i.e., 300 cpm $[^{14}C]$-albumin had passed into the lower compartment within 5 min. For $B = 9,850$, at 10 min there were 10,000 cpm/mL $[^{14}C]$-albumin in the upper compartment and 9,700 cpm/mL at time point 15 min $(10,000 + 9,700 = 19,700$ cpm $\div 2 = 9,850$ cpm$)$. For $C = 600$, there was an increase of 60 cpm/mL ^3H_2O in the lower compartment between 10 and 15 min. The volume of the lower system is 10 mL, i.e., 600 cpm ^3H_2O had passed into the lower compartment within 5 min. For $D = 9,700$, at 10 min there were 10,000 cpm/mL ^3H_2O in the upper compartment and 9,400 cpm/mL at 15 min $(10,000 + 9,400 = 19,400$ cpm $\div 2 = 9,700$ cpm$)$.

Thus $RC = 1 - (300 \div 9,850) \times (9,700 \div 600) = 1 - 0.49 = 0.51$.

4. Notes

1. It is critical to exclude all factors which could reduce growth and adherence of endothelial cells on the polycarbonate filter membrane. Toxic factors can be released from polycarbonate filter membranes. Therefore, membranes from dif-

ferent suppliers have to be tested for optimum growth of endothelial cells. Note that even different batches from the same supplier may vary.

2. Endothelial cells in confluent culture display the characteristic cobble-stoned pattern. Growing endothelial cells show a rather irregular pattern. To confirm the mesenchymal nature of the cells isolated, specific markers, such as vimentin, have to be demonstrated. In contrast to endothelial cells of human origin, porcine endothelial cells express very low levels of the endothelial-specific von Willebrand factor *(13)*.

3. It is crucial to pipet the cell suspension in a small volume ($\leq$500 µL) on the filter membrane only.

4. Petri dishes are recommended, whose surface prevents cells from crawling from the filter membrane to the Petri dish. It is important to test Petri dishes from different sources to avoid this problem. We obtained good results with Falcon 1016 Petri dishes.

5. Cells must form a confluent monolayer to allow sealing of the filters. Sealing, a prerequisite for the experiment, needs to occur under continuous exposure to a hydrostatic pressure of 10 cm H_2O (i.e., the initial filtration rate of 50–150 µL/min should decrease within 30–60 min to reach a nadir of 10–20 µL/min. Unsealed filters cannot be used for permeability experiments.

6. The system **(Fig.1)** must be warmed to 37°C prior to the experiment.

7. Roller pumps should be used which provide a pulse-free flow.

8. The hydrostatic pressure should be calibrated in the absence of the filter membrane prior to the experiment.

9. The reference point is the filter membrane level.

10. Air in the system must be avoided under any circumstances during the entire experiment.

References

1. Van Hinsbergh, V. W. M., van Nieuw Amerongen, G. P., and Draijer, R. (1997) Regulation of the permeability of human endothelial cell monolayers In *Vascular endothelium: Physiology, pathology, and therapeutic opportunities.* (Born, G. V. R., and Schwartz, C. V., ed.), Schattauer, Stuttgart, Germany pp. 61–76.

2. Suttorp, N., Hessz, T., Seeger, W., Wilke, A., Koob, R., Lutz, F., and Drenckhahn, D. (1988) Bacterial exotoxins and endothelial permeability for water and albumin in vitro. *Am. J. Physiol.* **255,** C368–C376.

3. Shasby, D. M. and Roberts, R. L. (1987) Transendothelial transfer of macromolecules in vitro. *Fed. Proc.* **46,** 2506–2510.

4. Lum, H., and Malik, A. B. (1994) Regulation of vascular endothelial barrier function. *Am. J. Physiol.* **267,** L223–L241.

5. Garcia, J. G., Verin, A. D., and Schaphorst, K. L. (1996) Regulation of thrombin-mediated endothelial cell contraction and permeability. *Semin. Thromb. Hemost.* **22,** 309–315.

6. Michel, J. B., Feron, O., Sacks, D., and Michel, T. (1997) Pathways through microvascular endothelium of normal and increased permeability. In *Vascular*

endothelium: Physiology, pathology, and therapeutic opportunities. (Born, G. V. R., and Schwartz, C. V. ed.), Schattauer, Stuttgart, Germany, pp. 61–76.

7. Jaffe, E. A., Nachman, R. L., Becker, C. G., and Minick, C. R. (1973) Culture of human endothelial cells derived from umbilical veins. Identification by morphologic and immunologic criteria. *J. Clin. Invest.* **52,** 2745–2756.

8. Ryan, U. S., Clements, E., Habliston, D., and Ryan, J. W. (1978) Isolation and culture of pulmonary artery endothelial cells. *Tissue Cell* **10,** 535–554.

9. Suttorp, N., Polley, M., Seybold, J., Schnittler, H., Seeger, W., Grimminger, F., and Aktories, K. (1991) Adenosine diphosphate-ribosylation of G-actin by botulinum C2 toxin increases endothelial permeability in vitro. *J. Clin. Invest.* **87,** 1575–1584.

10. Suttorp, N., Weber, U., Welsch, T., and Schudt, C. (1993) Role of phosphodiesterases in the regulation of endothelial permeability in vitro. *J. Clin. Invest.* **91,** 1421–1428.

11. Robinson, L. A., Tu, L., Steeber, D. A., Preis, O., Platt, J. L., and Tedder, T. F. (1998) The role of adhesion molecules in human leukocyte attachment to porcine vascular endothelium: implications for xenotransplantation. *J. Immunol.,* **161,** 6931-6938.

12. Kopp, C. W., Grey, S. T., Siegel, J. B., McShea, A., Vetr, H., Wrighton, C J., Schulte am Esch, J. II, Bach, F. H., and Robson, S. C. (1998) Expression of human thrombomodulin cofactor activity in porcine endothelial cells. *Transplantation* **66,** 244–251.

13. Rosenthal, A.M. and Gotlieb, A. I. (1990) Macrovascular endothelial cells from porcine aorta. In *Cell culture techniques in heart and vessel research* (Piper, H. M. ed.), Springer Berlin, Heidelberg, New York, pp. 117–129.

13

Isolation and Culture
of Human Airway Smooth Muscle Cells

Aili L. Lazaar and Reynold A. Panettieri, Jr.

1. Introduction

Airway smooth muscle (ASM) cells may be considered an important modulator of airway inflammatory responses, since they synthesize cytokines, chemokines, growth factors and metalloproteinases as well as support the adhesion of activated T lymphocytes. The study of the cellular and molecular mechanisms of inflammatory mediators on airway smooth muscle was initially hampered by the inability to prepare pure populations of cells that retained the phenotypic characteristics of the differentiated cell. The study of smooth muscle cell immunobiology has been facilitated by the development of a technique for isolating and maintaining nontransformed human airway smooth muscle cells *(1)*. These cells retain the physiologic responsiveness to a wide range of stimuli including inflammatory mediators, growth factors, contractile agonists and immune receptor crosslinking. Studies have shown that, although there is some phenotypic modulation, these cultured cells are stable over many population doublings and express smooth muscle cell-specific markers such as myosin heavy chain, myosin light chain kinase, α-actin, caldesmon, and SM22α. In addition, the synthetic function of these cells appears to be comparable to those studied in vivo. Here, we describe in detail our method for the isolation of human airway smooth muscle cells.

2. Materials

2.1. Reagents

1. Media 199 (Gibco-BRL): store at 4°C.
2. Ham's F12 (Gibco-BRL): store at 4°C.

From: *Methods in Molecular Medicine, vol. 56:*
Human Airway Inflammation: Sampling Techniques and Analytical Protocols
Edited by: D. F. Rogers and L. E. Donnelly © Humana Press Inc., Totowa, NJ

3. EGTA (ethyleneglycol-bis(betaaminoethylether)-N,N,N^1,N^1-tetraacetic acid) (Sigma).
4. Collagenase (Boehringer Mannheim, Indianapolis, IN): store desiccated at 4°C.
5. Soybean trypsin inhibitor (Sigma): store dessicated at 4°C.
6. Elastase (Worthington Biochemical, Freehold, NJ): store dessicated at 4°C.
7. Fetal calf serum (FCS) (Hyclone, Logan, UT): aliquot and store at –20°C.
8. CaCl$_2$ (JT Baker, Phillipsburg, NJ).
9. Penicillin/Streptomycin (stock contains 10,000 U/mL penicillin G and 10,000 mg/mL streptomycin) (Gibco-BRL): aliquot and store at –20°C.
10. Amphotericin.
11. 0.05% (w/v) Trypsin/0.53 mM EDTA (Gibco): store at –20°C.
12. Polypropylene mesh 105 µm (Spectrum, Houston, TX).
13. Tissue culture plates.

2.2 Media Preparation

1. Digestion media contains M199 supplemented with 1.7 mM EGTA, 640 U/mL collagenase, 1-mg/mL soybean trypsin inhibitor, and 10-U/mL elastase. This media needs to be made fresh on the experimental day and should not be stored. After adding the protease inhibitors and enzymes, pH the media to 7.4 (at 37°C) with NaOH, sterile filter and place on ice until use. The media needs to be at pH 7.4 to allow the enzymes to go into solution.
2. Complete Ham's F12 contains Ham's F12 supplemented with 10% (v/v) FCS (not heat-inactivated), 2 mM glutamine, 25 mM HEPES, 12 mM NaOH, 1.5 mM CaCl$_2$, 100-U/mL penicillin, 100-µg/mL streptomycin. This media can be prepared beforehand and should be stored at 4°C.

3. Methods

3.1. Culture of Human Airway Smooth Muscle Cells

Human ASM can be isolated from the trachea of lung transplant donors, from segments of bronchus resected for peripheral carcinoma, or from post-mortem specimens (*see* **Note 1**).

1. The muscle is dissected free with forceps and scissors using aseptic technique in phosphate buffered saline (PBS) (*see* **Note 2**). Transfer the muscle to a sterile Petri dish. Mince the tissue into small (1 mm or less) pieces while maintaining sterile conditions. Transfer the fragments to a sterile screw-top Erlenmeyer flask and resuspend in 10 mL of digestion media. Digest the tissue for 30–60 min in a shaking water bath at 37°C. Monitor the progression of the digestion by removing a small aliquot to look for the presence of individual cells. Stop the reaction by adding 1.5 vol of complete Ham's F12.
2. Filter the cell suspension through a sterile larger bore mesh to remove the large undigested pieces of tissue, then through the sterile 105 µm mesh. Centrifuge the cells at 1100g for 10 min and resuspend in a small vol (2–3 mL) of complete Ham's F12 plus 2.5 µg/mL amphotericin. Plate the cell suspension in a 6-well

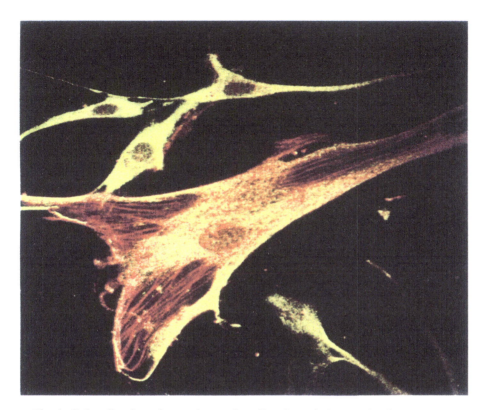

Fig. 1. Colocalization of smooth muscle cell actin and phosphatidylinositol 3-kinase (PI3K). ASM cells were incubated with mouse antihuman smooth muscle cell actin followed by Texas red-conjugated goat antimouse IgG. The p85 subunit of PI3K was visualized using rabbit anti-p85 and fluorescein isothiocyanate (FITC)-conjugated goat antirabbit IgG. Cells were visualized using a fluorescent microscope.

tissue culture plate at a density of 2×10^4 cells/cm^2. Media should be aspirated and replaced every 72 h. Grow the cells for 2–3 wk until they appear confluent (*see* **Note 3**).

3. To passage the cells, aspirate off the media and add one-half volume of Trypsin/ EDTA at 37°C (*see* **Note 4**). Incubate the cells for 7 min at 37°C in a CO_2 incubator. Remove the cells using a pipet and add to an equal volume of complete Ham's F12. Cells that are to be maintained as stock cultures should remain in Ham's F12 plus amphotericin. Cells that are being plated for experiments can be maintained in complete Ham's F12 *without* amphotericin. Determine the cell number using either a Coulter counter or a hemocytometer and replate at the required density (*see* **Note 5**).

Cells isolated in this manner represent a pure population of smooth muscle cells. These cells stain uniformly for smooth muscle cell-specific actin and retain their responsiveness to contractile agonists, as has been described by

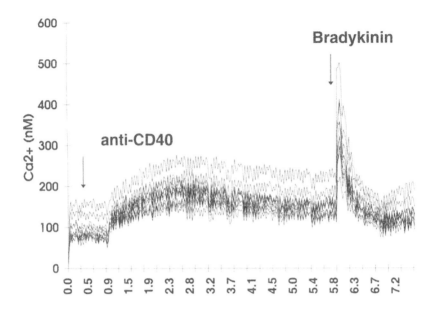

Fig. 2. The kinetics of CD40-induced cytosolic calcium response in human ASM cells. Each cell is represented as a single tracing that demonstrates a gradual and sustained rise in intracellular calcium. The subsequent addition of bradykinin evokes a larger, more rapid, calcium transient (From **ref.** *3* with permission. Copyright 1998, *The American Association of Immunologists*).

Panettieri et al *(1)*. Ideally, cells should be used between the third and sixth passage in order to retain these characteristics.

3.2. Experiments Using Human Airway Smooth Muscle Cells

In this section, typical examples of experiments that can be performed using ASM cells are shown.

1. *Immunofluorescence*: ASM cells are easily stained for either cell surface receptors, such as cell adhesion molecules, or for intracellular proteins, such as cytokines or cytoskeletal proteins. In **Fig. 1**, ASM cells have been stained simultaneously for smooth muscle-specific α-actin and phosphatidylinositol 3-kinase (PI3K). This demonstrates the structure of the actin cytoskeleton in ASM cells, as well as the diffuse distribution of PI3K within the cytoplasm.

2. *Measurements of intracellular calcium*: Using dyes such as fura-2/AM, intracellular calcium measurements can be performed at the single cell level. In this example, ASM cells were stimulated with antibodies specific for CD40, a costimulatory molecule that is present on the surface of human ASM cells *(3)*. This treatment induced a gradual and sustained increase in intracellular calcium *(see* **Fig. 2**) that differed from the rapid and larger increase in intracellular calcium following stimulation with bradykinin, a smooth muscle contractile agonist.

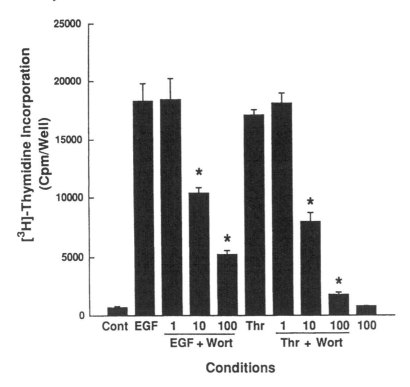

Fig. 3. Inhibition of phosphatidylinositol 3-kinase activity abolishes the effects of EGF and thrombin on ASM cell proliferation. Confluent ASM cells were pretreated with increasing doses of wortmannin (wort), then stimulated with EGF (10 ng/mL) or thrombin (Thr, 1 U/mL). DNA synthesis was measured as incorporation of [3H]-thymidine (From **ref.** *4* with permission. Copyright 1999, *American Physiological Society*).

3. *Proliferation assays*: A useful tool for determining smooth muscle cell growth is the incorporation of tritiated thymidine ([^{3}H]-TdR), as a measure of DNA synthesis in response to a stimulus. In this example (*see* **Fig. 3**), cells were growth arrested for 24 h in serum-free media, then stimulated with epidermal growth factor (EGF) or thrombin (Thr) for 36 h. [^{3}H]-TdR was added for the final 18 h of mitogen stimulation. In order to determine the role of PI3K in the mitogenic response to EGF or thrombin, cells were pretreated with wortmannin, a PI3K inhibitor. The adherent cells were lysed and the proteins and DNA precipitated in 10% (w/v) TCA. Precipitates were aspirated onto glass filters and counted (data from **ref.** *4*). These data suggest that mitogen-induced smooth muscle cell proliferation is dependent on PI3K activation.

4. Notes

1. Bronchial smooth muscle cells are available commercially (e.g., Clonetics). However, these cells are highly passaged and therefore, may not retain all the characteristics of freshly isolated cells.

2. This process should be completed in less than 30 min.

3. The initial population of cells obtained after digestion contains several cell types including smooth muscle, fibroblasts, and epithelial cells. After several weeks, the epithelial cells will be overgrown by the smooth muscle. As it can sometimes be difficult to distinguish fibroblasts and smooth muscle cells, it is important to perform staining for a smooth muscle-specific marker (such as α-actin) in order to ascertain that the population is pure.

4. Because ASM cells are adherent, it is necessary to remove them from the plate prior to some applications, such as flow cytometry. Usually cells are removed using trypsin/EDTA; however, trypsin can cleave certain cell surface receptors, such as ICAM-1 (although this is more of a problem with murine, rather than human, cells). If there is a concern regarding the stability of the receptor in the presence of trypsin, ASM cells can be lifted by incubating them in 5 m*M* EDTA in calcium/magnesium-free PBS for 10 min at 37°C.

5. Typically, cells are plated at $1 \times 10^4/cm^2$ (single density or 1D) and are allowed to grow for about 7 d before use in adhesion, proliferation or kinase assays, or for flow cytometry. In contrast, cells that will be transfected are plated at 1D, then transfected the following day.

References

1. Panettieri, R. A., Murray, R. K., DePalo, L. R., Yadvish, P. A., and Kotlikoff, M. I. (1989) A human airway smooth muscle cell line that retains physiological responsiveness. *Amer. J. Physiol.* **256,** C329–C335.

2. Solway, J., Forsythe, S. M., Halayko, A. J., Vieira, J. E., Hershenson, M. B., and Camoretti-Mercado, B. (1998) Transcriptional regulation of smooth muscle contractile apparatus expression. *Amer. J. Respir. Crit. Care Med.* **158,** S100–S108.

3. Lazaar, A. L., Amrani, Y., Hsu, J., Panettieri, Jr., R. A., Fanslow, W. C., Albelda, S. M., and Puré, E. (1998) CD40-mediated signal transduction in human airway smooth muscle. *J. Immunol.* **161,** 3120–3127.

4. Krymskaya, V. P., Penn, R. B., Orsini, M. J., Scott, P. H., Plevin, R. J., Walker, T. R., et al. (1999) Phosphatidylinositol 3-kinase mediates mitogen-induced human airway smooth muscle cell proliferation. *Amer. J. Physiol.* **277,** L65–L78.

14

Isolation and Purification
of Human Mast Cells and Basophils

Bernhard F. Gibbs and Madeleine Ennis

1. Introduction

Mast cells were once thought to represent a single population of highly granulated secretory cells. However, with the development of mast cell isolation techniques for a diverse range of tissues, it became apparent that mast cells from different species and those from different tissues within the same species exhibit variations in their biochemical, histochemical, and functional properties. The functional heterogeneity of mast cells has important implications for studies of the response of mast cells to secretory stimuli, antiallergic drugs, or drugs that have the potential to produce adverse responses.

Given the heterogeneous properties of mast cells from different origins, it is often imperative to use primary human mast cells rather than a rodent or cell line alternative. Furthermore, even studies of human mast cells from one tissue type may not be applicable to the target mast cell populations. Compound 48/80 causes histamine release from human skin mast cells but adenoidal, colonic, lung and tonsillar mast cells are unresponsive *(1–4)*. Although the neuropeptide substance P activates both human skin and bronchoalveolar lavage (BAL) mast cells, it has no effect on mast cells from most other human tissues including those enzymatically dispersed from human lung *(5)*. The antiallergic drugs sodium cromoglycate and nedocromil sodium exhibit a range of efficacies in inhibiting mediator release from human mast cells from different tissue sites. In mast cells dispersed from human lung, tonsillar and adenoidal tissue, both drugs inhibit IgE mediated histamine and PGD_2 release *(6)*. However, human skin mast cells and basophils are unresponsive to both these agents *(6,7)*. Sodium cromoglycate and nedocromil sodium exhibit tachyphylaxis in lung

From: *Methods in Molecular Medicine, vol. 56:*
Human Airway Inflammation: Sampling Techniques and Analytical Protocols
Edited by: D. F. Rogers and L. E. Donnelly © Humana Press Inc., Totowa, NJ

and tonsillar mast cells but not in mast cells dispersed from adenoidal and intestinal tissue *(6)*. This heterogeneous response is also observed in different mast cell populations in the lung. Nedocromil sodium is an order of magnitude more effective in suppressing histamine release from BAL mast cells than from mast cells dispersed from lung tissue *(8)*. Furthermore tachyphylaxis to the inhibitory effects of drugs sodium cromoglycate and nedocromil sodium occurs only in the dispersed lung mast cell population *(8)*.

The response of human mast cells to stimuli varies from donor to donor. Thus, although adenosine alone can induce histamine release from human BAL mast cells obtained from subjects attending for a clinically indicated bronchoscopy, the response was not universal with cells only from 37 of 54 subjects exhibiting histamine release *(9)*. We also found a remarkable degree of inter-donor variation in both the degrees of response and the concentration of adenosine eliciting maximal release. The underlying disease can also modify the response of mast cells to stimuli. Mild asthmatics not only have a greater histamine release response to anti-IgE but also to neuropeptides *(10–12)*. Human tissue mast cells are obtained from surgical specimens and thus the researcher is limited in his/her choice of material (e.g., if working with human lung, very few patients with asthma will undergo a lung resection). In contrast, patients can be specifically recruited for BAL studies or for blood sampling for basophil studies. The number of mast cells obtained by lavage is small and suitable purification methods have not yet been published. For this reason, we will also describe how to obtain pure basophil populations in this chapter.

There are a number of problems associated with using human mast cells such as lack of availability, time and cost intensive isolation and enrichment, as well as a large biological variation of mast cell reactivity between donors. The enzymatic dispersion techniques for the isolation of skin and lung mast cells are relatively well-established. However, methods are not yet available to purify these cells sufficiently for current molecular biology techniques to be employed. This is primarily owing to the lack of known specific extracellular markers for mast cells.

In terms of total tissue cells, isolated following enzymatic dispersion, mast cell purities range from 1–5% (both lung and skin) and only a small proportion of cellular contaminants are known to express high affinity IgE receptors or c-kit, both of which are characteristically, but not exclusively, expressed on mast cells. Thus, anti-IgE or stem cell factor (SCF) induced histamine (a mediator almost exclusively mast cell derived) release experiments from mast cells may be performed without further purification whereas other mediators (eicosanoids, cytokines) measured may be derived from other cellular sources. Ideally, mast cells should be enriched involving the removal of contaminants by negative selection (Percoll gradients, elutriation or immunomagnetic beads), a process which should not impair their final function. However, current protocols are not quite effective enough in terms of reaching total purity, without the costly repetition of existing methods. Here positive selection via either c-kit or FceRI following initial negative selection may be necessary but since both receptors are classical activation routes in mast cells functional changes cannot be ruled out. We have summarized the existing strategies below based on both previous reports and our own observations.

2. Materials
2.1. Bronchoalveolar Lavage Mast Cells

1. Tyrode's buffer: NaCl 137.0 mM (8.0 g/L); glucose 5.6 mM (1.0 g/L); KCl 2.7 mM (201 mg/L); $CaCl_2 \cdot 2H_2O$ 1.0 mM (147 mg/L); $MgCl_2 \cdot 6H_2O$ 1.0 mM (203 mg/L); N-2-hydroxyethylpiperazine-N-2-ethanesulphonic acid [HEPES] 10.0 mM (2.9 g/L); $NaH_2PO_4 \cdot 2H_2O$ 0.4 mM (62.5 mg/L). The pH is adjusted to 7.4 with NaOH (1 M). This buffer will keep for 1 wk at 4°C.
2. Calcium-magnesium-free Tyrode's buffer (CMF): prepare as above without $CaCl_2$ or $MgCl_2$.
3. Tyrode's bovine serum albumin (BSA) contains 1 mg/mL bovine serum albumin (Fraction V; 96.99 % albumin) (Sigma Chemicals Co.) (*see* **Note 1**).
4. Glucose free Tyrode's is prepared as for Tyrode's buffer, with the omission of glucose.
5. For studies on the calcium dependence of mediator release modified Tyrode's buffers are used with varying concentrations of calcium (*see* **Subheading 3.1.3.2**).
6. Trypan blue dye (0.1 mg/mL 0.9% NaCl) is stored at 4°C and then filtered through filter paper prior to use. Trypan blue (0.4%) can also be purchased from Sigma.
7. Toluidine blue is used as 0.5% toluidine blue in 0.5 M HCl and must be filtered before being used for staining.
8. Carnoy's fixative: this should be prepared in a fume cupboard. It is a mixture of absolute alcohol (6 parts), chloroform (3 parts), and glacial acetic acid (1 part). This can be stored at room temperature.

2.2. Human Skin and Lung Mast Cells

All buffers should be stored at 4°C and used within 1 wk. Purchased media and reagents should be used within the period given by the manufacturer.

1. Tyrode's buffer (*see* **Subheading 2.1., step 1**).
2. CMF Tyrode's buffer: (*see* **Subheading 2.1., step 2**).
3. RPMI 1640 with l-glutamine; penicillin-streptomycin 5000 IU/mL – 5000 UG/mL (Gibco-BRL).
4. Percoll (Pharmacia biotech).
5. BSA, fraction V (Sigma).

6. Enzymes: Lung mast cells: Collagenase type 1a (Sigma); Skin mast cells: Collagenase type 2 (Worthington), hyaluronidase (Sigma).

7. Alcian blue solution (adapted from *[13]*): Dissolve the following in distilled H_2O: cetyl pyridinium chloride (76 mg), lanthanum chloride (700 mg), NaCl (900 mg), Tween-20 (21 µL), and Alcian blue (143 mg). Stir for 2 h at room temperature and filter using a 1 µM filter. The solution is stable for at least 1 yr at 4°C.

3. Methods

3.1. Bronchoalveolar Lavage Mast Cells

3.1.1. Sample Preparation

1. The BAL fluid is placed in plastic pots (*see* **Note 2**) and immediately stored on ice. It should be transported from the bronchscopy suite as quickly as possible to the laboratory.

2. Where necessary the sample is pooled in a plastic beaker and then the total volume recorded. If sample has a particularly high mucus content, it should be filtered through two layers of absorbent gauze moistened with Tyrode's prior to being aliquoted. However, we do not routinely filter our samples, as this can give rise to cell losses. An aliquot (3–6 mL) should be removed for cell counting and preparation of slides and kept on ice until required.

3. Dispense the samples into conical polystyrene test tubes (e.g., Sarstedt number 57.469) and centrifuge (200*g*, 10 min, 4°C).

4. Remove the supernatant down to the fine line at bottom of the test tube (use a 5mL Gilson pipet or similar; *see* **Note 3**).

5. Resuspend the cell pellets with the appropriate buffer (3 mL). This is usually Tyrode's or Tyrode's BSA. Gently mix the cells using a 5 mL Gilson pipet or similar. Combine the resuspended cells from several tubes to reduce total tube number. Rinse the empty tubes with buffer and add this wash to the cell suspensions.

6. Centrifuge the samples as for step 3 above.

7. Repeat the washing step (step 5 above) and resuspend the cells in the final volume required for the experiment (*see* **Note 4**).

3.1.2. Cell Counts

1. Total cell numbers in the unprocessed lavage fluid are counted using a phase contrast microscope (magnification 40X) and an improved Neubauer hemocytometer.

2. Cellular viability is studied using the Trypan blue exclusion test. An aliquot of the Trypan blue solution is prewarmed to 37°C and then incubated with the cell suspension at 1:2 dilution for 5 min at 37°C. Cells which stain dark blue are not viable.

3. Differential cell counting is performed using the glass coverslip method *(14)* using the modification of Walters & Gardiner *(15)* (*see* **Note 5**). Place a 13-mm circular glass coverslip on the bottom of a flat bottomed test tube. Add 0.5-mL unprocessed BAL fluid to test tube and centrifuge (50*g*, 5 min, 4°C). Remove the fluid carefully using e.g., a 1-mL Gilson pipet. The coverslips are gently removed from the test tube using a needle (e.g., green needle with tip slightly bent) and

fixed onto glass microscope slides using clear nail varnish as an adhesive and allowed to set. In order to count all cells except mast cells, the Diff-Quik® staining set (Baxter Diagnostics AG, Switzerland) is used. Slides are dipped into Diff-Quik fixative (5 × 1 s), excess fixative is removed and the slide immersed in eosin (3 × 1 s). Excess dye is removed with blotting paper and the slide then immersed in hematoxylin (3 × 1 s). The slide is washed in distilled water to remove excess dye and allowed to dry. A drop of Styrolite® mounting medium is placed onto the slide and a square coverslip is carefully lowered on top of the circular glass coverslip (avoiding air bubbles). At least 500 cells are counted at a magnification of 1000 × under oil.

To enumerate mast cells, the slides are fixed in Carnoy's fixative (2.5 h). After fixation, the slides are washed in distilled water (1 min) and then immersed in a trough of filtered Toluidine blue for 90 min. The slides are washed in distilled water (1 min) and allowed to dry. Mounting can be performed as for differential cell counts, although routinely we do not mount these preparations. As the percentage of mast cells in the lavage fluid is less than 1% of the total cell population in the lavage fluid, at least 3000–5000 cells are counted at a magnification of 40×.

3.1.3. Histamine Release Studies

The method described below is also suitable for the measurement of other mast cell derived mediators (e.g., prostaglandin D_2). However, it must be remembered that contaminating cells may also release eicosanoids.

1. Prewarm the cells for 5 min at 37°C either in a polystyrene conical testtube or in a plastic beaker in a shaking water bath.
2. Add the cells (100 μL) to prepared prewarmed tubes containing Tyrode's buffer and the stimuli to give a final volume of 500 μL. Two tubes without stimulus should be included to give the spontaneous release and an extra tube without stimulus is required to give a value for total histamine content, in order to calibrate the autoanalyzer (if used) *(16)*. The total volume for these tubes should also be 500 μL. Histamine can also be reliably measured using radioimmunoassay kits from Immunotech S.A (France).
3. Allow the reactions to proceed for 20 min at 37°C.
4. Quench the reactions by placing the tubes in ice-water baths and adding 0.5 mL of ice-cold Tyrode's buffer.
5. Centrifuge the suspensions (200*g*, 10 min, 4°C).
6. Remove the supernatants using a Gilson pipet (or equivalent) into new tubes and resuspend the cell pellets in Tyrode's buffer (1 mL). We routinely label our supernatant tubes in red and our cell tubes in black with the same number.
7. The tubes can be stored at −20°C until ready for assay. In order to release the residual histamine in the cells, perchloric acid (0.4 *M* final concentration) should be added to both cells and supernatants for the autoanalyzer method of histamine analysis *only*. For other analysis methods, the tubes can be boiled for 10 min (put marbles on the top of the tubes to prevent loss of fluid) or a single freeze thaw cycle can be employed.

8. Histamine release is calculated as:

   Percentage histamine release = $[(H^s/H^s + H^c) \times 100]$

   where H^s and H^c are the histamine content in supernatant fractions and cell pellets, respectively.

   Corrected release = [percentage histamine release] - basal histamine release

   where basal (or spontaneous) histamine release is the percentage histamine release occurring in the absence of any stimuli.

3.1.3.1. ENERGY DEPENDENCE STUDIES

1. After the final wash in Tyrode's (**Subheading 3.1.1., step 7**), resuspend the cell pellet in glucose free Tyrode's and centrifuge as before. Do not perform the entire experiment isolation procedure in glucose-free buffers.
2. Resuspend the cell pellet in glucose free Tyrode's in an adequate volume for the experiment and aliquot the cells into the polystyrene tubes containing antimycin A ($1 \mu M$) and 2-deoxyglucose ($5 mM$). Preincubate the cells with these metabolic inhibitors for 20 min at 37°C.
3. Stimulate the cells with the secretagogues of interest (which have been dissolved in glucose-free Tyrode's) and continue as above. (*see* **Subheading 3.1.3., step 3**)

3.1.3.2. CALCIUM DEPENDENCE STUDIES

1. After the final wash in full Tyrode's (**Subheading 3.1.1., step 7**), resuspend the cells in CMF Tyrode's and centrifuge as before. Do not do the entire process in CMF (*see* **Note 6**).
2. Resuspend the cell pellet in CMF in an adequate volume for the experiment and aliquot the cells into the polystyrene tubes containing equal volumes of appropriately modified Tyrode's buffer. These modified Tyrode's buffers can contain either; CMF, 2×0.1 mM ethylerediaminetetraacetic acid (EDTA), 2×0.1 mM Ca^{2+}, 2×0.6 mM Ca^{2+} or 2×1.0 mM Ca^{2+}, or twice the calcium concentration of interest. High calcium concentrations, (e.g., final concentrations 10–20 mM), are usually inhibitory.
3. Prewarm the cells for 5 min at 37°C.
4. Stimulate the cells with the secretagogues of interest (which have been dissolved in CMF) and continue as above (**Subheading 3.1.3., step 3**).

3.2. Human Skin Mast Cells

3.2.1. Sample Preparation

1. Human skin should be placed in plastic pots containing CMF Tyrode's buffer cooled to 4°C and immediately transported to the laboratory.
2. Place the skin sample in a large plastic Petri dish, cut away fatty tissues and wash several times with CMF to remove erythrocytes.
3. Briefly blot the skin onto filter paper and weigh the tissue and then return the tissue into a plastic Petri dish containing CMF.

4. Cut the skin into strips (ca. 0.5 cm diameter) with scissors and then chop the strips finely so that the tissue is less than 2 mm³. The chopped tissue should be immediately placed in a plastic pot containing CMF (at 4°C). Do not allow the tissue to stand without being immersed in CMF.

3.2.2. Enzymatic Dispersion

1. Dilute the skin fragments with CMF (containing 1% BSA and 1% penicillinstreptomycin solution) by 10 mL per gram of skin (*see* **Notes 7** and **8**).
2. Add 2500 U of collagenase (e.g., Type 2; Worthington) per gram skin.
3. Add 2240 U of hyaluronidase per gram skin.
4. Cover the beaker and stir slowly on a heated magnetic plate stirrer, warming the contents to 37°C, for 4 h. Care must be taken to ensure that the temperature does not exceed 37°C.
5. Disrupt the tissue by expressing it through a large syringe (50 mL) and filter the suspension through gauze (pore size 100 μm). Place the undispersed tissue back into the beaker.
6. Centrifuge the filtrate (300*g*, 10 min, 37°C) and pour the supernatant back into the beaker containing the remaining tissue and repeat the dispersion as in **step 4**.
7. Resuspend the pelleted cells obtained above with CMF and centrifuge (300*g*, 10 min, 20°C), discard the supernatant and repeat. Afterwards resuspend the cells in CMF containing BSA (1 mg/mL) and keep at room temperature.
8. Repeat **steps 5–7** for the remaining dispersate, but discard undispersed material and finally pool the isolated cells obtained from both dispersions.

3.2.3. Cell Counts

1. Add 10 μL isolated skin cells to a mixture containing: 65 μL alcian blue solution (see **materials**), 65 μL physiological saline with 0.1% EDTA and 5 μL HCl (1 *M*). Leave for 10 min at room temperature and count using a hemocytometer. Mast cells will stain blue, exclusively, and the purity is usually between 1 and 5% with a yield of 150,000–400,000 mast cells per gram tissue.
2. Cell viability can be assessed using the Trypan blue exclusion test as described in **Subheading 3.1.2 step 2**.

3.2.4. Overnight Culture

1. Given both the time required for the enzymatic dispersion of the skin and the harsh conditions which may affect mast cell function (*see* **Notes 7** and **8**), it is often useful to incubate the cells overnight in order for them to recover full responsiveness. The cells should be centrifuged (300g, 10 min 10°C), resuspended in RPMI 1640 containing 1–2% penicillin-streptomycin solution and either human serum (1%, heat inactivated) or fetal calf serum (FCS) (1%). The cell density should not exceed $2 \leftrightarrow 10^6$ cells per mL.
2. Pipet the cells into a suitable plastic flask and place in a humidified incubator set to 37°C and 5% CO_2. The culture period should last for at least 12–14 h.
3. After culture, the cells are resuspended in the flask, aliquoted into 50-mL plastic

centrifugation tubes and centrifuged (500g, 10 min, 10°C). The pellets should be resuspended in CMF containing BSA (1 mg/mL) and the mast cell numbers as well as viability assessed as before.

3.2.5. Skin Mast Cell Purification

1. Prepare an isotonic Percoll solution by diluting 45 mL Percoll with 5 mL 10X concentrated CMF. Label as 100% Percoll and make the following dilutions: 80% (8 mL 100% Percoll + 2 mL CMF), 60% (6 mL 100% Percoll + 4 mL CMF), 50% (5 mL Percoll + 5 mL CMF) and 40% (4 mL 100% Percoll + 6 mL CMF).
2. In a 50-mL plastic centrifugation tube add the 80% Percoll solution (10 mL). Then carefully layer the next solution (60% Percoll, 10 mL) followed by the 50% Percoll (10 mL). Do not allow the various dilutions to mix, pipet carefully so that an interface is clearly visible between the various layers.
3. Centrifuge the cells (300g, 10 min, 4°C), resuspend in the 40% Percoll solution and carefully layer over the 50% fraction. Finally, layer 5 mL CMF over the 40% fraction containing the cells. Directly afterwards place the tube carefully into the centrifuge and centrifuge (850g, 20 min, 4°C).
4. After centrifugation, carefully remove each fraction (top-40%, 40–50%, 50–60%, 60–80%) and pipet into fresh 50-mL tubes containing 40 mL CMF. Resuspend and centrifuge (500g, 10 min, 4°C) and repeat the wash twice (centrifuging at 300g, 10 min, 10°C) to ensure the remaining Percoll is removed. Finally resuspend in 20 mL CMF and count the various fractions as described earlier. Skin mast cells are usually found at the 50–60% and 60–80% interfaces. Highest purities range from 35–75% using breast skin; whhereas superior purities can be expected with foreskin.
5. Depending on the mast cell number required pool the fractions with the highest purities. Mast cells can then be further enriched by negative selection using immunomagnetic beads coated with monoclonal antibodies directed against T cells (CD2, Dynabeads), monocytes (CD14, Dynabeads), and B cells (CD 19, Dynabeads). These are commercially available from Dynal with comprehensive instructions. In addition to the above, immunomagnetic beads against fibroblasts and neutrophils may be prepared by incubating sheep antimouse IgG-coated Dynabeads (M-450, Dynal) with mouse antihuman fibroblast antibodies (ASO2 Mouse IgG1-ab, Dianova), and mouse antihuman CD16 antibodies (Cymbus Biotechnology). Incubate the latter antibodies with Dynabeads for at least 2 h and remove the unbound antibodies according to the instructions. The various immunomagnetic beads prepared are then added simultaneously to the cells (in 2 mL CMF with 1mg/mL BSA) at a bead:cell ratio of 1:1 for each type. Incubate at 4°C with gentle agitation (rotor) for 30 min and separate the bound contaminants using the magnet supplied by the manufacturer and according to their instructions. These protocols, though commercially widely available, usually give rise to only a limited improvement of mast cell purity. Alternatively, skin mast cells may be enriched to near homogeneity by positive selection using immunomagnetic beads directed against CD117 (c-kit receptor) (Pharmingen) (*17*). It is, however, pos-

sible that this positive selection procedure may alter the functioning of the cells. Commercial kits specially produced for the positive or negative selection of human mast cells are currently under development and may soon be more readily accessible.

6. Count the purified cells using Alcian blue (*see* **Subheading 3.2.3, step 1**) and determine viability.

3.2.6. Histamine Release from Human Skin Mast Cells (High Purity not Required)

1. Cells are washed and resuspended in either Tyrode's buffer or RPMI 1640 medium and aliquoted (450 µL) in polystyrene conical testtubes at a density of ca. 200,000 mast cells/mL.
2. Place the tubes in a water bath set at 37°C and allow to equilibrate for 15 min.
3. Add either 50 µL of prewarmed stimulus or 50 µl of prewarmed buffer to the tubes and allow the reactions to proceed for 30 min (*see* **Note 9**).
4. Quench the reactions by adding 500 µL ice-cold CMF into each tube and centrifuge immediately (500g, 2 min, 4°C).
5. Decant the supernatants into fresh tubes and add 1 mL CMF to the pellet tubes. Lyse the pellet tubes by 3x freeze/thaw cycles. Alternatively add 50 µl Perchloric acid (70%), this is only suitable for the autoanalyzer method of histamine analysis. Vortex the pellet tubes and centrifuge (850g, 10 min, 4°C) to remove debris. If perchloric acid is used for pellet lysis, the supernatants should be treated likewise.
6. The tubes can be stored at –20°C until ready for assay.
7. Assay for histamine (either using commercial kits or fluorometric analysis see **Subheading 3.1.3 step 2**).
8. Histamine release is calculated as shown in **Subheading 3.1.3 step 8**.

3.2.7. Eicosanoid and Cytokine Production by Human Mast Cells

Unlike histamine, which is almost exclusively found in mast cells and the circulatory equivalent basophil leukocyte, the release of eicosanoids (mainly LTC_4 and PGD_2) and cytokines from mast cells may not be limited to these cells alone, thus requiring purified mast cell suspensions. This is still problematical given the lack of inexpensive and effective negative selection procedures which, in most cases, do not give rise to purities of more than 90%. However, with purities of over 50%, IgE-dependent stimulation is unlikely to cause considerable mediator release from other cell contaminants since there are few such cells in skin or lung cell isolates which express a functionally active high affinity IgE receptor as found on mast cells. Nontheless, it is strongly recommended that in initial experiments both purified and unpurified mast cell fractions are compared in order to observe any contribution of mediator release from nonmast cell contaminants. Studies requiring homogeneous human mast cell populations, such as gene expression, unavoidably necessitate the employment of positive selection procedures, which may alter mast cell function considerably.

1. Experimental conditions are the same as previously shown above (**Subheading 3.2.6, steps 1–3**) except for the variable incubation periods (see **Subheading 3.2.7, steps 2 and 3**) and termination of reactions. Unless the mast cell density is very high (e.g., 200,000 mast cells in 500μL total reaction volume), it is not recommended to quench with chilled CMF (since the factors of interest may then be too diluted to detect) but briefly place all tubes in ice-water and centrifuge immediately ($850g$, 2 min, 4°C). Decant the supernatants into fresh test tubes and freeze immediately (–30 °C or lower) until ready for assay.

2. Eicosanoid release is usually complete after 30 min stimulation and is measured in the supernatants only.

3. Cytokine production from mast cells is usually rapid (within 4–6 h), however their ability to produce these factors over 24 h periods has not been fully elucidated. Furthermore, some preformed cytokines may be released very rapidly (within the first 30 min). It is therefore recommended to use several stimulation periods e.g., 10 min, 30 min, 1 h, 2 h, 4 h, 6 h, and more in order to establish the kinetics of both preformed and *de novo* generated cytokine mediators. At the end of each time point, harvest the supernatants as described earlier and freeze immediately for storage before assaying cytokine release.

3.3. Human Lung Mast Cells

3.3.1. Sample Preparation

1. Human lung should be placed in plastic pots containing CMF Tyrode's buffer cooled to 4°C and immediately transported to the laboratory.

2. Place the lung sample in a large plastic Petri dish, cut away major airways and blood vessels and wash in CMF.

3. Briefly blot the lung tissue onto filter paper and weigh after which place the tissue back into a plastic beaker containing CMF.

4. Cut the lung into small fragments (ca. 0.5 cm diameter) with scissors and filter over gauze (pore size 100 μ*m*). Wash fragments with CMF, stir slowly for 10 min and repeat the filtration until the filtrate is clear (of blood) and then chop the fragments finely so that the tissue particle size is less than 1 mm^3. The chopped tissue should be immediately placed in a plastic pot containing CMF (at 4°C). Do not allow the tissue to stand without being immersed in CMF.

3.3.2. Enzymatic Dispersion

1. Place the lung fragments in CMF (containing 1 mg/mL bovine serum albumin and 1% penicillin-streptomycin solution) using 10 mL per gram lung.

2. Add 160 U of collagenase (e.g., Type 1a; Sigma) per gram lung.

3. Cover the beaker and stir slowly on a heatable magnetic plate stirrer, warming the contents to 37°C, for 1.5 h. Care must be taken to ensure that the temperature does not exceed 37°C. A shaking water bath set at 37°C may also be used for the lung preparations.

4. Disrupt the tissue by expressing through a large syringe (50 mL) and filter the suspension through gauze (pore size 100 μm). Place the undispersed tissue back into the beaker.

5. Centrifuge the filtrate (300*g*, 10 min, 37°C) and pour the supernatant back into the beaker containing the remaining tissue and repeat the dispersion as in **step 4**.
6. Resuspend the pelleted cells obtained above with CMF and centrifuge (300*g*, 10 min, 20°C), discard the supernatant and repeat. Afterwards resuspend the cells in CMF containing bovine serum albumin (1 mg/mL) and keep at room temperature.
7. Repeat steps 4–6 for the remaining dispersate but discard undispersed material and finally pool the isolated cells obtained from both dispersions.

3.3.3. Cell Counts

1. Procedures identical as for skin mast cells described in **Subheading 3.2.3**. Lung mast cell yield is usually greater than for skin, typically ranging from 500,000–1,000,000 mast cells per gram.

3.3.4. Overnight Culture

1. Isolated human lung mast cells usually respond adequately to various secretagogues without the need for overnight culture. However, should culturing be deemed necessary the same protocol may be used as described earlier for isolated skin mast cells (**Subheading 3.2.4**).

3.3.5. Lung Mast Cell Purification

Unlike skin mast cell, isolated human lung mast cells are easily enriched by counter current centrifugal elutriation (described below). However, if no elutriator is available the cells may be enriched using the Percoll density centrifugation technique described for skin under the same conditions except the centrifugation step is run at 200*g*, for 20 min at 4°C.
Elutriation (adapted from *[18]*):

1. Slowly cool the lung mast cell suspension (in CMF containing 1 mg/mL BSA) to 4°C.
2. Pump the suspension, at a flow rate of 12 mL/min, into a Beckman counter current elutriation chamber (JE 6B) rotating at 1025 r.p.m and set to 4°C. Avoid air bubbles (use the bubble trap supplied) and after loading the cells place the inlet tube into a beaker containing CMF with 1 mg/mL BSA (2 L).
3. Collect at least 100 mL and then raise the flow rate by 3 mL/min.
4. Collect 100 mL and increase the flow rate by another 3 mL/min.
5. Repeat these steps until the final flow is at 26 mL/min.
6. Switch off the rotor and collect the cells remaining in the chamber.
7. Centrifuge all tubes (300*g*, 10 min, 10°C).
8. Count the lung mast cell number and determine the purity using alcian blue (described in **Subheading 3.2.3, step 1**) for each fraction. Mast cells are usually found in later fractions or withheld in the chamber. Maximum purities of ca. 80% can be expected.

9. Pool the purest fractions. If the further purification is required a Percoll gradient or immunomagnetic selection may be employed as described earlier.
   Experimental conditions for mediator secretion are as described in **Subheadings 3.2.6 and 3.2.7**.

3.4. Human Basophils

3.4.1. Sample Preparation

1. Dilute freshly drawn blood immediately with CMF (containing $1M$ EDTA) by 9:1. For extensive functional studies, about 500-mL blood is required. Freshly prepared buffy coat blood (leukocyte concentrate from normal blood donation) may also be used.
2. In 50 mL plastic centrifugation tubes, add 15 mL Ficoll-Paque (Pharmacia-Biotech) and carefully layer 25 mL blood over the Ficoll.
3. Centrifuge at $460g$ for 20 min at 4°C.
4. Carefully harvest the basophil-rich interface. Dilute with CMF (room temperature) and centrifuge ($300g$, 10 min, 20°C). Resuspend in CMF, repeat the centrifugation and resuspend in 20 mL CMF for counting.

3.4.2. Cell Counts

1. Procedures identical as for skin mast cells described in **Subheading 3.2.3**. Basophil yield varies considerably between donors, typically ranging from 10,000–100,000 basophils per mL blood with purities of 0.5–4 % of all nucleated cells.

3.4.3. Purification

Basophil enrichment is now easily achieved using commercial reagents or specially developed kits for negative selection (*19,20*). However, final purity following negative selection is cheaper and more successful following an initial enrichment of the basophils to over 10%.

1. Slowly cool the basophil suspension (in CMF containing 2 mg/mL BSA) to 4°C.
2. Pump the suspension, at a flow rate of 20 mL/min, into a Beckman counter current elutriation chamber (JE 6B) rotating at 2450 r.p.m and set to 4°C. Avoid air bubbles (use the bubble trap supplied) and after loading the cells place the inlet tube into a beaker containing CMF with 2 mg/mL BSA (2 L).
3. Collect at least 100 mL and then lower the speed by 50 r.p.m.
4. Collect 100 ml and then lower the speed by a further 50 r.p.m
5. Repeat these steps until the final speed is 2250 r.p.m..
6. Switch off the rotor and collect the cells remaining in the chamber.
7. Centrifuge all tubes ($300g$, 10 min, 10°C).
8. Count the basophil number and determine the purity using Alcian blue (described in **Subheading 3.2.3, step 1**) for each fraction. Basophils are usually found in later fractions but this may vary considerably and must be determined for each individual preparation. Maximum purities of ca. 40% can be expected but are generally between 10–30%. Pool the purest fractions.

9. Further purification is performed using the MACS basophil isolation kit (Miltenyi Biotec) according to the manufacturer's protocol. Purities of over 90% are generally achieved (*19*) with prior enrichment described above. This commercially available kit is also suitable for enriching basophils after the Ficoll step but costly and results is lower purities (range 66–95%) than basophil suspensions enriched by elutriation.

Experimental conditions for mediator secretion are as described in **Subheadings 3.2.6** and **3.2.7**.

4. Notes

1. When using buffers containing BSA (Fraction V; 96.99% albumin) (Sigma Chemicals Co.,UK), the BSA (1 mg/mL) is sprinkled on top of Tyrode's buffer and allowed to dissolve slowly. It must be made freshly each day. The spontaneous release of histamine is lower in buffers containing BSA but it can modify mediator release by some stimuli.
2. Mast cells adhere to glass surfaces. All tubes and vessels used should be made of plastic. Some plastic materials will cause histamine release. We have obtained good results using Sarstedt test tubes (number 57.469).
3. When handling the cell suspensions, it is necessary to pipet very gently. When pipeting small volumes, cutting the tip of the pipet can help reduce spontaneous histamine release.
4. Spontaneous histamine release is usually greater at low cell density, which also varies depending on the mast cell type and their state of releasability to immunologic activation (*21*). It is recommended to keep spontaneous histamine release low (below 10%), as greater release may mask the releases caused by various secretagogues. However, the spontaneous histamine release may be higher in samples obtained from patients with inflammatory airway disease.
5. If you intend to use the slides (**Subheading 3.1.2, step 3**) for immunocytochemistry, then instead of nail varnish use Loctite Glass Bond, as acetone often used for immunocytochemistry will dissolve the nail varnish and you will lose your coverslip.
6. Mast cell isolation and purification techniques may damage the cells obtained from tissues. Therefore, and in order to reduce cell activity during these processes, it is essential to work in CMF conditions. Lowering the buffer temperature may further protect the cells but for long periods reduces their final activity. Therefore we recommend keeping the cells cool (4°C) during transport of undigested tissues and purification stages, keeping them at 10–20°C at other times (except during dispersion or overnight culture), although time periods must be kept at a minimum. For periods longer than 4 h, cells should be cultured as described. Before the experiment, cells should be allowed to equilibrate slowly to 37°C in buffers containing calcium and magnesium.
7. Enzymes used for tissue dispersion may contain impurities which affect mast cell responsiveness to various stimuli and these effects often vary considerably from batch to batch. It is therefore highly recommended to order small quantities of

several batches from the same company and compare which enzyme batch gives rise to not only best mast cell yields but also best releasability (in particular to anti-IgE) before ordering larger quantities.

8. Isolated mast cell suspensions often clump (especially just after enzymatic dispersion or following culture) and this seriously reduces the success of enrichment techniques. Therefore do not allow the cells to stand for long periods without intermittent resuspension. If clumping occurs resuspend relatively vigorously and filter through gauze (100-μ*m* pore size).

9. BAL and skin mast cells respond to high concentrations of neuropeptides (25, 50 μ*M*) e.g., substance P, neurokinin A, calcitonin gene related peptide (CGRP) and bradykinin *(22–24)*. They also respond to the calcium ionophore A23187 (Calbiochem, 0.5-5 μ*M*), antihuman IgE (Dako, 18.75, 37.5, 75 ng/mL) and concanavalin A (Sigma, 5–50 μg/mL) *(7)*. Human lung mast cells and basophils are generally unresponsive to neuropeptides but are activated by anti-IgE and A23187 at similar concentrations as above. Both human skin and lung mast cells are also responsive to SCF. This cytokine, which plays a crucial role in mast cell development, induces low levels of histamine release at 10–100 ng/mL and potentiates IgE-dependent activation at concentrations as low as 0.1 ng/mL *(25,26)*. Basophils are unresponsive to SCF but are primed by IL-3, IL-5, GM-CSF and NGF. They are also responsive to *N*-formyl methionyl leucine phenylalanine and C5a. Antihuman IgE can produce bell shaped dose response curves. Some sources of antihuman IgE do not elicit very good release. We have found Dako to be reliable but other sources may also be suitable.

References

1. Galli, S. J. (1990) Biology of disease: New insights into "The riddle of the mast cells" Microenvironmental regulation of mast cell development and phenotypic heterogeneity. *Lab. Invest.* **62,** 5–33.

2. Barrett, K. E. and Pearce, F. L. (1994) Mast cell heterogeneity, in *Immunopharmacology of mast cells and basophils* (Foreman, J. C., ed.) Academic Press, London, p.29–39.

3. Pearce, F. L. (1986) Functional differences between mast cells from various locations. in *Mast cell differentiation and heterogeneity* (Befus, D. A. , Bienenstock, J., Denberg, J. A., eds.) Raven Press, New York, p. 215–222.

4. Church, M. K., Okayama, Y., and Bradding, P. (1995) Functional mast cell heterogeneity in *Asthma and Rhinitis* (Busse, W. W., Holgate, S. T., eds.) Blackwell Scientific Publications, London, p. 209–220.

5. Heaney, L. G., Cross, L. M. J., Stanford, C. F., and Ennis, M. (1995) Substance P induces histamine release from human pulmonary mast cells. *Clin. Exp. Allergy* **25,** 179–186.

6. Okayama, Y., Benyon, R. C., Rees, P. H., Lowman, M. A., Hillier, K., and Church, M. K. (1991) Inhibition profiles of sodium cromoglycate and nedocromil sodium on mediator release from mast cells of human skin, lung, tonsil, adenoid and intestine. *Clin. Exp. Allergy* **22,** 401–409.

7. Pearce, F. L., Boulos, P. B., Lau, H. Y. A., Liu, W. L., and Tainsh, K. R. (1991) Functional heterogeneity of human mast cells. *Int. Arch. Allergy Appl. Immunol.* **94,** 239–240.

8. Leung, K. B. P., Flint, K. C., Brostoff, J., Hudspith, B. N., Johnson, N. McI., Lau, H. Y. A., et al.,(1988) Effects of sodium cromoglycate on histamine secretion from human lung mast cells. *Thorax* **43,** 756–761.

9. Forsythe, P., McGarvey, L. P. A., Heaney, L. G., MacMahon, J., and Ennis, M. (1999) Adenosine induces histamine release from human bronchoalveolar lavage mast cells. *Clin. Sci.,* **96,** 349–355.

10. Heaney, L. G., Cross, L. M. J., Stanford, C. F., and Ennis. M. (1995) Substance P induces histamine release from human pulmonary mast cells. *Clin. Exp. Allergy* **25,** 179–186.

11. Flint, K. C., Leung, K. B. P., Brostoff, J., Hudspith, B.N., Pearce, F. L. and Johnson, N. Mcl. (1985) Bronchoalveolar mast cells in extrinsic asthma: a mechanism for the initiation of antigen specific bronchoconstriction. *Br. Med. J.* **291,** 923–926.

12. Casolaro, V., Galeone, D., Giacummo, A., Sanduzzi, A., Melillo, G. and Marone, G. (1989) Human basophil/mast cell releasability. V Functional comparisons of cells obtained from peripheral blood, lung parenchyma, and bronchoalveolar lavage in asthmatics. *Am. Rev. Respir. Dis.* **139,** 1375–1382.

13. Gilbert, H. S. and Ornstein, L. (1975). Basophil counting with a new staining method using alcian blue. *Blood* **46,** 279–286.

14. Laviolette, M., Carreau, M. and Coulombe, R. (1988) Bronchoalveolar lavage differential on microscope glass cover. *Am. Rev. Respir. Dis.* **138,** 451–457.

15. Walters, E. H, and Gardiner, P. V. (1991) Bronchoalveolar lavage as a research tool. *Thorax* **46,** 613–618.

16. Ennis, M. (1991) Automated fluorometric assay in *Handbook of Histamine and Histamine Antagonists.* Exp. Pharmacol. vol. 97 (Uvnäs, B., ed.) Springer-Verlag, Berlin, p. 31–38.

17. Okayama, Y., Hunt, T. C., Kassel, O., Ashman, L.K. and Church, M. K. (1994) Assessment of the anti-c-kit monoclonal antibody YB5.B8 in affinity magnetic enrichment of human lung mast cells. *J. Immunol. Methods* **169,** 153–161.

18. Schulman, E. S., MacGlashan, D. W. Jr., Peters, S. P., Schleimer, R. P., Newball, H. H., and Lichtenstein, L. M. (1982). Human lung mast cells: purification and characterization. *J. Immunol.* **129,** 2662–2667.

19. Haisch, K., Gibbs, B. F., Korber, H., Ernst, M., Grage-Griebenow, E., Schlaak, M. and Haas, H. (1999). Purification of morphologically and functionally intact human basophils to near homogeneity. *J. Immunol. Methods* **226,** 129–137.

20. Gibbs, B. F., Noll, T., Falcone, F. H., Haas, H,. Vollmer, E., Vollrath, I., Wolff, H.H., and Amon, U. (1997). A three-step procedure for the purification of human basophils from buffy coat blood. *Inflamm. Res.* **46,** 137–142.

21. Gibbs. B. F., Amon, U., and Pearce, F. L. (1987) Spontaneous histamine release from mast cells and basophils is controlled by the cellular environment. *Inflamm. Res.* **46** Suppl 1, S25–S26.

22. Cross, L. M. J., Heaney, L. G., and Ennis, M. (1997) Histamine release from human bronchoalveolar lavage mast cells by neurokinin A and bradykinin. *Inflamm. Res.* **46,** 306–309.

23. Forsythe, P., McGarvey, L. P. A., Heaney, L. G., MacMahon, J., and Ennis, M. (2000) Sensory neuropeptides induce histamine release from bronchoalveolar lavage cells in both non-asthmatic coughers and cough variant asthmatics. *Clin. Exp. Allergy* **30,** 225–232.

24. Heaney, L. G., Cross, L. J. M., and Ennis, M. (1998). Histamine release from bronchoalveolar lavage cells from asthmatic subjects after allergen challenge and relationship to the late asthmatic response. *Clin. Exp. Allergy* **28,** 196–204

25. Frenz, A. M., Gibbs, B. F., and Pearce, F. L. (1997) The effect of recombinant stem cell factor on human skin and lung mast cells and basophil leukocytes. *Inflamm. Res.* **46,** 35–39.

26. Columbo, M., Horowitz, E. M., Botana, L. M., MacGlashan, D. W. Jr., Bochner, B. S., Gillis, S., et al.(1992). The human recombinant c-kit receptor ligand, rhSCF, induces mediator release from human cutaneous mast cells and enhances IgE-dependent mediator release from both skin mast cells and peripheral blood basophils. *J. Immunol.* **149,** 599–608.

15

Neutrophils

Collection, Separation, and Activation

Sarah V. Culpitt

1. Introduction

Neutrophils are manufactured in the bone marrow from stem cell precursors (myeloblasts) by a series of cell divisions. In healthy individuals only the mature neutrophils enter peripheral blood. They are the most numerous leukocyte subgroup, constituting half of the circulating white cell population. Healthy blood donors typically yield 1 million neutrophils per mL of venous blood.

Neutrophils have a characteristic dense nucleus consisting of between two and five lobes and a pale cytoplasm containing distinctive granules. Granules are classed as primary (azurophilic) and secondary (specific), both contributing to the armoury of enzymes, proteins, and glycosaminoglycans that participate in cell function. Primary granules contain myeloperoxidase (MPO), acid phosphatase, elastase, and other neutral serine proteases, and lysosomal acid hydrolases. Secondary granules, which predominate in the mature cell, contain collagenase, lactoferrin (LTF), lysozyme, adhesion molecules, and chemotactic factor receptors (e.g., the N-formyl-met-Leu-Phe receptor). The existence of a third (tertiary) granule population is disputed, but where a distinction is made the tertiary granules are those containing gelatinase (1).

The primary function of neutrophils is in host defense, specifically the phagocytosis and killing of pathogens in tissues. To fulfill this role, the cell must detect a signal from an infected tissue, move toward the wall of the postcapillary venule (marginate), interact with the endothelium (adhere), migrate to the site of infection (chemotaxis), and kill foreign cells. Each ele-

From: *Methods in Molecular Medicine, vol. 56:*
Human Airway Inflammation: Sampling Techniques and Analytical Protocols
Edited by: D. F. Rogers and L. E. Donnelly © Humana Press Inc., Totowa, NJ

ment of this response has been studied and some simple methods to assess neutrophil function are included in this chapter.

Cell adhesion molecules, in particular the selectin family, are important in initiating neutrophil sequestration. Chemoattractants are then required to change CD11/CD18 molecules to an adhesive conformation, enabling firm adhesion to ligands on endothelial cells (ICAM-1, ICAM-2). The process of chemotaxis along a concentration gradient of chemoattractant toward the pathogen (or host stimulus) can then occur. Neutrophils express numerous receptors for chemoattractants and although they are specific for different molecules they conform to a common pattern of seven transmembrane segments and G-protein coupling. Receptors for fMet-Leu-Phe (fMLP) *(2)*, interleukin-8 (IL-8) *(3)*, complement fragments (e.g., C5a) *(4)*, leukotriene B_4 (LTB_4) *(5)* and platelet activating factor (PAF) *(6)* have been identified on neutrophil cell membranes. The use of a microchemotaxis chamber to study neutrophil chemotaxis in vitro has been extensively validated (*7–9*, and *see* **Chapter 28**).

Once a neutrophil has migrated into the tissue, its primary purpose is to recognize, phagocytose, and destroy pathogens. Neutrophils recognize (bind) some materials on the surface of the foreign organism directly (e.g., lipopolysaccharide, LPS), but most particles require opsonization (e.g., with complement or immunoglobulin). Bound particles are then internalized into the phagosome where they are neutralized. Intracellular killing involves initiation of the respiratory burst with the intraphagosomal release of toxic oxygen metabolites. The respiratory burst can be indirectly measured by nicotinamide adenine dinucleotide phosphate (NADPH) oxidase activity, for example the production of formazan by the reduction of nitrobluetetrazolium *(10)*.

Neutrophils also secrete granule contents (e.g., MPO, LTF, elastase) and lipid mediators of inflammation (e.g., LTB_4) into surrounding tissues where they contribute to leukocyte recruitment and bacterial killing. Degranulation requires the neutrophil to be primed first, either by the action of phagocytosis or by mediators such as LPS. It is a controlled exocytotic release and the presence of granule constituents in biological samples therefore indicates that neutrophils are activated.

2. Materials

2.1. Reagents

All reagents were from Sigma-Aldrich (Dorset, UK), except where stated. Chemicals should be cell culture grade and endotoxin-free.

2.1.1. Neutrophil Collection (see **Note 1**)

1. Acid citrate dextran (ACD): 5 g glucose, 4.2 g di-sodium hydrogen citrate in 100-mL pyrogen-free water. The solution is filter sterilized by passing through a 0.2μm filter. ACD can be stored in 10 mL aliquots at –20°C.

2. ACD (as above) is used as an anticoagulant for venous blood, at a concentration of 10% (v/v); i.e., 1 mL ACD + 9 mL blood. ACD is drawn into the syringe used for venipuncture before blood is aspirated.

2.1.2. Neutrophil Separation by Percoll Gradient

1. On the day of the experiment a 10% ACD (v/v) solution is prepared, for use in sedimentation, by dilution of ACD (as above) with 0.9% (w/v) sterile sodium chloride (Baxter Healthcare Ltd, Norfolk, UK) e.g., 3 mL ACD + 27 mL NaCl.
2. 9% sodium chloride (w/v): 9 g sodium chloride in 100-mL pyrogen free water. Filter sterilize and store aliquots at −20°C.
3. elo-HAES: 6% (w/v) medium molecular weight HydroxyEthyl starch in 0.9% (w/v) sodium chloride (Fresnius Ltd, Basingstoke, UK). Store at 4°C.
4. Percoll (*see* **Note 2**): 100% percoll is prepared from the proprietary solution (Amersham Pharmacia Biotech, St Albans, Herts, UK) by diluting with 9% (w/v) sodium chloride in a 10:1 v/v ratio, e.g., 27 mL Percoll + 3 mL 9% (w/v) NaCl. This dilution should be freshly prepared on the day of the experiment.
5. Sterile phosphate buffered saline (PBS) without calcium and magnesium.
6. Hanks balanced salt solution (HBSS) without phenol red, buffered with HEPES (20 m*M*). Adjust pH to 7.2. This can be stored at 4°C for up to 1 mo.
7. Bovine serum albumin (BSA). Store at 4°C.

2.1.3. Neutrophil Separation by Ficoll-Hypaque

1. Ficoll-Hypaque (Amersham Pharmacia Biotech, St Albans, Herts, UK): store at 4°C.
2. Other reagents as above for blood sedimentation.

2.1.4. Markers of Neutrophil Activation in Biological Fluids

2.1.4.1. MYELOPEROXIDASE

1. Bioxytech MPO Enzyme Immunoassay (Oxis International, Portland, Oregon) or equivalent. Kit containing all necessary reagents for 96 assays of MPO. Store at 4°C. Paired antibodies are also available for enzyme linked immunosorbent assay (ELISA) and Western blotting.
2. Sample diluting buffer: PBS, containing 0.1% (v/v) Tween-20, 2% (w/v) BSA. Adjust pH to 7.4. Buffer is stable at 4°C for 1 mo, for longer storage add 0.2% (w/v) sodium azide. **Safety note:** Sodium azide may form explosive lead or copper azides in plumbing, so waste solutions should be diluted prior to disposal.

2.1.4.2. ACTOFERRIN

Bioxytech Lacto*f* Enzyme Immunoassay (Oxis International, Portland, Oregon) or equivalent. Kit containing all necessary reagents for 96 assays of MPO. Store at 4°C. Paired antibodies are also available for ELISA and Western blotting.

2.1.4.3. ELASTASE

1. Buffer: 100 m*M* Tris-HCl, pH 8.6, buffer in 300 m*M* NaCl. For 100 mL – 1.75 g NaCl, 1.211 g Trizma base in 100 mL distilled water. Adjust to pH 8.6. Store at 4°C for up to 1 mo.
2. Elastase substrate: N-methoxysuccinyl-ala-ala-pro-val p-nitroanilide. Dissolve in the smallest possible volume of 100% dimethylsulphoxide (DMSO). Make up to 14.16 mg/mL solution with pure water. Aliquot into 300 mL volumes and store at –20°C. This solution is stable for 1 y but avoid freeze-thaw cycles. On day of use, thaw and add 900 µL of pure water. Two aliquots are sufficient for one 96-well plate.
3. Elastase standards: select a standard comparable to the elastase present in your sample. A suitable elastase for human samples is Human Sputum Elastase (HSE). HSE is dissolved in tissue culture medium, e.g., Dulbecco's Modification of Eagle's Medium, to make a 1-mg/mL solution. Aliquot in 20 µL volumes and store at –20°C for up to 6 mo.
4. Pure water: cell culture grade sterile water. Store at 4°C.

2.1.5. Nitrobluetetrazolium Test

1. Aspirate heparin (100 iu per mL of blood, Leo Labs Ltd, Princes Risborough, Bucks, UK) into a syringe for venipuncture. 5 mL blood is ample for the experiment.
2. Nitrobluetetrazolium (NBT) solution: 0.15% NBT (v/v), 0.17% sucrose (w/v) in PBS. Store at 4°C for up to 1 wk.
3. Endotoxin: 200 µg/mL Escherichi coli endotoxin in RPMI medium. This solution can be stored at -70°C for 6 mo.
4. Giemsa stain (BDH, Poole, Dorset UK). Stable at room temperature (RT).

2.1.6. Neutrophil Chemotaxis

1. HBSS/HEPES/BSA: HBSS (*no* phenol red), 20 m*M* HEPES, 0.1% (w/v) BSA, adjust to pH 7.2. HBSS/HEPES can be stored at 4°C for 1 mo. BSA should be added on the day of the experiment.
2. Kimura stain: Toluidine blue 0.05% (w/v) (22 mL), Light Green 0.03% (w/v) (1.6 mL), Saponin 1.0 mL, 66 m*M* phosphate buffer (10 mL). Store at RT.
   a. 0.05% Toluidine blue: 0.05 g in NaCl 1.8% (50 mL), ethanol 96% (22 mL). Make up to 100 mL with distilled water.
   b. 0.03% Light Green: 0.03 g in 100 mL distilled water.
   c. Saponin: dissolve to saturation in 50% ethanol.
   d. Phosphate buffer: KH_2PO_4 9.023g/L, Na_2HPO_4 9.464g/L (mix 1:1 v/v).
3. N-formyl-met-leu-phe (fMLP): reconstitute in PBS and store at 10^{-3}M, -20°C for up to 6 mo. Dilute in HBSS/HEPES/BSA prior to use in chemotaxis. Suitable concentration curve is from 10^{-10}–$10^{-5}M$.
4. 100% ethanol (>99% purity, BDH, Poole, Dorset, UK): from this solution, prepare 70% (v/v) and 95% (v/v) solutions. Solutions should be prepared just before use. Industrial methylated spirits (IMS) is *not* a suitable alternative.

5. Butanol (>99% purity, BDH): prepare an 8:2 ethanol: butanol solution. Prepare fresh solution for each experiment.
6. Xylene (BDH): should be used in a glass dish as it dissolves plastic. Can be reused if stored in a lidded container, but evaporates over time.
7. Haematoxylin (BDH): filter through a 0.2 μm pore filter (Gelman, Northants, UK) before use. Stable at RT.
8. Depex (R.A. Lamb, London, UK): stable at RT.

2.2. Apparatus

2.2.1. Neutrophil Collection

1. Sterile 19-gage needles for venipuncture.
2. Sterile syringes for blood.
3. 50-mL Falcon tubes.

2.2.2. Neutrophil Separation by Percoll Gradient

1. 15-mL Falcon tubes.
2. Parafilm
3. Sterile 2-mL syringes.
4. Sterile 21-gage needles.

2.2.3. Neutrophil Separation by Ficoll-Hypaque

1. 50-mL Falcon tubes.

2.2.4. Markers of Neutrophil Activation in Biological Fluids

1. For ELISA: 96-well plates (Greiner, Gloucester, UK).
2. Microplate reader (Anthos Labtac Instruments) capable of absorbance measurements at 420 nm (lactoferrin and elastase) and 405 nm (MPO).

2.2.5. The Neutrophil Respiratory Burst

1. Luckhams tubes: Luckham (Hants, UK).
2. Microscope slides: BDH (Poole).
3. Waterbath (Grant, Cambridge, UK): for incubation at $37 \pm 1°C$.

2.2.6. Neutrophil Chemotaxis

1. 48-well modified Boyden chamber: Neuro Probe Inc. Gaithersburg, MD. Supplied by Receptor Technologies Limited, Oxon UK.
2. Cellulose nitrate 3 μ*m* pore filters: Receptor Technologies Limited.
3. 0.2 μ*m* pore filters: Gelman, Northants, UK.
4. Curved forceps (2 pairs): Interfocus, Suffolk, UK.
5. Petri dishes: Becton Dickinson, Oxford, UK.
6. Microscope slides and coverslips: R.A. Lamb, London, UK.

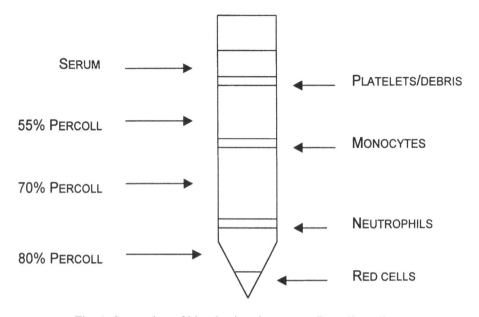

Fig. 1. Separation of blood using three-stage Percoll gradient.

3. Methods

3.1. Collection of Neutrophils

Neutrophils are obtained from peripheral venous blood. It is essential that venipuncture is performed by a qualified operator using aseptic technique. Neutrophils are easily activated by mechanical stress and therefore sampling should be as gentle as possible. Ideally, a 19-gage needle or butterfly is introduced into a large vein in the antecubital fossa (elbow) in a single movement. Blood is gently aspirated into a syringe, which has been prefilled with an appropriate volume of ACD (1 mL for every 10 mL of blood to be withdrawn). Where a 19-gage needle is too large (for example pediatric donors) aspiration should be slow to avoid turbulent blood flow. In every circumstance, the rate of aspiration should not cause bubbles to appear within the syringe as this inevitably leads to neutrophil activation.

Once the blood sample has been obtained, the syringe should be gently inverted several times to ensure thorough mixing of blood and ACD. The sample should be sedimented (*see* **Subheading 3.2.1.**) as soon as possible. Any delay in further processing requires the sample to be refrigerated. Neutrophils have a short half-life in the circulation, which is further reduced when ex vivo. Therefore cell viability will be reduced if the sample is not processed expediently.

3.2. Neutrophil Separation by Percoll Gradient

1. Blood anticoagulated with ACD is first sedimented: add 20 mL blood to 20 mL elo-HAES and 5 mL 10% ACD (v/v) in a 50-mL Falcon tube. Inversion mix and remove air bubbles with a pipet (to prevent neutrophil activation). Leave to sediment for 45 min.
2. Sedimentation results in buffy coat (top layer) and red cells (soft pellet). Carefully remove the buffy coat, taking care to avoid aspirating red cells.
3. Pellet white blood cells by centrifugation at 400g for 10 min at 4°C.
4. Prepare 100% (v/v) Percoll. From this solution prepare 80% (v/v), 70% (v/v) and 55% (v/v) by dilution with PBS without Ca/Mg.
5. Prepare the Percoll gradient in a 15-mL Falcon tube (**Fig. 1**): 4 mL of 80% (v/v) forms the lowest layer, 4 mL of 70% (v/v) the middle layer, and 3 mL of 55% (v/v) the top layer. The 80% (v/v) Percoll can be directly pipeted into the tube, but subsequent solutions must be carefully layered on top to prevent the solutions mixing. This can be achieved by allowing the solution to run slowly down the side of the tube (*see* **Note 3**).
6. Resuspend the white blood cell pellet in buffy coat and layer on top of the Percoll gradient.
7. Centrifuge the gradients at 500g for 25 min at 18°C.
8. White cells are separated as follows: neutrophils and eosinophils at the 70/80% (v/v) interface, peripheral blood mononuclear cells (lymphocytes and monocytes) at the 70/55% (v/v) interface.
9. Pipet the neutrophils into a 50-mL Falcon tube and wash with HBSS without Ca/Mg three times.

3.3. Neutrophil Separation by Ficoll-Hypaque

1. Anticoagulate and sediment the blood exactly as above (**steps 1–3**).
2. Resuspend the white blood cells in 2-mL buffy coat.
3. Place 5 mL of Ficoll-Hypaque in a 15-mL Falcon.
4. Carefully layer the white blood cells on top of the Ficoll-Hypaque.
5. Centrifuge at 500g for 30 min at 20°C.
6. White cells are separated as follows: peripheral blood mononuclear cells at the Ficoll/buffy coat interface, all other cells form a pellet at the bottom of the tube.
7. To obtain neutrophils, it is necessary to lyse the contaminating red blood cells: resuspend the cell pellet in 5-mL ice cold distilled water, keep on ice for 1 min.
8. Add HBSS without Ca/Mg (at room temperature). Centrifuge at 400g for 10 min at 4°C.
9. Wash 3 times in HBSS without Ca/Mg (*see* **Note 4**).

3.4. Markers of Neutrophil Activation in Biological Fluids

Neutrophil efficacy in self-defense depends on their ability to kill a wide range of microorganisms. This lethal activity is provided by a broad range of proteases, hydrolases, and cationic proteins located in intracellular granules, which are released from neutrophils when they are activated. Assays are available for many granule components: three simple, validated measures of neutrophil activation are provided below.

3.4.1. Myeloperoxidase

MPO can be measured by ELISA. Samples of bronchoalveolar lavage, cerebrospinal fluid, urine and cell culture supernatants can be assayed directly (*see* **Note 5**). For blood samples, it is necessary to separate cells from plasma by centrifugation of a heparinized sample at 3000*g* for 10 min at 4°C. Plasma samples usually require dilution 1:30 (v/v) with PBS/Tween containing 2% (w/v) BSA.

For cell assays, cells must first be homogenized. A suitable technique is:
1. Collect neutrophils as above. Count cells using Kimura stain.
2. Resuspend 2×10^6 cells in PBS and wash three times.
3. Resuspend the final pellet in 1mL PBS containing 0.1% (v/v) Tween-20.
4. Break the cells by freeze thawing 3 times at –70°C.
5. Centrifuge at 12,000*g* for 15 min at 4°C.
6. Remove supernatant. Dilute 1:10 with PBS/Tween containing 2% (w/v) BSA.

3.4.2. Lactoferrin

Lactoferrin (LTF) can be measured by ELISA. Samples of bronchoalveolar lavage, cerebrospinal fluid, urine, and cell culture supernatants can be assayed directly (*see* **Note 5**). Heparin may interfere with LTF assays so EDTA should be used as the anticoagulant. Prepare plasma from whole blood as above (**Subheading 3.4.1.**). Plasma samples should be diluted with PBS/Tween containing 2% BSA (w/v) before assay.

3.4.3. Elastase

This assay is suitable for the measurement of serine protease activity in biological fluids, cell homogenates (*see* **Subheading 3.4.1.** for suggested method of homogenization) and cell culture supernatants. Neutrophils also contain metalloproteinases with elastolytic activity, but they require an alternative substrate.

1. Prepare standards of elastase from the stock solution. The assay is linear in the range 0–2µg/mL.
2. Pipet into a 96-well plate (in the following order): 70-µL pure water, 100-µL Tris buffer, 10-µL sample (or standard), 20-µL elastase substrate (*see* **Note 6**).
3. Cover the plate with a plate sealer and shake for 1 min.
4. Centrifuge the plate at 200*g* for 2 min at RT.
5. Incubate the plate for a further 30 min at RT (*see* **Note 7**).
6. Read at 405 nm.

3.5. The Neutrophil Respiratory Burst

This assay provides a simple, whole blood measurement of oxidase activity, and thus indirectly, the respiratory burst. It is dependent on the production of formazan by the reduction of nitrobluetetrazolium. As described in **steps 3 and 4**, the method compares unstimulated blood with endotoxin-stimulated blood, but the same method can be used to compare unstimulated samples from different donors or different stimuli of the respiratory burst.

1. Collect a sample of blood with heparin as the anticoagulant. 100 µL is required for each sample and control.
2. Make nitrobluetetrazolium (NBT) solution.
3. In tube 1 (control): place 100 µL of blood, 100 µL of NBT solution, and 100 µL RPMI.
4. In tube 2 (stimulated): place 100 µL of blood, 100 µL of NBT solution, and 100 µL of RPMI containing endotoxin.
5. Mix samples and incubate in a water bath at 37°C for 20 min.
6. Incubate at RT for a further 20 min.
7. Make a blood smear from each sample by placing a drop of blood toward one end of a glass slide. Draw a second glass slide over the blood drop and spread thinly toward the other end of the slide. Allow the blood smear to air dry for a few minutes.
8. Fix slides in 100% (v/v) methanol for 3 min.
9. Stain slides in Giemsa for 20 min. Wash off excess stain with PBS.
10. Air-dry slides for 5 min.
11. Count 100 neutrophils and record the percentage containing blue formazan granules (*see* **Note 8**).

3.6. Neutrophil Chemotaxis

This method can be used to compare neutrophil response to a variety of chemoattractants. Neutrophils are first separated (**Subheading 3.1.**) then placed in the upper wells of a modified Boyden chamber with chemoattractant in the lower wells. Migrating neutrophils are counted within a filter placed between the upper and lower wells.

1. Resuspend the washed neutrophils in 2 mL HBSS/HEPES/BSA. Count the cells on a standard hemocytometer by staining with Kimura (10 µL of cell solution + 90 µL Kimura).
2. Dilute neutrophils to 2×10^6 per mL. For a 48-well chamber (with a capacity of 50 µL per upper well), 6 mL buffer containing 12 million neutrophils is sufficient.
3. Leave neutrophils to rest for 1 h at RT.
4. Add chemoattractant to the lower wells of the chemotaxis chamber. Include a negative control (HBSS/HEPES/BSA) and positive control (e.g., fMLP $10^{-7}M$). Adjust the volume according to the capacity of the wells (*see* **Note 9**).
5. Soak a filter (*see* **Note 10**) in HBSS/HEPES/BSA in a clean Petri dish. Cut off 1 mm of one corner of the filter: this enables subsequent orientation of the filter.

6. Carefully apply the filter to the lower wells, followed by the rubber seal and the upper part of the chamber. Tighten the screws to ensure the wells do not leak. Place a glass slide over the upper wells to prevent evaporation and consequent drying of the filter.
7. Allow to equilibrate to 37°C for 15 min.
8. Carefully pipet the neutrophils into the upper wells of the chamber, adjust the volume according to the capacity of the wells (*see* **Note 11**). Replace the glass slide on top of the chamber.
9. Incubate the chamber for 1 h at 37°C (*see* **Note 12**).
10. While the chamber is incubating, set up the solutions and stain needed for fixing the filter as follows:

    a. 70% (v/v) ethanol.
    b. Distilled H_2O.
    c. Hematoxylin.
    d. Distilled H_2O.
    e. Tap water.
    f. 70% (v/v) ethanol.
    g. 95% (v/v) ethanol.
    h. 8:2 (v/v) ethanol:butanol.
    i. Xylene (in a glass dish).

11. After the 1 h incubation, remove the chamber from the incubator, loosen the screws all round and then take them off. Turn the whole chamber upside down onto some tissue and bang firmly on the table. The filter should stick to the top half of the chamber. Immediately place the bottom half of the chamber into dH_2O. Begin the staining and fixing steps (**step 12**), place the other components of the chamber into dH_2O.
12. Staining and fixing:

    a. 70% (v/v) ethanol: 5 min.
    b. dH_2O: 1 min.
    c. Hematoxylin: 45 s.
    d. dH_2O: 1 min.
    e. Tap water: rinse under the tap for 3 min.
    f. 70% (v/v) ethanol: 2 min.
    g. 95% (v/v) ethanol: 2 min.
    h. 8:2 ethanol:butanol: 5 min.
    i. Xylene: at least 5 min (*see* **Note 13**).

13. Cut the filter vertically into four pieces to fit on four microscope slides.
14. Mount filters by placing a drop of Depex onto each slide. Place the filter on top, then another drop of Depex, then a coverslip. Manipulate the coverslip to expel air bubbles. Allow to dry for at least 2 h before counting the cells.
15. Count migrating neutrophils by light microscopy (40× magnification). Disregard cells in the top 30 μm and count all cells in the remaining thickness of filter (*see* **Note 14**).

4. Notes

1. The required purity of reagents for collection and separation of neutrophils depends on the subsequent experiments being planned. Where neutrophils are to be maintained in culture, tissue culture grade chemicals should be used, reagents should be prepared in a culture hood and filter sterilized before freezing. Neutrophils will be activated by reagents contaminated by endotoxin.

2. Percoll degrades on exposure to air. If the undiluted solution is to be opened and then stored for longer than 1 mo it should be divided into sterile airtight aliquots before storage at 4°C.

3. Separation of neutrophils will only be achieved if the Percoll solutions do not mix. If there are not discrete "bands" of cells at the interfaces, this suggests that the layering process is not working. An alternative method of achieving unmixed layers is to cover the top of the Falcon tube with parafilm and pierce the membrane with a 21-gage needle attached to a 2-mL syringe from which the barrel has been removed. With the tip of the needle wedged against the side of the tube, Percoll can be pipeted into the syringe and the desired slow rate of layering is achieved via the needle.

4. Neutrophils will be activated differently according to the method of separation used. For this reason it is recommended that the same method is used consistently for a set of experiments.

5. It may be necessary to dilute samples before assay. A suitable diluting buffer is PBS/Tween containing 2% (w/v) BSA.

6. The pure water/sample volumes may be altered according to the elastase levels in the sample, but the total volume of pure water/sample must be 80 µL.

7. Different samples may require different incubation times since the assay depends on the rate of degradation of the substrate by the elastase activity in the sample. To optimize conditions, start reading the plate at 15 min and read every 2 min for up to 1 h. Plot the peak absorbency at 405 nm and use this as the optimal time point.

8. Typical results (mean ± standard error) for the NBT test are 11 ± 2% for unstimulated cells and 71 ± 4% for stimulated cells. It is possible to adapt this technique for pure neutrophil preparations: resuspend 1×10^5 neutrophils in 100mL RPMI. Continue as per protocol, but instead of making a blood smear for staining, prepare a cytospin using 100 µL of the cell/NBT solution per slide. Spin slides at 40g for 5 min and count formazan positive cells as before. Neutrophils are activated by separation from whole blood and therefore results will be more reproducible if cells are left to "rest" in RPMI at RT for 1 h prior to the NBT test.

9. When loading the lower wells of the chemotaxis chamber it is essential that they are filled flush to the top so that no air bubble will be trapped between the fluid and filter. Allow the meniscus of the chemoattractant to rise above the top edge of the well.

10. Always handle the filter with clean forceps. Untoothed, curved forceps are preferable, to avoid ripping the filter.

11. The action of pipeting can activate neutrophils. To avoid this, it may be necessary to cut the ends off the pipet tips, creating a wider aperture for delivery of

neutrophils. It is essential that the pipet tip does not touch the filter, as this will damage it. However, any air trapped between cells and filter will prevent chemotaxis, so the cells must be introduced into the bottom of the well. Air bubbles are easily detected since they prevent the full volume of cells being pipeted into wells and they can be seen if the chamber is held horizontally at eye level.

12. It is not necessary to incubate the chamber in an incubator where CO_2/O_2 are controlled. This is because the incubation period is short and buffer will prevent acidosis developing over this period of time. It is a sensible precaution to place the chamber in a clean container lined with damp tissue paper and with a loose fitting lid. This keeps the outside of the chamber clean and maintains a humid atmosphere.

13. Xylene changes the filter from opaque to clear. It is not possible to count cells in an opaque filter so adequate "clearing" is essential. The filter can safely be left overnight in xylene to facilitate clearing.

14. It is necessary to know (from the manufacturer) the exact thickness of the filter in order to calibrate the microscope and disregard the cells in the top 30 μm. Focus the top of the filter, note the reading on the focus dial, then scroll the focus down through the filter to the bottom and note the reading again. Count the number of divisions on the focus dial corresponding to the full thickness of the filter: from this and the known thickness of the filter, calculate the depth of each division. It is then possible to move focus from the top of the filter to a depth of 30 μm just by scrolling down the corresponding number of divisions on each occasion. After these initial calculations, always use the same method to establish the starting point for counting.

Acknowledgments

Much credit is owed to Dr. L.E. Donnelly, Dr. J.R. Allport, and Mrs. Carmen deMatos for their technical ability in perfecting the methods described, and their help in the preparation of this chapter.

References

1. Baggiolini, M. (1980). *The Cell Biology of Inflammation* (Weissman, G., ed.), Elsevier/North Holland, NY, pp. 163–187.
2. Aswanikumar, S., Corcoran, B., Schiffman, E., Day, A. R., Freer, R. J., Showell, H. J., and Becker, E. L. (1977) Demonstration of a receptor on rabbit neutrophils for chemotactic peptides. *Biochem. Biophys. Res. Comm.* **74,** 810–817.
3. Grob, P. M., David, E., Warren, T. C., DeLeon, R. P., Farina, P. R., and Homon, C.A. (1990) Characterisation of a receptor for human monocyte-derived neutrophil chemotactic factor/ interleukin-8. *J. Biol. Chem.* **265,** 8311–8316.
4. Gerard, N.P. and Gerard, C. (1991) The chemotactic receptor for human C5a anaphylatoxin. *Nature.* **349,** 614–617.
5. Kreisle, R. A. and Parker, C. W. (1983) Specific binding of leukotriene B$_4$ to a receptor on human polymorphonuclear leukocytes. *J. Exp. Med.* **157,** 628–641.

6. Kunz, D., Gerard, N. P., and Gerard, C. (1992) The human leukocyte platelet-activating factor receptor. *J. Biol. Chem.* **267,** 9101–9106.
7. Falk, W., GoodwinJR., R. H., and Leonard, E. J. (1980) A 48-well micro-chemotaxis assembly for rapid and accurate measurement of leukocyte migration. *J. Immunol. Methods* **33,** 239–247.
8. Wilkinson, P. C. (1988) Micropore filter methods for leukocyte chemotaxis. *Methods Enzymol.* **162,** 38–50.
9. Allport, J. R., Donnelly, L. E., Hayes, B. P., Murray, S., Rendell, N. B., Ray, K. P., and MacDermot, J. M. (1996) Reduction by inhibitors of mono (ADP-ribosyl) transferase of chemotaxis in human neutrophil leucocytes by inhibition of the assembly of filamentous actin. *Br. J. Pharmacol.* **118,** 1111–1118.
10. Wolf, H., Fruhwirth, M., Ruedl, C., Oswald, H. P., Fischer, H., Bock, G., and Wick, G. (1995) Chronic granulomatous disease assessed by single call granulocyte oxidative burst activity. *Int. Arch. Allergy Immunol.* **106(4)** 425–427.

16

Macrophages

Identification, Separation, and Function

Leonard W. Poulter and C. M. Burke

1. Introduction

Within the human lung, macrophages can be found in the pleura, interstitium, alveoli, airways, vasculature, and walls of the bronchi and bronchiols. This distribution does not simply reflect the ubiquitous nature of these cells, as the macrophages found at these different sites show subtle distinctions in terms of cell physiology and phenotype *(1)*. Further, animal studies have revealed functional differences between macrophages from different lung compartments *(2)*. These differences may however be more apparent than real. Macrophages are motile cells and those, for example, present in the airways may arrive via the lung interstitium and are known to be capable of migrating back into the tissues of the lung. Thus, any observed differences between cells in different compartments are likely to be a reflection of the particular environment the cells find themselves in, rather than definitive distinctions between cell types (reviewed in *3*). The message is that macrophages are "plastic" in terms of their phenotype. As different phenotypes have been shown to reflect different functions, it would seem inevitable, therefore, that these cells also exhibit a diversity of function. Indeed, it is now recognized that the phagocytic scavenger or microbicidal effector cell, are just two of several roles these cells can play.

Macrophages may of course act as antigen presenting cells inducing T-cell responsiveness *(4)*. In contrast, they can act as suppressive cells turning off T cells *(5)*. They may also act as secretory cells producing a wide repertoire of cytokines, other immunomodulatory proteins, such as complement compo-

From: *Methods in Molecular Medicine, vol. 56:*
Human Airway Inflammation: Sampling Techniques and Analytical Protocols
Edited by: D. F. Rogers and L. E. Donnelly © Humana Press Inc., Totowa, NJ

nents, and products of arachidonic acid metabolism. It is clear that together these soluble factors can have a profound influence on local immune reactivity and of course the inflammatory process. What is important to recognize is that the overall function of the macrophage pool in any organ, or compartment within an organ, is inevitably a reflection of the balance between these diverse functional capabilities exhibited within the macrophage population. Thus, with any approach aimed to identify, separate, and/or determine macrophage function, it is important to preserve a concept of this diversity.

Realistically there are only two approaches to studying the macrophages of the human lung. Firstly they can be investigated *in situ* using immunohistologic techniques on tissue sections from biopsies or post-mortem samples. Secondly, cells can be obtained by bronchoalveolar lavage (BAL) whereby airway macrophages are washed from the lungs using a fiberoptic bronchoscope. There is arguably a third approach whereby lung tissues may be disaggregated and digested to a point where cell suspensions can be prepared. Although this approach has been shown to be of considerable value in obtaining lymphocytes, fibroblasts, and other cell types, it produces poor yields of macrophages and is not an approach favored by many. We have used such approaches to study lymphocytes from the lung *(6)*, but have not found this technique suitable for macrophages.

Both the other approaches have advantages and disadvantages. Using tissue sections you are able to visualize the precise disposition of cells in the tissues and reveal how they relate to other cell types. It is not possible however to study cell function in a tissue section. The use of monoclonal antibody (MoAb) probes for functionally relevant surface markers, and probes for cytokines in the body of the cell, might give you some idea of what the cell is capable of, no definitive tests for cell function are possible. BAL a possible approach to obtain significant numbers of viable macrophages from the lung, which can be maintained in vitro, and their functional capacity determined *(7)*. This approach, however, predominantly samples the alveolar macrophage pool and such cells may not reflect those in the bronchial wall, interstitium, or pleura.

What is clearly important, therefore, is to decide exactly what you wish to know and then pursue the appropriate approach that will answer that particular question. This chapter will concentrate on the techniques using tissue sections from the lung and those where airway cells obtained via BAL are used.

2. Materials

The biological material employed in the methods below will be derived from human subjects either at biopsy or postmortem. Acquisition of the material

Table 1
MoAbs used in the Identification of Monocyte and Macrophage Subsets

MoAbs	Class	Specificity	Source
CD14	IgG1	Monocytes	Dako
CD68	IgG1	All cells of monocyte/macrophage lineage	Dako
RFD1	IgM	MQ subset/APCs	Serotec UK Ltd
RFD7	IgG1	MQ subsets	Serotec UK Ltd
CD35	IgG2	CR1 complement receptor	Serotec UK Ltd
CD64	IgG1	FcγRI Fc receptor	Serotec UK Ltd
HLA-DR	IgM	Framework epitope HLA-DR	RF&UCMS

Table 2
Second-Layer Reagents for Immunohistology

Technique	Reagent(s)	Supplier
Immunoperoxidase	Goat anti and murine Ig Conjugated to HR peroxidase	Dako
APAAP	(I) G&M Ig AP conjugate	Dako
	(II) Mouse AAP-AP conjugate	Dako
Immunofluorescence	(I) G&M Ig . FITC	Cambridge Bio. Sci.
	(II) G&M Ig TRITC	Cambridge Bio. Sci.
N.B. FITC conjugate can be used for immuno-histology & indirect Immuno. fluorescence for flow cytometry	N.B. Isotype specific & subclass specific conjugates are also available, as are phycoerythrin conjugates for flow cytometry	

Table 3
Substrates/Chromogens for Immunohistology

Technique	Reagents	Source
Immunoperoxidase	Substrate:- hydrogen peroxide	B.D.H.
	Chromogen:- D.A.B.	Sigma Chem. Co.
APAAP	Substrate: +1 - Naphthol ASBI phosphate	Sigma Chem.Co.
	+2 - Naphthol ASMX phosphate	Sigma Chem.Co.
	Chromogen: 1 – Fast blue	Sigma Chem.Co.
	2 - Fast red	Sigma Chem.Co.
	Inhibitor: Levamisol	Sigma Chem.Co.

+ These are alterations and the choice of stain depends upon preference for blue or red colouration.

will require clinical procedures, which will not be detailed here (*see* Chapter 2). They may also require ethical approval and this possibility must be considered before any use is made of material derived from patients or from cadavers. In this regard attention should be drawn to the new guidelines published by the Royal College of Pathologists *(8)*.

2.1. Preparation of Tissue Sections

Samples are obtained from bronchoscopy, surgical resection, or postmortem. The size of the samples should be restricted to a maximum of 0.5 cm^3 if the tissue is to be frozen. There is no minimum size. We routinely cut cryostat sections from one mm^3 samples.

1. Optimum cutter temperature compound (OCT) Medium (Brights Instrument Company, UK).
2. Cork disks (Raymond A. Lamb Ltd., Eastbourne, UK).
3. Isopentane (BDH, Poole, UK).
4. Liquid nitrogen (Distillers Company, Guildford, UK).
5. Paraformaldehyde fixative (BDH).
6. Polysiloxane (Sigma Chemical Company, Poole, UK).

2.2. Immunohistology

1. PBS tablets (Sigma Chemical Company).
2. Normal rabbit serum (Gibco-BRL, Paisley, Scotland).
5. Monoclonal antibodies used are described in **Table 1**.
6. Second layer reagents for immunohistology are described in **Table 2**.
7. Chromogens and development solutions for immunohistology are described in **Table 3**.
8. Hematoxylin and "Diff-Quik" solution (BDH).

2.3. Flow Cytometry

1. Diluent for flow cytometry (Becton Dickinson, Oxford, UK).
2. Fluorescent reagents (*see* **Table 2**).
1. Permafix (Caltag Laboratories Ltd., Market Harborough, UK).
2. Crystal violet (Raymond A.Lamb Ltd).

2.4. Cell Separation

1. Lymphoprep (Nicomed UK, Oslo, Norway).
2. Culture medium, RPMI (GIBCO).
3. Metrizamide (Sigma Chemical Co.).
4. Microbeads & buffers for microbeads (Miltenyi Biotec, Bisley, UK).

2.5. Cell Culture and Functional Studies

1. AIM V. medium (Gibco-BRL).
2. All culture vessels and multiwelled plates (Costar Corning, New York).

3. Enzyme-linked imminosorbent assay (ELISA) kits (R&D Systems, Abingdon, UK).
4. Trititated thymidine (Amersham Radiochemicals, Amersham, UK).
5. Lipopolysaccaride (Sigma Chemical Co).

3. Methods
3.1. Preparing Tissue Sections

The freezing of fresh tissue should be done as soon as possible after collection of biopsies, ideally within 2 h. In the case of post-mortem material, it should be obtained from the cadaver within 18 h of death. In both cases:

1. Samples should be placed on moistened surgical gauze in sputum pots and transported to the laboratory.
2. A freezing bath is prepared by placing a 100 mL beaker half full of isopentane into a bath of liquid nitrogen held in a polystyrene container. The bath is ready to use when the isopentane begins to freeze. This is normally between –80°C and –90°C and can easily be seen as semisolid white isopentane begins to form in the base of the beaker. At the same time place forceps and a supply of universal tubes with holes punched in their caps into the liquid nitrogen.
3. Place a small blob of OCT (up to a half centimeter cube) onto a cork disc. Place the tissue sample on the OCT, orientate if required and allow it to sink into the OCT medium.
2. Drop the disc plus sample into the cold isopentane and leave immersed for 30 s.
3. Using the cooled forceps, remove the frozen sample from the isopentane and place in a precooled universal tube. Transfer immediately to a liquid nitrogen storage container (*see* **Note 1**).
4. When section cutting is required, remove sample from liquid nitrogen container and attach to cryostat chuck using OCT and a liquid nitrogen freezing bath (as above). Ensure tissue does not thaw in any way. Lock the 'chuck' plus sample onto the microtome in the cryostat.
5. With the cryostat at –25°C or below proceed to cut sections (normally 6 μm in thickness) which should be picked up onto microscope slides maintained at room temperature.
6. These should be air-dried for 1 h and fixed in chloroform-acetone for 5–10 min, wrapped in cling film and stored at –20°C until used (*see* **Notes 2** and **3**).

3.2. Immunohistology

There is a specific section on these techniques in the present volume (Chapter 30), and to avoid duplication we only summarize here the protocols currently in use in our laboratory.

3.2.1. Immunoperoxidase

This technique can be used to identify total macrophages (CD68+ cells) or monocytes (CD14+ cells) in both fresh, frozen, or paraformaldehyde-fixed material.

1. Ring sections with polysiloxane.
2. Apply 50 µL normal rabbit serum (NRS) (1:100 PBS) incubate for 10 min.
3. Drain off NRS solution.
4. Apply 50-µL monoclonal antibody at appropriate dilution, incubate for 45 min at room temperature.
5. Wash in PBS for 2 min.
6. Apply peroxidase conjugated antibody (*see* **Table 2**), incubate for 45 min.
7. Wash in PBS for 2 min.
8. Apply DAB substrate solution (*see* **Table 3**) for 5 min.
9. Wash in running tap water for 5 min.
10. Counter stain in hematoxylin.
11. Wash, dehydrate, and mount in DPX.

3.2.2. Alkaline Phosphatase Antialkaline Phosphatase Staining

The principles behind this approach are the same as those for immunoperoxidase staining. This technology would be used under similar circumstances to the above. However, the use of an extra layer allows the amplification of this immunocytochemical reaction to a point where antigens of low incidence may be detected which would not be clearly seen with the immunoperoxidase method (*see* **Note 4**).

1. Ring sections with polysiloxane.
2. Apply a first layer monoclonal antibody and incubate for 30 min at room temperature.
3. Wash in Tris buffered saline (TBS) for 2 min and apply the goat antimouse immunoglobulin for 30 min.
4. Wash again in TBS for 2 min and apply a mouse alkaline phosphatase antialkaline phosphatase complex and incubate for a further 30 min.
5. Wash in TBS for 2 min and apply substrate/chromogen (Fast Red or Fast Blue) solution and incubate at room temperature for 3–15 min.
6. Rinse slides in TBS followed by a rinse in water, and counterstain in hematoxylin.
7. Mount in PBS/glycerol 9:1.

3.2.3. Immunofluorescence

Often, two separate antigens need to be identified within the same section, for example either identification in two separate cells or localization of surface antigens (e.g., complement receptor on a particular cell type). The normal approach used is that of double immunofluorescence *(9)*. In this procedure two monoclonal antibodies are used that differ either in class or subclass and these can then be discriminated using second-layer reagents specific either for the class or subclass of these first layer reagents. The two second-layer reagents will be selectively conjugated with either fluorescein (FITC) or rhodamine (TRITC), thus offering a red and green fluorescent distinction between the two antigens identified. This is a standard procedure used on lung tissues.

1. Ring section with polysiloxane.
2. Apply a first layer combination of two appropriately diluted monoclonal antibodies.
3. Rinse in PBS for 2 min.
4. Apply a second layer combination of two fluorochrome-conjugated goat antimouse heteroantisera that can between them discriminate the classes or subclasses of the antibodies used in the first layer (e.g., G & M IgG FITC: G & M IgM – TRITC) (*see* **Table 2**).
5. Wash in PBS for 2 min.
6. Mount in 9:1 PBS/glycerol.

This preparation is observed with a fluorescence microscope with epi-illumination and appropriate barrier filters for FITC and TRITC. Such an approach is ideal for revealing the relative distribution of macrophages vs other immunocompetent cells in the section, or discriminating subpopulations of macrophages (e.g., using monoclonal antibodies RFD1 and RFD7) or identifying on macrophages specific functionally relevant surface molecules, such as F_cRI.

3.3. Flow Cytometry

The identification of lung macrophages from BAL using flow cytometry has been hampered by problems of autofluorescence within the macrophages. However, some workers *(10)* have been able to use the autofluorescence to discriminate using flow cytometry the alveolar macrophages from dendritic cells and thus investigate these two populations separately. Furthermore, there are now techniques that can quench the autofluorescence (*see* **Subheading 3.3.1.**). In our laboratory we have used flow cytometry to look at the subpopulations of macrophages identified by the monoclonal antibodies RFD1 and RFD7 *(11)*. These studies were performed on peripheral blood monocytes matured into macrophages in vitro. The method, however, for investigating macrophages in BAL would be the same.

The protocol used for the flow cytometer was standard. An analysis was performed using a live gate setting on the antigen presenting cells (APC) populations.

1. Cell suspensions are prepared in PBS at a concentration of 5×10^5 cells/100 μL.
3. All cell suspensions are permeabilised and fixed.
3. Monoclonal antibodies RFD1 (IgM 1:10) and RFD7 (IgG1 1:100) are used in combination to identify the macrophage subpopulations. This incubation is followed by a second layer containing appropriate phycoerythrin and/or FITC labeled goat antimouse antibodies at a dilution of 1:300.

4. Cell suspensions are centrifuged (300*g* for 5 min), washed and resuspended in PBS to apply to the flow cytometer.

3.3.1. Autofluorescence Quenching

The levels of auto-fluorescence are such that they may make it impossible to analyze macrophages by flowcytometry. Autofluorescence can be reduced using the following procedure.

1. After the second layer goat antimouse phycoerythrin or FITC labeled antibodies have been used the cells are washed with PBS and centrifuged at 300*g* for 5 min.
2. The cell pellets are resuspended in 0.2-mL saturated (2 mg per mL) crystal violet solution and incubated at room temperature for 5 min.
3. Cells are then washed with 2-mL PBS, centrifuged at 400*g* for 8 min and resuspended in 0.5-mL PBS. They are now ready for analysis (*see* **Note 5**).

3.4. Cell Separation

Separating macrophages and/or monocytes is traditionally done in one of two ways:

1. Adherence of macrophages and monocytes to glass or plastic substrates.
2. Separation using monoclonal antibody-labeled magnetic beads to either positively or negatively select cells from a mixed population.

3.4.1. Cell Separation Using Adherence

This method can be applied to BAL samples.

1. Pass the BAL through several layers of surgical gauze to remove any remaining mucus.
2. Centrifuge the lavage at 400*g* for 10 min and resuspend the cells in PBS. Repeat this washing procedure a second time and then resuspend the cells in RPMI medium supplemented with 10% fetal calf serum (FCS) at a cell concentration of 1-5 × 10⁶ cells per mL (*see* **Note 6**).
3. Place appropriate volumes of these cells into either Petri dishes or multi-welled plates allowing a cell concentration of approx 1 × 10⁶ cells per cm² and place in the incubator for 2 h in an atmosphere of 5% CO_2 at 37°C.
4. After 2 h the culture vessel should be removed and the supernatant aspirated.
5. The adherent cells should be washed gently with fresh RPMI at 37°C and after washing to remove nonadherent cells the adherent population should be covered with RPMI at 4°C and the culture vessel placed in the refrigerator for 30 min.
6. After this time in the cold, the adherent cells should be scraped off the base of the culture vessels using a cell scraper (a.k.a. "rubber policeman").
7. Harvested cells and supernatant are transferred to a fresh tube, kept on ice and centrifuged at 4°C at 400*g* for 10 min and resuspended in cold PBS (*see* **Note 7**).

3.4.2. Cell Separation using Magnetic Beads

Magnetic bead technology has by and large superseded the above method and allows separation of cells to a purity of over 95%. The procedure below can be used for up to a total of 10^9 positive cells.

1. Prepare a washed population of BAL cells.
2. Resuspend in 80 μL PBS supplemented with 0.5% BSA and 2 mM EDTA to a concentration of 10^7 total cells per 80 μL.
3. To this suspension add 20 μL MACS CD14 labeled or CD68 labeled micro beads per 10^7 total cells.
4. Mix well and incubate for 15 min at 4^0C.
5. Wash the cells by adding 10–20 × the labeling volume buffer and then recentrifuge them at 300g for 10 min.
6. Remove the supernatant and resuspend the cell pellet in 500 μL buffer for every 10^8 total cells.
   The cells are now ready to apply to the magnetic separation column (*see* **Note 8**).
7. Wash the column with 500 μL of appropriate buffer and apply the cell suspension in this buffer at a volume of 500–1000 μL.
8. Allow the negative cells to pass through the column and rinse with further buffer (3 × 500 μL).
9. Remove the column from the separator and place above a suitable collection tube.
10. Apply a further 1 mL buffer to the top of the column and flush out the positive cells using the plunger supplied.

With the combination of positive and negative selection described above, it is possible to isolate pure populations of not only monocytes and macrophages but also subpopulations within the macrophage pool, discriminated via their antigen phenotype.

3.5. Function of Macrophages

Macrophages are recognized as being multifunctional cells. Detailed below are techniques that can be applied to test some of this capacity. In the case of lung macrophages, one is normally interested in three specific functions:

1. Phagocytosis.
2. Regulation (in terms of the production of immunoregulatory cytokines).
3. Antigen presentation.

Methods to determine these functional characteristics are described below.

3.5.1. Phagocytosis

1. Prepare suspension of macrophages on monocytes to be tested as described above. 1×10^5 cells per mL in supplemented RPMI.
2. Place as 1 mL aliquots in each well of 24-well plates.

3. Add fluorescein-coated latex beads of 1 μM diameter at a relative concentration of 100 beads per cell.

4. To half the wells, add cytochalasin B at 2×10^5M in 0.2% dimethylsulphoxide to block phagocytosis *(13)*.

5. Incubate all cells for 2 h at 37°C in 5% CO_2 in a humidified incubator.

6. Harvest cells as described above for separation.

7. After harvest readjust concentration to 5×10^5 cells per mL and prepare cytospins with 50 μL aliquots of the suspension.

8. View the cytospins under a fluorescence microscope counting 100 cells and documenting the percentage of cells with five or more beads inside. Do this for both the test and the control cytospins and subtract any proportion of cells with five beads attached on the control from the figures derived from the test sample.

3.5.2. Cytokine Production

Production of cytokines by separated macrophages and monocytes can be determined either by methods of in situ hybridization which detect mRNA for specific cytokines or by quantification of the released cytokine in the culture supernatant. We have used both these approaches. Methods of in situ hybridization are best suited to the study of cells within tissue sections.

Where isolated cells in suspension are available the measurement of released cytokine using ELISA technology reflects better this functional capacity of the macrophage populations. We and others have found that IL-1, TNFα, and TGFβ levels show relevance to the regulatory role of macrophages, but many other cytokines produced by these cells are of considerable interest and can be quantified. The assay procedure is described in detail with the commercial kits used. Below we describe how the macrophages to test for cytokine production should be prepared.

1. Resuspend separated macrophages and monocytes (see above) in AIM V serum-free medium at a concentration of $1–3 \times 10^6$ cells per mL.

2. Culture the cells at 37°C for 24–48 h in humidified 5% CO_2 (*see* **Note 9**).

3. For activation of the cells lipopolysacharide may be added at the start of culture at aconcentration of $10^{-5} M$ *(13)*.

4. After 24 or 48 h, harvest the supernatants and centrifuge at 400g for 10 min. Aspirate the supernatants and apply these to the ELISA test kits purchased commercially (*see* **Note 10**).

3.5.3. Antigen Presentation

This is normally investigated using either one-way mixed lymphocyte reactions or antigen-driven lymphocyte transformation. The former test is used for routine analysis of macrophage APC capacity. The latter test is used if the presentation of a specific antigen is to be investigated.

1. Prepare peripheral blood lymphocyte suspensions using density centrifugation from a donor unrelated to the subject from which the macrophage/monocyte population under test is derived.
2. Place 100 μL peripheral blood mononuclear cells (PBMC) solution at a concentration of 5×10^6 cells per mL in supplemented RPMI into sufficient numbers of wells of a 96-well microtiter plate to ensure all tests and controls can be done in triplicate.
3. Prepare homogenous macrophage populations (separated as detailed above).
4. Add 100 μL macrophage suspension containing 5×10^5 macrophages to all but 3 of the wells containing the allogeneic lymphocytes.
5. To these 3 remaining wells add 100 μL of culture medium, as an autologous control.
6. To at least 1 triplicate set of macrophage/lymphocyte mix, add mitomycin C at a concentration of 1 mM to block any division and record nonspecific absorption of isotope.
7. Culture plates should be incubated for 6 d at 37°C in humidified 5% CO_2.
8. On day 6, add 10 μL tritiated thymidine (1 μCi, specific activity 5Ci mMol) to each well.
9. After 18 h, harvest all wells using an automated microtiter plate cell harvester. Levels of lymphocyte stimulation/APC capacity are determined by thymidine incorporation measured on a scintillation counter.

4. Notes

1. Using screw cap universal tubes and liquid nitrogen can be dangerous. If liquid nitrogen enters the tube the liquid gas can rapidly expand when the tube is removed from the N_2 container, causing an explosion. To avoid this, a hole must be punctured in the cap of the universal tube so that any liquid nitrogen inside the tube can rapidly escape as a gas on expansion. Small freezing tubes with screw caps are designed to avoid liquid nitrogen getting inside, however there is still a remote risk of explosion and extreme care should be taken when handling these, including the use of facemasks and gloves.
2. We prefer to store sections rather than tissue blocks and tend to cut significant numbers of sections and store these at –20°C. For the vast majority of monoclonal antibodies we may wish to use, we obtain good results even after 18 mo of storage. Less success is obtained if tissue blocks are stored for this time or if they are constantly removed from the liquid nitrogen for section cutting and replaced.
3. Frozen sections do not exhibit the clarity in terms of morphology that paraffin wax embedded samples do. To improve morphology, tissues may be fixed in paraformaldehyde prior to freezing, *(13)*.
4. On balance this alkaline phosphatase anti-alkaline phosphatase technique is the preferred approach if paraformaldehyde fixed sections are to be used.
5. Although the cells look purple and the suspension may still have some color, this procedure significantly quenches the autofluorescence within the macrophages.
6. The medium should be prewarmed to 37°C before the cells are suspended in it.

7. This procedure routinely generates an 80–95% pure population of monocytes/ macrophages the major contaminating cells being B cells but some T cells do remain in the suspension.
8. Column set up depends upon the total number of cells being used for the separation, the details given in the methods are for separation for up to 10^7 positive cells.
9. Culture times will vary depending on cytokine production tested and status of cells.
10. If necessary, supernatants may be concentrated. A 200 µL sample is normally required for the ELISA test. Thus, a 2-mL culture can be concentrated 10-fold before analysis. It is recommended, however, that all tests are performed in duplicate and it is important to ensure one has sufficient material before concentration is considered.

Acknowledgments

The authors are pleased to acknowledge the financial support of Glaxo Wellcome UK for their work on lung macrophages.

References

1. Mearlen, J., nan Hoorst, W., de Wit, H. J., et al. (1994) Distribution and immunophenotype of mononuclear phagocytes and dendritic cells in the human lung. *Am. Rev. Resp. Cell Mol. Biol.* **10,** 487–492.
2. Prokhorova, S., Lavnikova, N., and Laskin, D.L. (1994) Functional characterisation of interstitial macrophages and sub-populations of alveolar macrophages from rat lung. *J. Leuco.Biol.* **66,** 141–146.
3. Poulter, L. W. (1997) Pulmonary macrophages, in *Pulmonary Defences,* Stockley, R.A., ed., Wiley Publ., Chiclester, England, pp. 77–92.
4. Spiteri, M. A., Clarke, S. W.,and Poulter, L. W. (1994) The isolation of phenotypically and functionally distinct alveolar macrophages from human bronchoalveolar lavage. *Eur. Resp. J.* **5,** 717–726.
5. Spiteri, M. A. and Poulter, L. W. (1991) Characterisation of immune inducer and suppressor macrophages from normal human lung. *Clin. Exp. Immunol.* **83,** 157–163.
6. Lapa eSilva, J. R., Guerreiro, D., Munro, N.C., et al. (1990) Cell mediated immune kinetics in experimental Bronchiectasis, in: *Advances in Mucosal Immunology.* MacDonald, T. T, Challacombe, S. J.,Bland, P. W., Stokes, C. R., Heatley, R. V., Mowat, A. M ., eds., Kluwer Publishers, pp. 821–824.
7. Ainslie, G., Poulter, L. W., and duBois, R. M. (1989) Relation between immunocytological features of bronchoalveolar lavage fluid and clinical indices in sarcoidosis. *Thorax* **44,** 501.
8. Royal College of Pathologists. (March 2000) Guidelines for the retention of tissues and organs at post-mortem examination.
9. Janossy, G., Bofill, M., and Poulter, L. W. (1986) Two colour immuno-fluorescence analysis of the lymphoid system with monoclonal antibodies, in: *Immunocytochemistry Today.* Polak, J., Van Noorden, S. J., eds., Wright & Sons Bristol. 438–449.

10. Havenith, C. E., vanHaarst, J. M., Breedijt, S.. et al. (1994) Enrichment and characterisation of dendritic cells from human bronchoalveolar lavages. *Clin. Exp. Immunol.* **96,** 339–343.
11. Taams, L. S., Poulter, L. W., Rustin, M. H. A., and Akbar, A. N. (1999) Phenotypic analysis of IL10-treated macrophages using monoclonal antibodies RFD1 and RFD7. *Pathobiology* **67,** 249–252.
12. Axline, S., and Reaven, E. P. (1974) Inhibition of phagocytosis and plasma membrane motility of the cultivated macrophage by cytochalasin B. Role of subplasmalemmal microfilmaments. *J. Cell Biol.* 647–659.
13. Jeffrey, P. K. (1991) Morphology of the airway wall in asthma and in chronic obstructive pulmonary disease. *Am. Rev. Resp. 1Dis.* **143,** 1152–1158.

17

Collection, Separation, and Activation of Human T Lymphocytes

Yannis Sotsios and Stephen G. Ward

1. Introduction

There is increasing evidence that T lymphocytes play a central role in regulating both the initial and chronic inflammatory cascades of allergic asthma *(1,2)* and can also regulate baseline airway responsiveness in mouse models of asthma *(3)*. In particular, activation of antigen-specific CD4+ T cells of the Th2 subset in the lungs, resulting in interleukin (IL)-5 secretion, plays a major role in allergic inflammation of the airways *(4)*. T-cell activation requires two signals, one provided by interaction between the TCR and specific antigen in association with major histocompatability antigens (MHC) class II molecules, the other provided by costimulatory molecules *(5,6)*. CD28 is the best-characterized costimulatory molecule and is constitutively expressed on the surface of both CD4+ and CD8+ T lymphocytes *(5,6)*. CD28 and its homolog CTLA-4 bind the natural ligands B7.1 and B7.2 (also known as CD80 and CD86, respectively), which are present on antigen presenting cells *(APCs) (5,6)*. CD28 ligation provides cyclosporin A-resistant biochemical signals to T cells, which are an absolute requirement to drive proliferation and IL-2 production from CD3-stimulated T cells, as well as enhance cell survival *(5,6)*. In contrast, CTLA-4 negatively regulates the immune response *(7,8)*. Costimulation through B7.2 has been demonstrated to be required for the induction of lung mucosal Th2 immune response and altered airway responsiveness *(4)*, whereas B7.1 costimulation has been reported to be essential for the maintenance or amplification of lung inflammatory responses *(9)*. Hence, better understanding of the biochemical and functional effects of CD28 and CTLA-4 is essential to formulating better strategies aimed at inhibition of CD28 interaction with its

From: *Methods in Molecular Medicine, vol. 56:*
Human Airway Inflammation: Sampling Techniques and Analytical Protocols
Edited by: D. F. Rogers and L. E. Donnelly © Humana Press Inc., Totowa, NJ

ligands as these may represent a possible therapeutic target for the treatment of lung mucosal allergic inflammation.

This chapter will deal specifically with the collection, isolation, and activation of peripheral blood derived T lymphocytes, although most of the techniques described can just as easily be applied with some modifications to the isolation and activation of T cells in suspension derived from lymphoid tissues.

Two strategies for the purification of untouched CD3$^+$ T lymphocytes are described and both are negative selection systems in which the unwanted cells (e.g., B-cells, monocytes, NK cells, dendritic cells, early erythroid cells, platelets, and basophils) are immunomagnetically labeled using hapten-conjugated antibodies to specific cell markers and then bound to a magnetic column. The desired cells are collected in the column flowthrough and as such, these cells have not had antibody bound to their surface and are therefore suitable for further functional studies.

The research applications for isolated T lymphocytes include: functional studies on CD3$^+$ T cells; studies on signaling requirements for T-cell activation, T-cell proliferation or induction of anergy; studies on signal transduction in T cells; and studies on regulation of T-cell cytokine/chemokine expression.

2. Materials

2.1. Reagents

All reagents are from Sigma (Dorset, UK) unless otherwise stated; all cell culture media and supplements are from Life Technologies (Paisley, UK); materials and apparatus for MACS Microbead and Dynabead separation of T cells are from Miltenyi Biotec (Sunnyvale, CA) and Dynal (Dynal, Lake Success, NY), respectively.

1. Phosphate Buffered Saline (PBS) without Ca^{2+} ions: 155 mM NaCl, 1.5 mM KH$_2$PO$_4$, 3 mM Na$_2$HPO$_4$, adjust to pH 7.2–7.4 with HCl if necessary.
2. Buffer 1 (PBS containing 2 mM ethylenediaminetetraacetic acid(EDTA) and 1% BSA.
3. Tissue culture medium (RPMI-1640).
3. Heat-inactivated Fetal Calf Serum (FCS).
4. Penicillin and streptomycin for tissue culture (*see* **Note 1**).
5. Neubauer hemocytometer and glass coverslips.
6 Fluorochrome-conjugated antibodies for flow cytometric control of T-cell isolation.
7. Lymphoprep (density 1.077; Nycomed, Birmingham, UK).
8. Heparin solution (500 U/mL Monoparin; CP Pharmaceuticals, Wrexham, UK).
9. Phytohemagglutinin (5 mg/mL stock solution).

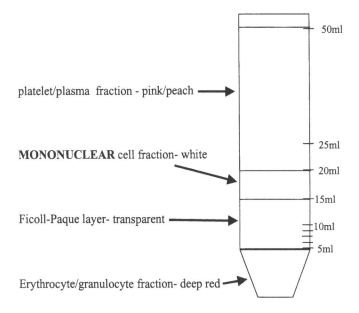

platelet/plasma fraction - pink/peach ⟶

MONONUCLEAR cell fraction- white

Ficoll-Paque layer- transparent ⟶

Erythrocyte/granulocyte fraction- deep red ⟶

50ml

25ml
20ml
15ml
10ml
5ml

Fig. 1. Schematic diagram of PBMC separation after centrifugation with Lymphoprep. The diagram is representative of the separated layers after centrifugation with Lymphoprep, as they appear ideally undisturbed in a transparent conical 50-mL tube.

10. Human recombinant IL-2 (1 mg/mL stock solution).
11. [^{3}H]-thymidine (2Ci/mmol; Amersham-Pharmacia Biotech, Bucks, UK).
12. MACS hapten-antibody cocktail or mouse anti-human antibodies against unwanted cell surface markers (e.g., anti-CD11b, anti-CD16, anti-CD19, anti-CD36, and anti-CD56).
13. MACS anti-hapten-coupled supramagnetic microbeads or magnetic Dynabeads M-450 covalently coupled to sheep anti-mouse IgG.
14. MACS separation column(s).
15. Fluorochrome conjugated antibodies for flow cytometrc control of T-cell isolation (e.g., anti-CD3-fluorescein isothiocyanate (FITC) and anti-CD2-FITC; Serotec, Oxford, UK).

2.2. Apparatus

1. MACS Magnetic Cell Separator or Dynal Magnetic Particle Concentrator.
2. Standard benchtop centrifuges and microfuges.
3. Flow cytometer for surface marker analysis.
4. Automated cell harvester.

3. Methods

3.1. Isolation of Peripheral Blood Mononuclear Cells (PBMC)

1. Start with fresh human peripheral blood treated with 10 U/mL heparin as an anti-coagulant or leukocyte buffy coat not older than 8 h (*see* **Note 2**).
2. Dilute blood with 2–4 vol of RPMI-1640 (*see* **Note 3**).
3. Carefully layer 35 mL of diluted cell suspension over 15-mL Lymphoprep (1.077 density) in a 50-mL transparent conical centrifuge tube and centrifuge at 400g for 30–40 min at 20°C without the brake (*see* **Note 4**).
4. After centrifugation, aspirate the upper layer (autologous serum that can be used as a buffer supplement) leaving the mononuclear cell layer undisturbed at the interphase (*see* **Fig. 1**) (*see* **Note 4**).
5. Carefully transfer the mononuclear cell layer (e.g., lymphocytes, monocytes) to a new 50-mL conical centrifuge tube.
6. Fill the conical tube with RPMI-1640 or PBS, mix and centrifuge at 400g for 10 min at 20°C. Carefully remove the supernatant either by decanting into an appropriate sterile waste container or by aspiration, taking care not to disturb the pellet. These washes are important to remove any Lymphoprep that may have been transferred with the peripheral blood mononuclear cells (PBMC) (*see* **Note 5**).
7. Resuspend the cell pellet in 50 mL of RPMI-1640/PBS and centrifuge at 400g for 10–15 min at 20°C. Carefully remove the supernatant completely and repeat this wash twice more.
8. Resuspend the cell pellet in an appropriate volume of RPMI-1640. Count the cells using Trypan blue and hemocytometer and proceed to the next step.

3.2. Preparation of PHA-Activated Human Lymphoblasts

Human PBMC are activated by culture with the mitogen phytohemagglutinin (PHA) for a total of 3 days, during which time the T cells become lymphoblasts. On day 3, the cultures are washed free of mitogen and IL-2 is added to promote lymphoblast proliferation. On day 5, the lymphoblasts are harvested, washed, and adjusted to the desired cell concentration.

1. Collect peripheral blood cells from normal donors as described in **Subheading 3.1**.
2. Suspend PBMC in 50-mL supplemented medium at 1×10^6/mL and add to a 80-cm^2 culture flask. Add 50 µL of 5 mg/mL PHA and shake flask to mix. Incubate horizontally for 3 d (*see* **Note 6**).
3. After 3 days in culture, decant the nonadherent cells into a 50-mL conical tube and centrifuge. Carefully remove the supernatant completely by decanting into waste container or by aspiration, taking care not to disturb the pellet.
4. Resuspend the cell pellet in 50-mL RPMI-1640 and centrifuge at 350g for 10–15 min at 20°C. Carefully remove the supernatant completely and repeat this wash 2 times. These washes remove residual mitogen or super-antigen (*see* **Note 7**).
5. Resuspend the cell pellet in 50-mL supplemented medium and transfer the cells to a clean 80-cm^2 flask. Add human recombinant IL-2 to flask to a final concentration of 20 ng/mL, then incubate for 48 h in a humidified CO_2 incubator.

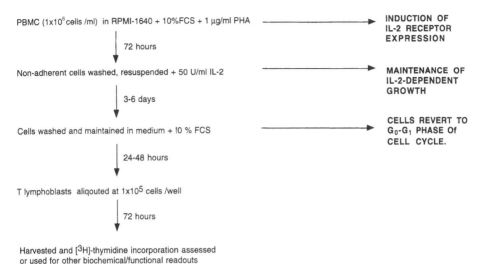

PBMC (1x10⁶ cells /ml) in RPMI-1640 + 10%FCS + 1 µg/ml PHA ⟶ **INDUCTION OF IL-2 RECEPTOR EXPRESSION**

↓ 72 hours

Non-adherent cells washed, resuspended + 50 U/ml IL-2 ⟶ **MAINTENANCE OF IL-2-DEPENDENT GROWTH**

↓ 3-6 days

Cells washed and maintained in medium + !0 % FCS ⟶ **CELLS REVERT TO G₀-G₁ PHASE Of CELL CYCLE.**

↓ 24-48 hours

T lymphoblasts aliqouted at 1x10⁵ cells /well

↓ 72 hours

Harvested and [³H]-thymidine incorporation assessed or used for other biochemical/functional readouts

Fig. 2. A schematic summary of the preparation of T lymphoblasts.

6. After another 48 h, the cell cultures can be expanded so that half of the cell suspension is removed into clean 80-cm^2 or 175-cm^2 flasks. Add two volumes of supplemented medium to each flask and 50 U/mL human recombinant IL-2. Repeat this step every 48 h up until day 10 (*see* **Fig. 2**).

7. The T lymphoblasts can be used for experimentation from day 8–14. Two days before experimentation, they are washed 3 times in serum-free medium and resuspended in supplemented medium without IL-2. This treatment ensures that the lymphocytes accumulate in the G_0-G_1 phase of the cell cycle. These cells have been stimulated to express the IL-2 receptor by PHA treatment and maintained in culture with IL-2. They will no longer produce endogenous IL-2 by the time of utilization in an assay, but they will respond to exogenous IL-2 and can be used for biochemical and functional analysis (*10*).

3.3. Preparation of Purified T Lymphocytes by Negative Selection

This method utilizes an indirect magnetic labeling system for the isolation of untouched CD3$^+$ T cells from human PBMC by magnetic depletion of B cells, monocytes, NK cells, dendritic cells, early erythroid cells, platelets, and basophils. A cocktail of hapten-conjugated CD11b, CD16, CD19, CD36, and CD56 antibodies in combination with MACS Microbeads coupled to an anti-hapten monoclonal antibody is used for the depletion of non-T cells. The magnetically labeled cells are depleted by retention on a MACS column in the magnetic field of a MACS magnetic cell separator. Isolation of highly pure T cells with excellent recoveries can be achieved using the above system which does not stain or activate the desired cell fraction.

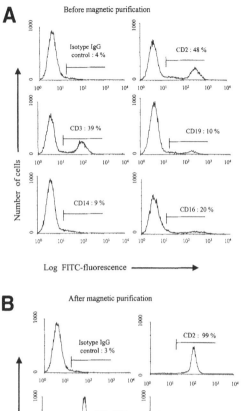

Fig. 3. Effect of magnetic Dynabead purification of T cells on the expression of PBMC surface markers. 1×10^5 freshly isolated PBMC cells/point were analyzed for surface expression of CD2, CD3, CD19, CD14, and CD16 with specific monoclonal primary antibodies or isotype-matched control antibodies, before (**A**), or immediately after (**B**), magnetic Dynabead purification of resting T cells. The cells were analyzed with an FITC-conjugated goat anti-mouse polyvalent (anti-IgM, IgG, IgA) secondary antibody on a Becton Dickinson FACS Vantage; excitation λ 488 nm, emission λ 530 nm. Expression percentages are indicated for each surface marker examined. Expression profiles shown are from one experiment representative of five other T-cell purifications.

1. Collect adherent cell-depleted PBMC from normal donor as described in **Sub-heading 3.1**.
2. Count the cells using trypan blue and wash them three times in calcium free PBS supplemented with 2 mM EDTA at 6–12°C.
3. Resuspend the cell pellet in 80 µL of PBS supplemented with 2 mM EDTA and 1% w/v bovine serum albumin (BSA) (Buffer 1) for 1×10^7 viable cells, always at 6–12°C.
4. Add 20 µL of MACS Hapten -Antibody Cocktail per 10^7 total cells (*see* **Note 8**).
5. Mix well and incubate for 10 min at 6–12°C (*see* **Note 9**).
6. Wash cells carefully with Buffer 1 by adding 10–20× the labeling volume, centrifuge and remove supernatant. Repeat this washing step.
7. Resuspend cell pellet carefully in 80 µL of Buffer 1 per 10^7 total cells. Add 20 µL of MACS Anti-hapten Microbeads per 10^7 total cells to label the cells magnetically.
8. Mix well and incubate for 15 min at 6–12°C with rotation.
9. Wash cells carefully with buffer by adding 10–20× the labeling volume, centrifuge and remove supernatant completely.
10. Resupend the pellet in 500 µL of Buffer 1 per 10^8 total cells (for less cells use 500 µL) (*see* **Note 10**).
11. Place a MACS separation column (e.g., column type CS) in the magnetic field of an appropriate MACS Magnetic Cell Separator (*see* **Note 11**).
12. Apply cell suspension onto the depletion column (*see* **Note 12**)
13. Let the unlabeled cells pass through and collect effluent as negative fraction, representing enriched T-cell fraction (*see* **Note 12**).
14. Rinse the column with 30 mL of Buffer 1 and collect effluent as negative fraction, representing the enriched T-cell fraction (*see* **Notes 12 and 13**).
15. The purity of the isolated T cells can be evaluated by staining aliquots of the cell fractions with a fluorochrome-conjugated antibody against T-cell surface molecules (e.g., CD2-FITC and CD3-FITC) and analysis by flow cytometry (**Fig. 3**) (*see* **Notes 13 and 14**).

3.4. Activation of Purified T Lymphocytes or T Lymphoblasts

Once T cells have been purified or they have been maintained in culture as T lymphoblasts in the presence of IL-2, they can be used for the appropriate biochemical and functional studies that are required. The most common measurement of lymphocyte function is the capacity to proliferate which can be assessed by incorporation of [^{3}H]-thymidine into T-lymphocyte DNA. The procedure below describes the use of purified T cells in assessing the role of CD28 in costimulation of T lymphocytes:

1. The isolated T lymphocytes or T lymphoblasts are aliquoted into 96-well, flat-bottomed microtiter plates at 6×10^4 cells/well in a final volume of 200 µL supplemented RPMI-1640.
2. If the effect of pharmacological inhibitors on T-cell proliferation is to be studied, the compounds should be applied to the aliquoted cells at the appropriate dilutions prior to proliferative stimulation (*see* **Note 15**).

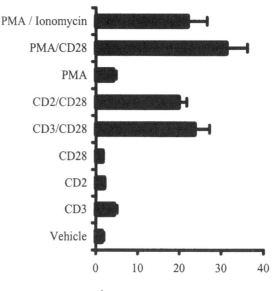

^{3}H-Thymidine incorporation (x 1000 cpm)

Fig. 4. [^{3}H]-thymidine incorporation by purified T lymphocytes. T cells were aliquoted (6×10^4 cells/well) in 96-well tissue culture plates and stimulated as indicated with either humanized anti-CD3 mAb OKT3, anti-CD28 mAb 9.3, or anti-CD2 mAbs 6F103 and 39Ci5, in the combinations described. The anti-CD3, anti-CD2, and anti-CD28 mAbs were covalently attached (either alone or in the combinations indicated) to tosylactivated M-450 Dynabeads at 1 µg/mL each and used at a density of 1 bead/cell. Alternatively, T cells were stimulated with 5 ng/mL PMA (Sigma) alone or in combination with 1 µM ionomycin (Calbiochem, Nottingham, UK) or anti-CD28-coated Ab beads as indicated. Data are the mean ± S.E.M. of quintuplicate samples from a single representative experiment.

3. Quintuplicate aliquots are then treated with 1 µg/mL anti-CD3 Ab (e.g., UCHT1) either in the absence or presence of 1 µg/mL anti-CD28 -Ab (e.g., mAb 9.3). Antibodies are presented either as soluble antibodies that are crosslinked by the addition of a crosslinking anti-mouse Ig antibody or are covalently coupled to tosylactivated M-450 Dynabeads at 1 µg/mL each and used at a density of 1 bead/cell (*see* **Note 16**).
4. The treated plates can be incubated for 54–60 h in a humidified 37°C, 5% CO_2 incubator and then pulsed with 1 µCi/well of sterile [^{3}H]-thymidine diluted in RPMI-1640.
5. After 12–18 h of ^{3}H-thymidine incorporation, or when the total period of cellular incubation has reached 72 h, the plates are ready for harvesting onto GF/A filter paper (Whatman, Maidstone, UK) using a multiple automated cell harvester followed by β-scintillation counting (**Fig. 4**).

4. Notes

1. All incubations are performed in a humidified 37°C, 5% CO_2 incubator unless otherwise noted. All solutions used should be filter-sterilized to minimize contamination. Cell culture medium (e.g., RPMI-1640) is supplemented with 10% heat-inactivated fetal calf serum (FCS), as well as the antibiotics streptomycin (50 µg/mL) and penicillin (50 U/mL).

2. Other anticoagulants such as citrate, acid citrate dextrose, or citrate phosphate dextrose may also be used.

3. Alternatively, blood may be diluted with PBS, which is cheaper.

4. It is important to avoid shaking or any disturbance (such as brake-on deceleration), to the tubes after centrifugation. Precise visual identification of the mononuclear interphase is necessary for optimum purification and depends on transparent conical centrifuge tubes. The bouyant mononuclear cell fraction should be opaque, off-white in color, and located between the 15-mL and 20-mL tube marks. A representative diagram of the separated layers after centrifugation with Lymphoprep, as they appear ideally undisturbed in a transparent conical 50-mL tube, is shown in **Fig. 1.**

5. Prolonged exposure to Lymphoprep can be deleterious to T cells in culture, this is why extensive washing is required.

6. For T-cell lymphoblastic transformation from isolated PBMCs, other mitogenic stimuli such as Concanavalin A, phorbol ester (e.g., 5 ng/mL PMA) in combination with 1 µ*M* ionomycin can be used. Alternativley, super-antigens such as 1µg/mL of the superantigen Staphylococcal Enterotoxin B (SEB) may also be used.

7. Activated T cells such as T-lymphoblasts exposed to mitogen in combination with further stimulation such as IL-2 or CD3 ligation can undergo programmed cell death or become unresponsive. Hence, mitogen has to be removed after 3 days with extensive washing.

8. Avoid capping of antibodies on the cell surface during labeling by working fast and keeping cells cold. Use cold solutions only.

9. Increased temperature and prolonged incubation time for labeling may lead to nonspecific T-cell labeling and hence lower T-cell yields.

10. Use degassed buffer only. Degassing can be achieved by applying vacuum or sonication. Excess of gas in buffer will form bubbles in the matrix of the column during separation. This may lead to clogging of the column and decreases the quality of the separation.

11. A range of MACS columns are available. The type of column should be selected according to individual needs and the column(s) should be prepared according to manufacturer's specifications. For larger cell numbers (up to 2×10^8 magnetically labeled cells), use a MACS column type CS.

12. Loading of column, washing and elution of enriched T cells takes 10–20 min. To increase sensitivity, cells can be passed over the depletion column a second time.

13. The purity of T cells obtained by depletion on non-T cells is strongly dependent on the quality of the PBMC preparation. Contamination with erythrocytes may cause decreases in the purity of the T-cell yield. Remaining erythrocytes can be

lysed by incubation with excess volume of isotonic ammonium chloride buffer (155 mM NH$_4$Cl, 10 mM KHCO$_3$ and 0.1 mM EDTA) for 5–7 min at room temperature. Cells are then centrifuged at 300g for 15 min at 20°C and washed twice with buffer, resuspending the cell pellet in buffer. Alternatively, remaining erythrocytes can be removed by density gradient centrifugation using Lymphoprep (density 1.077). A typical profile of cellular markers before and after magnetic T-cell purification is shown in **Fig. 3**.

14. An alternative to MACS column separation is to aliquot the PBMC fraction resuspended in supplemented medium into Petri dishes, and incubate for 2 h at 37°C to allow adherence of monocytes to the plastic surface of the plates. After 2 h at 37°C, nonadherent cells are removed using a pipet and placed into a clean conical tube. The plastic-adhered cells can be discarded. Nonadherent cells are incubated with 1 µg/mL anti-CD19, anti-CD14, and anti-MHC-II antibodies for 1 h at 4°C with rotation. Following a thorough wash with RPMI-1640, M450 Dynabeads covalently coupled to sheep anti-mouse IgG are added to PBMC in suspension (2 mL suspension volume per 10^8 cells). Dynabeads should be added to antibody-coated cells to a final concentration of 1–2 × 10^7 Dynabeads per mL of sample and at least four Dynabeads per estimated target cell (always refer to manufacturer's specifications for advice on titration and optimal use of the Dynabead product). Incubate for 30 min at 4°C with rotation. Bound monocytes and B cells, as well as any potential APCs expressing MHC-II are removed by magnetic separation using a Dynal Magnetic Particle Concentrator. This Dynabead separation has the advantage of using a cheaper magnet than the MACS magnetic separator, and the primary antibody composition can be custom-designed according to individual requirements. Use of the Dynal Magnetic Particle Concentrators ensures reliable isolation of cells within 2 min.

15. Most inhibitors require a certain time of incubation to take effect and should not be administered at the same time as the proliferative stimulations.

16. Alternatively, microtiter plates can be precoated with antibodies prior to the addition of T cells. In this case, 1 µg/mL of the appropriate anti-CD3 and/or anti-CD28 antibodies are aliquoted in 200 µL PBS into the 96-well plate and incubated overnight at 37°C. The plate is then washed twice in RPMI-1640 prior to the addition of cells. An alternative to using anti-CD28 Abs is to use the natural ligand for CD28 namely B7.1/B7.2 that has been stably transfected into chinese hamster ovary (CHO) cells *(11)*. These cells are paraformaldehyde fixed and 2 × 10^4 cells are added to the T cells (i.e., 1 CHO-B7$^+$ cells : 3 T cells). Finally, T cells may be activated by the addition of phorbol ester (e.g., 5 ng/mL PMA) either in combination with 1 µM ionomycin or with anti-CD28 Abs or CHO-B7.1$^+$ cells. A proliferation profile measuring [^{3}H]-thymidine incorporation after 72 h in culture is shown in **Fig. 4**.

References

1. Azzawi, M., Bradley, B., Jeffery, P. K., Frew, A. J., Wardlaw, A. J., Knowles, G., et al. (1990) Identification of activated T lymphocytes and eosinophils in bronchial biopsies in stable atopic asthma. *Am. Rev. Resp. Dis*. **142,** 1407–1413.

2. Walker, C., Bode, E., Boer, L., Hansel, T. T., Blaser, K., and Virchow, J. C. (1992) Allergic and nonallergic asthmatics have distinct patterns of T cell activation and cytokine production in peripheral-blood and bronchoalveolar lavage. *Am. Rev. Resp. Dis.* **146,** 109–115.

3. De Sanctis, G. T., Itoh, A., Green, F. H. Y., Qin, S., Kimura, T., Grobholz, J. K., et al. (1997) T lymphocytes regulate genetically determined airway hyperresponsiveness in mice. *Nature Med.* **3,** 460–462.

4. Tsuyuki, S., Tsuyuki, J., Einsle, K., Kopf, M. and Coyle, A. J. (1997) Costimulation through B7.2 (CD86) is required for the induction of a lung mucosal T helper cell 2 (Th2) immune response and altered airway responsiveness. *J. Exp. Med.* **185,** 1671–1679.

5. Ward, SG. (1996) CD28: A signalling perspective. *Biochem J.* **318,** 361–377.

6. Ward SG., June CH., and Olive, D. (1996) PI 3-kinase: A pivotal pathway in T cell activation? *Immunol.Today* **17,** 187–197.

7. Tivol, E. A., Borriello, F., Schweitzer, A. N., Lynch, W. P., Bluestone, J. A., and Sharpe A. H. (1996) Loss of CTLA-4 leads to massive lymphoproliferation and fatal multi-organ tissue destruction, revealing a critical negative regulatory role of CTLA-4. *Immunity* **3,** 541–547.

8. Waterhouse, P., Penninger, J.M,. Timms, E., Wakeham, A., Shahinian, A., Lee, K.P., et al. (1996) Lymphoproliferative disorders with early lethality in mice deficient in CTLA-4. *Science* **270,** 985–988

9. Harris, N., Peach, R., Naemura, J., Linsley, P.S., Le Gros, G., and Ronchese, F. (1997) CD80 costimulation is essential for the induction of airway eosinophilia. *J. Exp. Med.* **185,** 177–182.

10. Cantrell, D. A. and Smith, K. A. (1984) The interleukin 2 T cell system: a new cell growth model. *Science* **224,** 1312–1315.

11. Ward, S. G., Wilson, A., Turner, L., Westwick, J., and Sansom, D. M. (1995) Inhibition of CD28-mediated T cell costimulation by the phosphoinositide 3-kinase inhibitor wortmannin. *Eur. J. Immunol.* **25,** 526–532.

18

Eosinophils

Collection, Separation, and Activation

Leo Koenderman, Jan van der Linden, Laurien Ulfman, and Paul Coffer

1. Introduction

Granulocytes play an important role in the host defense against invading microorganisms such as bacteria and fungi *(1,2)*. For the killing reaction, these cells have an extensive machinery of cytotoxic effector mechanisms including phagocytosis, production of toxic oxygen metabolites, initiated by a membrane bound nicotinamide adenine dinucleotide phosphate (NADPH)-oxidase, and degranulation of cytotoxic proteins (for reviews *see 1,2*). Apart from being cytotoxic, these cells are also involved in maintaining inflammatory reactions by the release of cytokines and bioactive lipids such as platelet-activating factor and arachidonic acid metabolites. Uncontrolled activation of neutrophils plays an important role in the pathogenesis of diseases like acute respiratory distress syndrome (ARDS) and septic shock. Syndromes associated with granulocyte dysfunctions can cause severe clinical conditions *(1,2)*.

Granulocyte activation is a multistep process. It is widely accepted now that optimal activation of granulocytes by semiphysiological activators requires priming by chemotaxins or cytokines. This priming of functional responses in vitro has been described in detail during the last decade *(3)*. Priming of granulocytes in vivo has been made plausible for eosinophils isolated from the blood of patients with allergic diseases *(4,5)*. Despite the recognition of the importance

From: *Methods in Molecular Medicine, vol. 56:*
Human Airway Inflammation: Sampling Techniques and Analytical Protocols
Edited by: D. F. Rogers and L. E. Donnelly © Humana Press Inc., Totowa, NJ

of priming for neutrophil responses relatively little is known about the intracellular signals responsible for this process.

Priming is also poorly defined in the context of expression of cell surface markers. Some studies describe upregulation of MAC-1, CD66b and downregulation of L-selectin in response to cytokines and chemotaxins *(6,7)*. The interpretation of these studies is hampered by the fact that priming and activation are poorly defined. Low doses of cytokines (pM range) do not cause activation of the respiratory burst and degranulation of azurophil and specific granules. Instead, they preactivate or prime these responses in the context of formylpeptides *(8)* and opsonized particles *(9)*. Another important drawback for the study of granulocyte priming in vitro in the context of cell surface marker expression is the induction of marker expression caused by isolation artefacts *(10)*.

Eosinophils can be isolated from the peripheral blood by several methods. However, most laboratories isolate eosinophils from the peripheral blood with the use of procedures that are based on negative selection with the use of immunomagnetic beads *(11,12)*. The advantages are several: easy, reproducible, high yield, and purity. One of the procedures will be described in detail below (*see* **Subheading 3.1.2.1**). Isolation of eosinophils with the use of these beads has one important drawback. The cells exhibit a relatively high background in several assays designed for the study of cytokine-induced preactivation of eosinophils *(13)*. This finding makes the latter method less appealing when pre-activation processes are subject of study. Consequently, an alternative method will be described which results in the isolation of eosinophils with low background priming (*14, see* **Subheading 3.1.2.2.**).

Motility is one of the responses of eosinophils that is most sensitive for priming by cytokines; migration of eosinophils has been studied in detail. Activated cells crawl through the tissue to the site of infection, guided by certain molecules that are secreted by the invading parasites, or secreted by other cells of the host immune system. Many studies have dealt with the ability of granulocytes to migrate through the tissues and their directional response to these molecules *(15,16)*. Although much detail is known, the more fundamental knowledge of how cells move and how they hone in on the infected site is still missing. Therefore, further methods to study cell migration can be useful. As of old, directed movement of granulocytes (chemotaxis) has been separated from nondirected (random) movement (chemokinesis). We will discuss a method to study both random and directed movement with the use of image analysis.

2. Materials

2.1. Eosinophil Isolation

1. Ficoll paque (1.077g/mL, Pharmacia-Upjohn, Uppsala, Sweden).
2. Percoll (Pharmacia-Upjohn).
3. Pasteurized human plasma solution (GPO, CLB, Amsterdam, The Netherlands).
4. Human serum albumin solution (20% wt/vol, CLB, Amsterdam, The Netherlands).
5. 'Concentrated phosphate-buffered saline (PBS) (dissolve NaCl (90 g/L) and $NaH_2PO_4.H_2O$ (13.8 g/L) in water: *do not adjust pH!*).
6. 10X trisodium citrate (TSC, 38 g/L).
7. RPMI culture medium (Gibco-BRL).
8. CD16 coupled immunomagnetic microspheres (Miltenyi Biotec, Bergisch Gladbach, Germany).
9. HEPES incubation medium: 20 mM HEPES, 132 mM NaCl, 6.0 mM KCl, 1.0 mM $MgSO_4$, 1.2 mM KH_2PO_4, supplemented with 5 mM glucose, 1.0 mM $CaCl_2$, and 0.5% (w/v) human serum albumin (HSA).
10. PBS: NaCl 8.2 g/l, $Na_2HPO_4.12H_2O$ 3.1 g/l, $NaH_2PO_4.2H_2O$ 0.2 g/l, pH 7.4 at 20°C.
11. PBS 2+: PBS supplemented with 10% pasturized plasma solution GPO (v/v) and 10% 10X trisodium citrate (v/v).
12. NH_4Cl lysis solution: NH_4Cl 8.3 g/l, $KHCO_3$ 1.0 g/l, Na_2 ethylenediaminetetraacetic acid (EDTA) 37.2 mg/l, phenol red 10 mg/l, pH 7.4 at 4°C.

2.2. Cell Migration

1. Different buffers can be used for measuring migration including HEPES buffered RPMI or HEPES buffered salt medium: 20 mM HEPES, 132 mM NACl, 6.0 mM KCl, 1.0 mM $MgSO_4$, 1.2 mM KH_2PO_4, supplemented with 5 mM glucose, 1.0 mM $CaCl_2$, and 0.5% (w/v) HSA.
2. Chemoattractants to be tested are dissolved in HEPES buffer in the appropriate concentration. Some experimenting is necessary to obtain correct testing concentrations, too high will sometimes give the same negative results as do too low concentrations.
3. Coatings: In two dimensional assays, several coatings can be applied to the glass substrate. Much used compounds are: poly-L-lysine, fibronectin, laminin, and several forms of collagen. The precise coating conditions of these compounds are, however, beyond the scope of the present chapter. In addition, granulocytes can also be made to move on confluently grown cell layers such as HUVEC and other cell lines.

2.3. Percoll Solutions

First, a Percoll stock solution is prepared [703.9 mL Percoll 1.130 g/mL, 57.5 mL concentrated PBS, 39 mL PBS, 100 mL GPO and 100 mL trisodium citrate(TSC.)] Check whether the density of this stock solution is 1.100 g/mL by a densitometer (e.g., DMA46, Mettler/Paar), pH 7.2 and osmolarity 285–300 mOsm. From this point different Percoll solutions can be made: 1.082 g/mL

(94.5 mL Percoll stock (1.100 g/mL) + 5.5 mL PBS2+) and 1.085 g/mL (83.5 mL Percoll stock (1.100 g/mL) + 16.5 mL PBS 2+).

2.4. Apparatus

To study the directed movement of eosinophils toward cellular stimulants, we use an automated microscope, coupled to a Leica Quantimet 570 Image Analyzer. The Image Analyzer controls a Leica DM-RXE upright microscope equipped with an eight slide scanning stage (Märzhäuser Wetzlar Germany) and a video camera (Sony XC-75CE). Because of the possibility of visiting the same spot over and over again, we can make time lapse sequences of several areas in one same experiment, the inter-image interval being specified by the number of areas imaged, and the speed of the scanning stage. Alternatively, time lapse recordings are made with the use of a black and white framegrabber (Pulsar, Matrox Electronic Systems Ltd., Dorval Quebec, Canada) in a standard PC (PII, 266 MHz, Windows NT,128 Mbyte Memory), running Image Analysis software (Optimas 6.1, Media Cybernetics, Silver Spring, MD). With this setup, of course, experiments are performed sequentially.

3. Methods

3.1 Collection and Isolation of Human Eosinophils

3.1.1. Collection of Blood Samples

Eosinophils are isolated from the peripheral blood anticoagulated with sodium heparin or sodium citrate (0.42% wt/v) and the blood must be kept at room temperature. Avoid at this stage, cooling of samples to limit activation of blood platelets. Ideally, do not store blood samples for longer periods of time (>3 h). Hereafter, the cells are isolated according to the following procedure:

3.1.2. Isolation Procedure

1. Mix whole blood with PBS2+ (1:1) or the buffy coat with PBS2+ (1:3).
2. Layer 25 mL of diluted blood solution on top of 15-mL ficoll paque and spin down (20 min, 1 000g_{avg} at room temp).
3. Remove mononuclear cells and lyse the erythrocytes in the pellet fraction with ice-cold and isotonic NH_4Cl solution (45mL) for 15 min on ice.
4. Spin granulocytes down (5 min 700g) and repeat the lysis procedure in the presence of 0.5% HSA for 5 min on ice.
5. Spin down the cells (5 min 700g) and wash the pellet with ice-cold PBS2+ (isolation procedure **Subheading 3.1.2.1.**) or with PBS2+ at room temperature (isolation procedure **Subheading 3.1.2.2.**).

3.1.2.1. ISOLATION PROCEDURE 1: IMMUNOMAGNETIC BEADS
(*SEE* **REFS. *11, 12*)**

1. Wash 25 µL CD16 coated beads per 100×10^6 granulocytes by adding the beads to the magnetic column (type AS, BS, CS) , add 10 mL PBS2+, remove the column from the Supermacs (Miltenyi Biotec, Bergisch Gladbach, Germany) and collect the fraction with beads in 4 times the starting volume (= 100 µL beads solution)
2. Add anti-CD16 beads to granulocyte fraction: 100×10^6 cells / 100 mL beads solution
3. Incubate for 30 min, 4°C.
4. Dilute the cell-beads suspension 10 times and put on the column, when cell/beads suspension has almost run through, add 3 times 1 mL PBS2+ then add 3 times a column volume PBS2+.
5. Collect the eosinophil solution, spin down the eosinophils (5 min 700*g*). Resuspend in buffer of choice (*see* **Notes 1–4**).

3.1.2.2. ISOLATION PROCEDURE 2: FMLP METHOD (*SEE* **REF. *14*)**

1. Resuspend cells in HEPES buffered RPMI/0.5% HSA and incubate the cells for 30 min at 37°C to restore initial densities of the eosinophils.
2. Spin down the cells and resuspend the cells in PBS2+ (75.106 cells/mL) and incubate the cells for 5 min at 37°C.
3. Add FMLP (10 n*M* final concentration) and continue the incubation for 10 min at 37°C.
4. Layer 1 mL of the cells on a discontinuous Percoll gradient (4 mL Percoll 1.082 g/mL on top of 1 mL Percoll 1.100 g/mL).
5. Spin down the cells (20 min, $1000g_{avg}$ room temperature)
6. Collect the cells from the interface between Percoll 1.082 g/mL and Percoll 1.100 g/mL.
7. Wash the cells with buffer of choice (*see* **Notes 5–7**).

3.2. Chemotaxis/Chemokinesis

3.2.1. Random Movement (Chemokinesis)

Freshly isolated Eosinophils (*see* **Subheading 3.1.2**), are resuspended in appropriate buffer and brought to adhere on the substrate being tested. This is performed by pipeting small drops (about 30–50 mL) on cover slips, and incubating them in a moist environment (water bath at 37°C). After 15 min, nonadhering cells are washed away with buffer, and the cover slips are mounted upside-down on firmer carriers (slide glass or Dunn Chamber slide). The so-formed micro chambers are then sealed with a mixture of paraffin, bees wax, and petroleum jelly (1:1:1 w/w/w). When only two opposite sides are sealed, additional fluids can be brought into the chamber by putting a drop at one of the unsealed sides, and then with a tissue, remove fluid from the opposite side. In this way, cells at rest can be stimulated with a certain agent. When long-term experiments are performed (hours) and temperatures are higher (i.e., 37°C; warming stages), the free chamber sides have to be sealed as well, avoiding evaporation and subsequent defocusing of the image by caving in of the cover slip (*see* **Note 8**).

3.2.2. Directed Movement (chemotaxis)

Dunn chamber (17). To overcome difficulties in creating a gradient of a diffusable chemoattractant on a 2D surface, a variety of chemotactic chambers have been designed, one of the most recent being the Dunn Chamber (*17*). In this ingenious device, circular compartments are separated by a fluid bridge of defined proportions, the ceiling of which consists of a cover slip with attached cells. The circular compartments are filled with standard cell buffer or a dilution of the chemoattractant being tested. It was demonstrated that after a certain time a stable standing gradient of small molecular substances (i.e., chemoattractants) forms in the fluid bridge. Sometimes, these gradients are stable for up to 24 h, permitting very long time lapse sequences of moving cells. This Dunn chamber can be used to assay the directed motility of eosinophils on bare or coated glass substrates.

3.2.3. Time Lapse for Cell Tracking

Time lapse recordings are also made with the use of a black and white framegrabber in a standard PC running Image Analysis software (*see* **Subheading 2.2.**). In this application, standard bright field microscopy is used with 10 × and 20 × lenses. To facilitate later analysis, cells are slightly defocused, thereby creating dark blotches on a white background. Series of 50 images are created with an average inter-image interval of 20 s. An Optimas macro was written for analysis of the image series, which works as follows:

First, the sequence of images is loaded into computer memory and the first image (t=1) is measured for cell positions.

Then for each cell present in the first image, a box with appropriate dimension is drawn centered at the cell position in the next image (t=2), and all cell positions in this box are measured. A nearest neighbor algorithm is then used to find the position closest to the center of the box, and this position is taken as the new cell position itself. The procedure is carried out for all cells, and for all the remaining images (t=3 to 50), generating a position list of each cell throughout the sequence. The connected coordinates can be drawn on screen to create a track for each cell or, alternatively, vectors of final displacement can be plotted (*see* **Notes 9–11**).

After spatial and temporal calibration, the tracks can be measured for length and direction, and appropriate statistics can be used to extract significant distance — (speed) and direction differences between various experimental conditions (*17*).

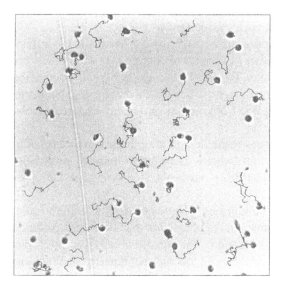

Dunn, RPMI + 20% S
Eotaxin $(10^{-7}M)$
gradient

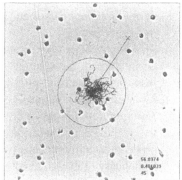

Fig. 1. Cell tracks of eosinophils moving in a gradient of eotaxin. The Dunn chamber was assembled as described in Materials and Methods. Movement of the eosinophils was measured starting 15 min after sealing of the chamber. Cell movement was monitored for 15 min several times within a 2 h period. Analysis of the cell tracks included direction measurement, as seen in the smaller panels. Centered tracks show the directional movement of the cells. The mean direction is indicated by a straight line toward an x. If a probability of 0.95 is reached, the straight line crosses the circle. Next to this panel the direction of the *applied* gradient is indicated with an arrow.

Another way to analyze granulocyte motility is the method of Gail and Boone *(18)* which uses rigid mathematical modeling to calculate a Diffusion Constant for the whole cell population. For a representative experiment, see **Fig. 1**.

4. Notes

1. *Mononuclear cells contaminate eosinophil preparation during isolation procedure 1.* The first Ficoll paque step is very important to remove all mononuclear cells. A small contamination with CD16- mononuclear cells in the granulocyte preparation will result in accumulation of these cells in the final eosinophil preparations. This problem can be minimized by avoiding overloading of the Ficoll gradients. An alternative is the additional use of beads coupled to CD14 and CD3 antibodies to remove contaminating monocytes and lymphocytes, respectively. The amount of these latter beads can be small and should be adjusted to the amount of contaminating mononuclear cells.
2. *Platelets contaminate eosinophil preparations.* Prevent storing of whole blood in cold conditions, which can cause platelet agglutination. Avoid overloading of Ficoll gradients. Too many platelets on the interface might lead to platelet acti-

vation. Include beads coupled to antibodies directed against IIb/IIIa or P-selectin and deplete for platelets and monocytes associated with platelets.

3. *Eosinophil preparations are not pure and have a low yield.* Activation of inflammatory cells during isolation is always a matter of concern. As soon as eosinophils physically interact with other CD16+ cells because of aspecific activation they will be depleted by the immunomagnetic bead method. This also holds true when clumping (e.g., induced by free DNA) occurs during any step in the isolation procedure.

4. *Air bubbles in column.* Disturbances in the flow of the column can be a result of air bubbles in the column: avoid air bubbles at all times. Remove air bubbles from the column by pushing cold PBS2+ out of the side syringe in the upper reservoir of the column.

5. *Eosinophil preparations are not pure during isolation procedure 2.* a) The quality of the Percoll solutions is absolutely critical for the success of isolation procedures applying density centrifugation. The percoll should have the correct osmolarity (290 +/– 10 mOsm), pH 7.0–7.2, and correct density. b) When the amount of eosinophils is around or below 1 % of total leukocytes methods utilizing density gradient centrifugation will lead to only moderate success.

6. *The eosinophil preparation has a low yield.* Cells can be activated and have changed their density or clump. This will obviously lead to poor results. Pay particular attention to the contamination of bacterial products such as lipopolysaccacharides which are potent preactivating substances for monocytes and polymorphonuclear leukocytes (PMNs).

7. *Eosinophils stay on the interface between buffer and Percoll or neutrophils pass the 1.082 g/mL layer.* Increase or decrease the density of the Percoll solution until a good separation is achieved. Do not overload the gradients!

8. Contrast between cells and background must be large enough to permit automated recognition of the cells during image analysis. Phase - and interference contrast images of cells are difficult to segment, and painstaking manual editing must then be performed. This can be avoided by defocusing in normal bright field mode or, alternatively, by using fluorescence microscopy. The latter method, of course, has its own problems and shortcomings such as the obligation to label the cells and to reduce bleaching (shuttering of the excitation light).

9. Series of images must be large enough to show movement during the given time course. Also, inter-image intervals must be long enough to allow for movement between time points. When intervals are used that are too long, difficulties arise with the analysis procedure. As explained above in **Subheading 3.2.3.**, cell identification is based on a nearest neighbor search in a restricted area. The cells are lost when they move out of this area during the inter-image interval. Some experimentation will deliver optimal time course parameters.

10. Noncontrolled (drifting) defocusing of the image is a great nuisance since it jeopardizes the correct Image Analysis of the cell's motion. Every precaution should be taken to avoid this. If defocusing occurs, manual Image Restoration must be performed and this can be really time consuming.

11. *Cells do not move because of lack of rear release.* It is often seen with eosinophils that the cells irreversibly adhere to the surface with the rear end of the cell. This absence of "rear-release" can be overcome by adding serum to the chemotaxis buffer.

References

1. Haslett, C., Savill, J. S., and Meagher, L. (1989) The neutrophil. *Curr. Opin. Immunol.* **2,** 10–18.
2. Gleich, G. J., Adolphson, C. R., and Leiferman, K. M. (1993) The biology of the eosinophilic leukocyte. *Annu. Rev. Med.* **44,** 85–101.
3. Coffer, P. J. and Koenderman, L. (1997) Granulocyte signal transduction and priming: cause without effect? *Immunol Lett* **57,** 27–31.
4. Warringa, R.A., Mengelers, H.J., Kuijper, P.H., Raaijmakers, J.A., Bruijnzeel, P.L., and Koenderman, L. (1992) In vivo priming of platelet-activating factor-induced eosinophil chemotaxis in allergic asthmatic individuals. *Blood* **79,** 1836–1841
5. Sehmi, R., Wardlaw, A. J., Cromwell, O., Kurihara, K., Waltmann, P., and Kay, A. B. (1992) Interleukin-5 selectively enhances the chemotactic response of eosinophils obtained from normal but not eosinophilic subjects. *Blood* **79,** 2952–2959.
6. Spoelstra, F. M., Hovenga, H., Noordhoek, J. A., Postma, D. S., and Kauffman, H. F. (1998) Changes in CD11b and L-selectin expression on eosinophils are mediated by human lung fibroblasts in vitro. *Am. J. Respir. Crit. Care Med.* **158,** 769–777.
7. Mengelers, H. J., Maikoe, T., Hooibrink, B., Kuypers, T. W., Kreukniet, J., Lammers, J. W., and Koenderman, L. (1993) Down modulation of L-Selectin expression on eosinophils recovered from bronchoalveolar lavage fluid after allergen provocation. *Clin. Exp. Allergy* **23,** 196–204.
8. Khwaja, A., Carver, J. E., and Linch, D. C. (1992) Interactions of granulocyte-macrophage colony-stimulating factor (CSF), granulocyte CSF, and tumor necrosis factor alpha in the priming of the neutrophil respiratory burst. *Blood* **79,** 745–753.
9. van der Bruggen, T., Kanters, D., Tool, A. T., Raaijmakers, J. A., Lammers, J. W., Verhoeven, A. J., and Koenderman, L. (1998) Cytokine-induced protein tyrosine phosphorylation is essential for cytokine priming of human eosinophils. *J. Allergy Clin. Immunol.* **101,** 103–109.
10. Kuijpers, T. W., Tool, A. T., van der Schoot, C. E., Ginsel, L. A., Onderwater, J. J., Roos, D., and Verhoeven, A. J. (1991) Membrane surface antigen expression on neutrophils: a reappraisal of the use of surface markers for neutrophil activation. *Blood* **78,** 1105–1111.
11. Hansel, T. T., Pound, J. D., and Thompson, R. A. (1990) Isolation of eosinophils from human blood. *J. Immunol. Methods* **127,** 153–164.
12. Hansel, T. T., De Vries, I J., Iff, T., Rihs, S., Wandzilak, M., Betz, S., Blaser, K., and Walker, C. (1991) An improved immunomagnetic procedure for the isolation of highly purified human blood eosinophils. *J. Immunol. Methods* **145,** 105–110.

13. Blom, M., Tool, A. T., Mul, F. P., Knol, E. F., Roos, D., and Verhoeven, A. J. (1995) Eosinophils isolated with two different methods show different characteristics of activation. *J. Immunol. Methods* **178,** 183–193.
14. Koenderman, L., Kok, P. T., Hamelink, M. L., Verhoeven, A. J., and Bruijnzeel, P. L. (1988) An improved method for the isolation of eosinophilic granulocytes from peripheral blood of normal individuals. *J. Leukoc. Biol.* **44,** 79–86.
15. Gail, M. H. and Boone, C. W. (1970) The locomotion of mouse fibroblasts in tissueculture. *Biophysical journal.* **10,** 980–993.
16. Hallet, M. B. (1887) Controlling the molecular motor of neutrophil chemotaxis. *BioEssays* **19,** 615–621.
17. Lauffenburger, D. A. and Horwitz, A. F. (1996) Cell Migration: A physically Integrated Molecular Process. *Cell* **84,** 359–369.
18. Zicha, D., Dunn, G. A., and Brown, A. F. (1991) A new direct-viewing chemotaxis chamber. *J. Cell Science* **99,** 769–775.

IV

GENE EXPRESSION / REGULATION

19

Analysis of Gene Expression

Reverse Transcription-Polymerase Chain Reaction

El-Bdaoui Haddad and Jonathan Rousell

1. Introduction

Numerous techniques have been developed to measure gene expression in tissues and cells. These include coupled reverse transcription and polymerase chain reaction amplification (RT-PCR), Northern blot (*see* Chapter 20), *in situ* hybridization (*see* Chapter 21), RNase protection assays, dot blots, and S1 nuclease assays. Of these methods, RT-PCR is the most sensitive and versatile *(1–5)*. PCR allows amplification of a DNA or cDNA template by greater than one million-fold quickly and reliably *(6)*. Starting with minute amounts of DNA, PCR generates sufficient material for subsequent experimental analyses such as cloning, restriction digestion, electrophoresis, and sequencing. The entire amplification process is performed in just a few hours.

As originally developed, the PCR process amplified short (approx 100–500 base pair (bp)) segments of a longer DNA molecule *(1)*. A typical amplification reaction includes the sample of target DNA, a thermostable DNA polymerase, two oligonucleotide primers, deoxynucleotide triphosphates (dNTPs), reaction buffer, magnesium, and optional additives. The components of the reaction are mixed and placed in a thermal cycler, which is an automated instrument that "cycles" the reaction through a predetermined series of specific temperatures and times. Each cycle of PCR amplification consists of a defined number of reaction steps. The steps are designed using temperature and duration time to denature the template, anneal the two oligonucleotide primers and extend the new complementary DNA strands by polymerization. These steps can be optimized for each template and primer pair combination.

From: *Methods in Molecular Medicine, vol. 56:*
Human Airway Inflammation: Sampling Techniques and Analytical Protocols
Edited by: D. F. Rogers and L. E. Donnelly © Humana Press Inc., Totowa, NJ

The amplified nucleic acid may then be analyzed (e.g., for size, quantity or sequence), or it may be used in further experimental procedures (e.g., cloning or mutagenesis).

Many variations of the original PCR method now exist and numerous critical factors for successful amplification under a variety of conditions have been delineated. The present chapter describes a protocol for routine PCR sufficient for many applications. During the last decade, the applications of PCR have been updated *(7,8)*:

1. Combining reverse transcription and PCR into the RT-PCR technique brought the benefits of PCR to analysis of RNA.
2. Using primers containing sequences that were not completely complementary to the template turned PCR into a tool for in vitro mutagenesis.
3. Replacing a single polymerase with a blend of thermostable polymerase (*Taq* DNA Polymerase) and proofreading polymerase (Two DNA Polymerase) made PCR an indispensable tool in the analysis and mapping of entire genomes by:
   a. Greatly extending the length of the sequence that could be amplified.
   b. Increasing the amount of PCR product.
   c. Providing higher fidelity during PCR.
4. Using a "Hot Start" (*see* **Subheading 3.4**) approach minimized the formation of primer-dimers during PCR.
5. Using short primers to produce a genomic "fingerprint" allowed analysis of organisms in which genomic sequences are largely unknown (e.g., differential display, random amplified polymorphic DNA).
6. Introducing molecular "tags", such as digoxigenin (DIG) or biotin-labeled dUTP into the PCR product, as it was amplified made PCR an invaluable tool for medical diagnostics. Such labeled PCR products may either be used as hybridization probes or be detected by use of capture probes. For instance, with PCR-generated DIG-labeled hybridization probes, it was possible to detect and quantify minute amounts of a pathogen.
7. Combining *in situ* hybridization with PCR (*in situ* PCR) made possible the localization of single nucleic acid sequences on one chromosome within a eukaryotic organism.
8. Extending PCR to the amplification of more than one sequence at a time (multiplex PCR) made it possible to compare two or more complex genomes, for instance to detect chromosomal imbalances.
9. Combining online detection and continuous fluorescence monitoring (kinetic PCR) allowed more rapid quantification of PCR products.

The ability of PCR to amplify a single molecule means that trace amounts of DNA contaminants could serve as templates, resulting in amplification of the wrong template (false positives). The points mentioned in **Notes 1–8** should be considered to avoid PCR contamination from sources such as laboratory benches, equipment, and pipeting devices, which can be contaminated by previous DNA preparations, by plasmid DNA, or by purified restriction fragments, products from previous PCR amplifications *(9)*.

2. Materials
2.1. Reagents

All reagents were from Sigma (Poole, Dorset), unless stated otherwise. All solutions must be sterilized by autoclaving.

1. Nuclease-free water (Promega or Ambion).
2. 0.5 *M* ethylenediaminetetraacetic acid (EDTA), pH8.
3. Tris-acetate-EDTA (TAE) buffer: 0.04 *M* Tris-acetate and 0.001 *M* EDTA. Prepare a 50X stock solution: Add 242 g Tris to 57.1mL glacial acetic acid and 100 mL 0.5 *M* EDTA (pH 8.0). Add deionized water to 1 liter. The working solution is 1X TAE and is made directly from the stock solution.
4. DEPC-treated water: 0.1% (v/v) diethyl pyrocarbonate (DEPC) in sterile water. To fully dissolve the DEPC it should be left at room temperature overnight (*see* **Note 9**). DEPC traces are removed by autoclaving. DEPC is a possible carcinogen.
5. Reverse transcriptase, e.g., avian myeloblastosis virus (AMV)-RT (Promega) (*see* **Note 10**). These enzymes are supplied with the appropriate reaction buffers.
6. RT primers, e.g., random hexamers (Promega) (*see* **Note 11**).
7. dNTP mixture, containing dATP, dGTP, dTTP, and dCTP; 25 µmol each (Bioline, London, UK) (*see* **Note 12**).
8. RNase inhibitor (e.g., RNasin: Promega).
9. PCR buffer: there are several types commercially available, for example the 10X KCl buffer from Bioline: 500 m*M* KCl, 100 m*M* Tris-HCl (pH 8.8), 15 m*M* MgCl$_2$, 1% (v/v) Triton X100 (*see* **Note 13**).
10. *Taq* polymerases: there are several types commercially available, for example Biotaq from Bioline (*see* **Note 14**).
11. Magnesium chloride: 50 m*M* stock solution (Bioline) (*see* **Note 15**).
12. PCR primers: these can be custom synthesized by a number of companies (e.g., Promega, Bioline, and Amersham-Pharmacia) (*see* **Note 16**).
13. Ethidium bromide (EtBr): Prepare as a 10 mg/mL solution in DEPC-treated water (*see* **Note 17**).
14. Agarose DNA gel: Mix the appropriate amount of agarose (*see* **Note 18**) with 1X TAE buffer and heat in a microwave for 1–2 min until the agarose is completely melted. Cool the solution to ~50°C and add 0.5µg/mL of ethidium bromide prior to gel casting.
15. Gel loading buffer (*see* **Note 19**): Add 0.08 g of orange G dye to 10 mL glycerol, 10 mL DEPC water and 40 µl EDTA (0.5 *M*). The solution can be autoclaved and stored in 0.5–1 mL aliquots at room temperature (or frozen if preferred).

2.2. Apparatus

1. Thermal cycler (*see* **Note 20**): there are several types commercially available, for example from Stratagene or Techne.

Table 1
Reaction Mixture for RT Reaction

Component	Volume/reaction	Final concentration
Master Mix		
10X Reaction Buffer	2μL	1X
dNTP Mix (10 mM of each dNTP)	1μL	0.5 mM each
Oligo(dT) primer (10 μM)	2	1μM
Rnase Inhibitor (10 units/μL)	1μL	0.5 units/μL
Reverse transcriptase	1μL	4units/20-μLreaction
RNase-Free Water	Variable	
Template		
Template RNA (0.5 mg/mL)	Variable	Up to 2 μg
Total volume	20μL	

2. Reaction tubes (*see* **Note 21**): there are several types commercially available, for example from Laser.
3. Agarose gel electrophoresis equipment (e.g., Submarine electrophoresis system from Bio-Rad).

3. Methods

RNA cannot serve as a template for PCR, so it must first be reverse transcribed into cDNA (e.g., with reverse transcriptase from Moloney murine leukemia virus (M-MuLV) or AMV).

3.1. First-Strand cDNA Synthesis (Reverse Transcription)

Procedures for creating and maintaining an RNase-free environment *(9,10)* as well as the protocol for extracting total or mRNA are described in Chapters 20 (for cells in culture) and 22 (for lung tissue) (*see* **Note 22**).

1. Prepare the reaction mix by combining the components indicated in **Table 1**. The table gives the volumes for one tube, and can be scaled up as appropriate (*see* **Note 16** concerning running of a "no-RT" negative control). Gently vortex the tube for 10 s to mix the components.
2. The RT reaction may require a template denaturation step prior to initiation: incubate the primers and RNA template at 65°C for 5 min or 94°C for 2 min (do not incubate the AMV-RT at 94°C because it will be inactivated). The template/primer mixture can then be added to the RT-reaction mix for the standard RT incubation at 42°C.
3. Initiate the reaction by adding the reaction mix to the template.
4. Incubate at 37°–48°C for 45–60 min for efficient first-strand cDNA synthesis.
5. Following first-strand cDNA synthesis, the RT is inactivated using a 2 min incubation at 94°C (*see* **Note 23**).

Table 2
Reaction Mixture for PCR

Component	Volume/reaction	Final concentration
Master Mix		
10X Reaction Buffer	5μL	1X
MgCl$_2$ (25 m*M*)	3μL	1.5 m*M*
dNTP Mix (10 m*M* each)	1μL	0.2 m*M* each
Forward Primer (20 m*M*)	1.25μL	0.5 μ*M*
Reverse Primer(20 m*M*)	1.25μ	0.5 μ*M*
Taq DNA Polymerase (5U/μL)	0.25μL	0.025u/μL
RNase-Free Water	34.25μL	
Template		
Template DNA	4μL	1/10 of the RT reaction
Total volume	50μL	

6. Dilute with 80 μL nuclease-free water. The cDNA can now be stored at –20°C until required.

3.2. Second Strand cDNA Synthesis (PCR)

Although PCR is simple in theory, it can benefit from optimization of several parameters *(11–15)*. RT-PCR amplification of a particular mRNA sequence requires two PCR primers that are specific for the mRNA sequence. Primers for quantitative experiments are designed to amplify a target of between 200 and 600 bp. Targets smaller than 200 bp are difficult to resolve on agarose gels and larger targets place a greater burden on the investigator to optimize PCR conditions. In most PCR applications, it is the sequence and the concentration of the primers that determine the overall assay success.

The PCR cycling profile provided below should serve as a guideline for initial experiments. We recommend optimizing the parameters for each target RNA.

1. Place the reagents on ice and prepare the reaction mix by combining the components indicated in **Table 2** (*see* **Note 24**).
2. Initiate the reaction by adding the DNA template (*see* **Note 25**) and gently vortex the tubes for 10 s.
3. Place a layer of light mineral oil over the reaction mixture to prevent evaporation during PCR (if the thermal cycler has a heated lid, oil overlay is not necessary).
4. Program the thermal cycler according to the manufacturer's instructions. A typical PCR cycling program is outlined in **Fig. 1**.
5. After amplification, samples can be stored overnight at 4°C (or longer at –20°C) before analysis by agarose gel electrophoresis.

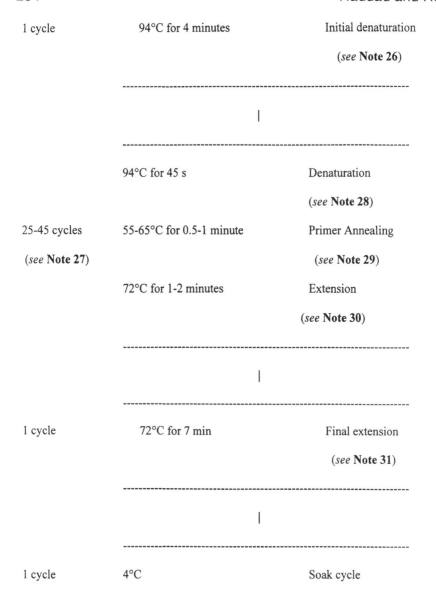

| 1 cycle | 94°C for 4 minutes | Initial denaturation |
| | | (*see* **Note 26**) |

25-45 cycles	94°C for 45 s	Denaturation
(*see* **Note 27**)		(*see* **Note 28**)
	55-65°C for 0.5-1 minute	Primer Annealing
		(*see* **Note 29**)
	72°C for 1-2 minutes	Extension
		(*see* **Note 30**)

| 1 cycle | 72°C for 7 min | Final extension |
| | | (*see* **Note 31**) |

| 1 cycle | 4°C | Soak cycle |

Fig. 1. Typical PCR cycling program. The sequences of the primers are a major consideration in determining the temperature of the PCR amplification cycles *(22–24)*. An amplification cycle typically consists of a denaturation step (94°C), a template/ primer annealing step (42°–60°C), and an extension step (72°C). For primers with a high T_m, it may be advantageous to increase the suggested annealing and extension temperatures. The higher temperature minimizes nonspecific primer annealing, which increases the amount of specific product produced. For primers with a low T_m, it may be necessary to decrease the annealing temperature to allow the primer to anneal to the target template.

6. Prepare the appropriate agarose DNA gel using 1X TAE (*see* **Subheading 2.1., step 14,** and **Note 18**).
7. Mix 10 µL PCR product with 4 µL orange G dye, and load the samples and DNA markers (chosen to suit the fragment sizes generated). Fragment sizes are calculated by extrapolation from a standard curve of the mobility of DNA fragments.
8. Make sure the gel is completely covered with running buffer (1X TAE) and electrophorese at 5 V/cm. The gel should be run until the band of interest has migrated 40–60% down the length of the gel. Longer electrophoretic times result in greater separation between fragments.
9. The products can be visualised using ultraviolet transillumination and captured using Polaroid film or digital camera.
10. Quantification (*see* **Subheading 3.5**).

An example of an RT-PCR analysis is shown in **Fig. 2**.

3.3. Single- and Two-Step RT-PCR

RT-PCR can be performed as either a two-step or a one-step procedure *(16–18)*.

3.3.1. One-Step Procedure or Coupled RT-PCR

Both cDNA synthesis and PCR amplification are performed with the same buffer and site-specific primers, eliminating the need to open the reaction tube between the RT and PCR steps. The advantages of one-step RT-PCR procedures are:

1. Higher sensitivity than the one tube, two-step reaction because the entire cDNA sample is used as template for PCR (*see* **Subheading 3.3.2.**).
2. Fewer pipeting steps than the two-step reaction, significantly reducing the time needed to perform RT-PCR and eliminating pipeting errors.
3. Minimizes the chance of contamination, since the entire reaction is performed with minimal pipeting steps and without opening the tube.
4. Permits direct analysis of a specific transcript, since the primers used in both steps are sequence-specific.
5. The thermoactive reverse transcriptase used in this procedure allows a high RT reaction temperature (50°–72°C), which reduces false priming and increases the specificity of the reaction by eliminating secondary mRNA structure *(16–18)*.

3.3.2. Two-Step Procedures

The advantages of two-step RT-PCR procedures are:

1. Optimizes reaction conditions. The two-step format allows both RT and PCR to be performed under optimal conditions, to ensure efficient and accurate amplification.
2. Provides flexibility. Two-step procedures allow the product of a single cDNA synthesis reaction to be used for analysis of multiple transcripts. This flexibility

is valuable for specialized applications such as rapid amplification of cDNA ends (RACE) and Differential Display Reverse Transcription (DDRT).

3. Amplifies long sequences. With the right combination of reverse transcriptase and thermostable DNA polymerase, two-step RT-PCR can amplify RNA sequences up to 14 kb long.

Two tube, two-step procedure: Useful for experiments where multiple transcripts are to be analyzed from the same RT reaction or for specific applications such as DDRT or RACE (see above). Since the RT reaction is performed under optimal conditions, this approach produces the longest RT-PCR products (up to 14 kb in length, with the appropriate enzymes). In the first tube, first-strand cDNA synthesis is performed under optimal conditions, using either random hexamers, oligo(dT) primers (generating a cDNA pool), or sequence-specific primers. An aliquot of the RT reaction is then transferred to another tube (containing thermostable DNA polymerase, DNA polymerase buffer, and PCR primers) for PCR.

One tube, two-step procedure: Useful when template amounts are limited, since the entire RT reaction is used in the subsequent PCR. In the first step, reverse transcriptase produces first-strand cDNA in the presence of Mg^{2+} ions, high concentrations of dNTPs, and either specific or nonspecific oligo(dT) primers. Following the RT reaction, an optimized PCR buffer (without Mg^{2+} ions), a thermostable DNA polymerase, and specific primers are added to the tube and PCR is performed.

3.4. Hot Start PCR

Hot start PCR protocols increase amplification specificity and product yield by creating conditions which minimize the possibility of nonspecific priming, primer-dimer formation or other reactions which can occur at low temperatures once all the PCR reaction components are mixed. In general, hot start techniques limit the availability of one necessary reaction component until a temperature >60°C is reached (19). This can be performed manually by the addition of the critical component once the reaction mixture reaches the higher temperature (20,21). However, this is tedious and can increase the chances of introducing contaminants into the reaction. Other approaches include using an antibody to inactivate the polymerase at lower temperatures. At higher temperatures, the antibody is denatured and binding is reversed, releasing a functional polymerase (22). Another method uses a wax bead to sequester the critical substance until the higher temperature is reached, at which point the missing component is released (23).

3.5. Quantification of RT-PCR Reactions

Quantification of PCR can be achieved using a number of methodologies. Some rely on the premise that DNA product is doubled with each round of

PCR producing a linear relationship between starting material and PCR product. In theory, doubling will occur until primer or nucleotide is exhausted or the enzymatic activity of the polymerase is lost. In practice, doubling occurs only for a limited number of cycles because of incomplete elongation of strands and competition by nonspecific products. Within a limited number of cycles, the PCR reaches a plateau phase where little further PCR product accumulates. It is important, to determine where the linear phase of the PCR reaction occurs. Semi-quantitative PCR may be performed to determine when it is first possible to visualise the PCR product on ethidium bromide-stained gels by sampling product after various cycles of PCR.

Measurement of the incorporation of a labeled nucleotide into the PCR product at various cycle numbers is more readily quantifiable but is a more time consuming approach. Incorporation of label into the PCR product after various cycle numbers is compared to that of a standard mRNA such as β-actin allowing the generation of a ratio of expression.

Quantification that relies on the PCR being in the linear phase can, however, suffer from major problems that are symptomatic of the sensitive nature of PCR. Mispriming in the early cycles of PCR or minute differences in pipeting may have dramatic effects on the subsequent accumulation of PCR product. Using an internal standard (i.e., where control and target RNAs are amplified in the same tube) can prevent spurious results caused by pipeting errors and other tube effects. However, competition between the PCR reactions of the internal standards and target DNA can have fundamental effects on the quantification. Primer annealing and chain elongation may favor amplification of one of the templates leading to preferential accumulation of the product.

An approach that attempts to resolve the above problems is "competitive" or "multiplex" PCR. PCR is performed with a range of known quantities of a PCR competitor (such as a synthetic RNA) that is added to the RT reaction in increasing molar amounts until the yield of product made from this synthetic transcript matches the yield from the endogenous target in the same sample. This approach does not require the PCR reaction to be in the linear phase of amplification, but it is important to obtain equal amplification efficiencies of the endogenous and exogenous targets for accurate quantification. This is normally achieved by using an altered form of the exogenous target (e.g., through deletion or addition of a restriction site), so that its product is distinguishable from that produced by the endogenous target. Comparison of the amount of endogenous product needed to give the same yield as the exogenous product indicates the amount of exogenous product in each sample.

4. Notes

1. At a minimum, set up physically separated workstations.
   a. Template preparation before PCR.
   b. Setting up PCR reactions.
   c. Post-PCR analysis.
2. Care must be taken to minimize the potential for cross-contamination between samples and prevent carryover of nucleic acid (RNA and DNA) from one experiment to the next. Use positive displacement pipetes or aerosol resistant tips to reduce cross-contamination during pipeting.
3. Wear gloves and change them often.
4. UV irradiation may be considered to eliminate contamination/carryover. Mix all components, except template DNA, irradiate in clear 0.5-mL polypropylene tubes in direct contact with glass transilluminator (254 and 300 nm UV bulbs) for 5 min. If possible, set up PCR reactions under a fume hood that is equipped with UV light.
5. Under the fume hood, store a microcentrifuge and disposable gloves, which are used only for PCR.
6. Always use new and/or sterilized glassware, plasticware, and pipetes to prepare PCR reagents and template DNA.
7. Have your own set of PCR reagents and solutions that are used only for PCR. Store these reagents in small aliquots.
8. Contaminating DNA in RNA preparations can produce incorrect results because of its potential to act as a second competitor *(24,25)*. This is a frequent cause of concern among investigators, because PCR is such a sensitive technique, a single copy of a gene can, theoretically, be detected. Genomic DNA false positive signals are easily identified by performing a "no-RT" control during RT-PCR. RNase-free DNase I treatment can be used to reduce genomic DNA contamination *(26)*. DNase is an endonuclease that cleaves DNA by breaking phosphodiester bonds. It must be inactivated or removed from the reaction prior to PCR, otherwise, it may digest newly amplified DNA and thus compromise the performance of the RT-PCR reactions. Problems that may arise using DNase I treatment may be traced to the extreme temperatures (95°C for 5 min) used to inactivate the DNase I prior to reverse transcription *(27)*. The enzyme can be removed using proteinase K digestion and phenol/chloroform extraction that partitions protein and DNA into the organic phase. The RNA is recovered by alcohol precipitation in the presence of sodium acetate (*see* Chapter 20). As an alternative to DNase treatment, RNA can be extracted using two rounds of phenol/chloroform extraction. Finally, it should be noted that DNase I treatment does not relieve the investigator of the burden of sensible primer design (*see* **Note 14**) or the necessity of performing the appropriate "no-RT" controls.
9. DEPC has a half-life of approx 30 min in water and, at a concentration of 0.1%, solutions autoclaved for 15 min/liter can be assumed to be DEPC-free.
10. A major factor to consider in RT-PCR is the choice of reverse transcriptase (RT) used to synthesize cDNA. Since each of the available enzymes has different

enzymatic properties, one may be more suitable for a specific experiment than the others. Among the enzyme properties to consider are:

  a. Temperature optima: higher incubation temperatures can eliminate problems of template secondary structure, and improves the specificity of reverse tran scription by decreasing false priming. Thus, thermoactive RTs that can be incubated at high temperatures (50°–70°C) are more likely to accurately tran scribe the RNA, especially if the template has a high GC content. At high temperatures, use only specific primers; do not use oligo(dT) or random hexamer primers.

  b. RNase H activity: in contrast to Tth DNA Polymerase, AMV, and M-MuLV RTs have RNase H activity. This activity will specifically degrade RNA in an RNA:cDNA hybrid. This can be detrimental if degradation of template RNA competes with DNA synthesis during production of first-strand cDNA. M-MuLV RT has lower RNase H activity than AMV RT. Mutated enzymes without RNase H activity are also available.

  c. Divalent ion requirement: most RTs require a divalent ion for activity. Enzymes that use Mg^{2+} are likely to produce more accurate cDNA copies than those that use Mn^{2+}, since Mn^{2+} adversely affects the fidelity of DNA synthesis.

  d. Specificity and sensitivity: RTs have different capacities to copy small amounts of template (sensitivity). They also differ in their ability to tran scribe RNA secondary structures accurately (specificity).

11. Priming affects the size and specificity of the cDNA produced. There are three types of primers that can be used for reverse transcription:

  a. Oligo(dT)12–18: binds to the endogenous poly(A)+ tail at the 3' end of mam malian mRNA. This primer often produces a full-length cDNA.

  b. Random hexanucleotides: bind to mRNA at a variety of complementary sites and lead to partial length (short) cDNAs. Random hexanucleotides can be ideal for overcoming the difficulties presented by extensive secondary struc ture in the template. These primers can also transcribe more efficiently 5' regions of the mRNA.

  c. Specific oligonucleotide primers: selectively prime the mRNA of interest. This type of primer has been used successfully in diagnostic assays.

12. Always use balanced solutions of all four dNTPs to minimize polymerase error rate. Imbalanced dNTP mixtures reduce *Taq* DNA Polymerase fidelity. Increases in dNTP concentration reduce free Mg^{2+}, thus interfering with polymerase activity and decreasing primer annealing. Thus, increases in concentration of dNTPs require increases in Mg^{2+} concentration. The final dNTP concentration should be 50–500 μM (each dNTP). The most commonly used dNTP concentration is 200 μM.

13. Generally, the pH of the reaction buffer supplied with the corresponding thermo stable DNA polymerase (pH 8.3–9.0) will give optimal results. However, for some systems, raising the pH may stabilize the template and enhance results.

14. The choice of a DNA polymerase can affect the outcome of the PCR reaction *(28)*. The primary requirements for a DNA polymerase used in PCR are optimal

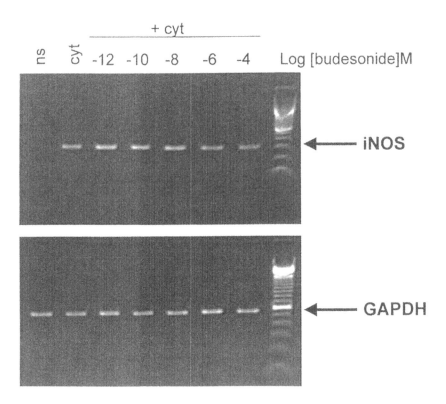

Fig. 2. PCR of human primary epithelial cells. Cells were cultured in supplement-free media (ns) or 50 ng/mL IL-1β, TNF-α and IFN-γ (cyt) in the absence or presence of increasing concentrations of budesonide. The cells were harvested, RNA extracted, and RT-PCR performed for iNOS and GAPDH.

activity at temperatures around 75°C, and the ability to retain activity after pro-longed incubation at higher temperatures (95°C). For most assays, the optimum amount of thermostable DNA polymerase (or a blend of polymerases) is 0.5–2.5 units/50 µl reaction volume. More enzyme will not significantly increase product yield. Increased amounts of enzyme and excessively long extension times increase the likelihood of generating artefacts owing to the intrinsic 5´—>3´ exo-nuclease activity of *Taq* DNA Polymerase. Artefacts can be seen as smeared bands in ethidium bromide-stained agarose gels *(29,30)*. The most frequent cause of excessive enzyme levels is pipeting errors. Accurate dispensing of submicroliter (<1 µL) volumes of enzyme solutions in 50% glycerol is difficult. We recommend the use of reaction master mixes sufficient for the number of reactions being performed to obviate this problem. A master mix increases the volumes of pipeted reagents and reduces pipeting errors.

15. Magnesium chloride solutions form a concentration gradient when frozen. It is important to completely thaw the $MgCl_2$ solution prior to use and vortex it prior

to pipeting. Magnesium concentration is a crucial factor affecting the performance of *Taq* DNA Polymerase. Reaction components, including template DNA, chelating agents (e.g., EDTA or citrate), dNTPs and proteins, all affect the amount of free magnesium in the PCR reaction mixture. In the absence of adequate-free magnesium, *Taq* DNA Polymerase is inactive. Conversely, excess-free magnesium reduces enzyme fidelity *(31,32)* and may increase the level of nonspecific amplification *(12,33)*. For these reasons, it is important to empirically determine the optimal $MgCl_2$ concentration for each reaction. To do so, prepare a reaction series containing 1.5–3.0 m*M* Mg^{2+} in 0.5 m*M* increments by adding 3, 4, 5, or 6 µl of the 25 m*M* $MgCl_2$ stock to 50µl reactions. The most commonly used Mg^{2+} concentration is 1.5 m*M* (with dNTPs at a concentration of 200 µ*M* each).

16. Several primer design software programs are available. These can be used to ensure that the primer sequences have the following general characteristics:
    a. Are 18–24 bases long.
    b. Contain no internal secondary structure.
    c. Contain 40–60% G/C.
    d. Have a balanced distribution of G/C and A/T rich domains. Avoid three G or C nucleotides in a row near the 3´-end of the primer as this may result in nonspecific primer annealing, increasing the synthesis of undesirable reaction products.
    e. Are not complementary to each other at the 3' ends, so primer-dimers will not form. Primer-dimers unnecessarily delete primers from the reaction and result in an unwanted polymerase reaction that competes with the desired reaction.
    f. Have a melting temperature (T_m) that allows annealing temperatures of 55°–65°C (for maximum specificity use temperatures of 62°–65°C).

Numerous formulas exist to determine the theoretical T_m of nucleic acids *(11,34)*. These may serve as a useful starting point for optimizing annealing conditions. It is best to optimize the annealing conditions by performing the reaction at several temperatures, starting approx 5°C below any calculated T_m. The formula below can be used to estimate the melting temperature for oligonucleotides:

$T_m = 81.5 + 16.6 \times (\log10[Na^+]) + 0.41 \times (\%G+C) - 675/n$

where $[Na^+]$ is the molar salt concentration ($[K^+] = [Na^+]$) and n = number of bases in the oligonucleotide.

The primer design should also allow differentiation between the amplified product of DNA and an amplified product derived from contaminating genomic DNA. An amplification product derived from genomic DNA will be much larger than the product of the RT-PCR reaction. This size difference not only makes it possible to differentiate the two products by gel electrophoresis, it also favors the synthesis of the smaller cDNA derived product (PCR favors the amplification of smaller fragments). There are two approaches to designing the required primers:

a. Make primers that anneal to sequences in exons on both sides of an intron.
b. Make primers that span exon/exon boundaries on the mRNA. Such primers should not amplify genomic DNA.

If the intron-exon structure is unknown, primers can be synthesized in different regions of the cDNA sequence and tried in combinations on both cDNA and genomic DNA. It should be possible to choose a primer combination that yields either no product (additional intron sequence produces too long target for efficient PCR) or an easily distinguishable product when amplifying from genomic DNA. An additional problem is that pseudogenes exist in the mammalian genome for many genes, including the most commonly used internal controls (ß-actin, GAPDH, cyclophilin). These sequences, arising from integration of an RT product into the genome, do not have introns. Thus, the size of a PCR product amplified from a pseudogene may be identical to that produced from a cDNA copy. The only way to identify these products is to perform a "no-RT" control.

Regardless of primer choice, the final concentration of primers in the reaction must be optimized. Primer concentrations between 0.1 and 0.6 µ*M* are generally optimal. Higher primer concentrations may promote mispriming and accumulation of non-specific product. Lower primer concentrations may be exhausted before the reaction is completed, resulting in lower yields of desired product. For some systems, a higher primer concentration (up to 1 µ*M*) may improve results. When testing new primers, always include a positive control reaction with a template that has been tested for function in PCR. This control shows whether the primers are working. The sequence of the primers can also include regions at the 5´-ends that may prove useful for downstream applications. For example, restriction enzyme sites can be designed at the 5´-end of primer pairs if the desired PCR product is to be subsequently cloned. Caution should be used however, since all restriction enzymes may not cut efficiently close to the end of DNA fragments.

17. Ethidium bromide should be handled with care, as it is a known carcinogen.
18. The percentage of agarose gel used will depend on the size of the fragment to be separated. Agarose concentrations vary from 0.6% (w/v) for large fragment separation to 2% (w/v) for small fragments. Gel thickness has a profound effect on the resolution of smaller fragments.
19. Gel loading buffers serve three purposes in DNA electrophoresis:
    a. Increase the density of the sample to ensure that the DNA will drop evenly into the well.
    b. Color the sample to simplify loading.
    c. Enable monitoring of the electrophoretic process (by observation of movement of the dye front).
20. A thermal cycler must accurately and reproducibly maintain the three PCR incubation temperatures, change from one temperature to another ("ramp") over a definable time, arrive at the selected temperatures without significant over- or undershoot. Cycling conditions have to be adjusted depending on the respective thermal cycler or primer/template combinations.
21. The reaction tubes affect the rate at which heat transfers from the thermal cycler to the reaction mixture. Therefore, preferably use thin-walled reaction tubes that are designed for PCR and that fit precisely into the wells of the particular brand of thermal cycler you are using.
22. Successful RT is dependent on the integrity and purity of the mRNA used as the template. The use of purified mRNA as template, rather than total RNA, will

greatly increase the likelihood of successful amplification of rare mRNAs, since the proportion of mRNA in a total RNA preparation is low (typically, 1–5% of total RNA from a mammalian cell). When using mRNA as template, check its integrity by gel electrophoresis before use in the RT-PCR. The mRNA should appear as a smear between approx 500 bp and 8 kb. The minimum amount of RNA that can be amplified using RT-PCR is both template and primer dependent. Excellent amplification results can be obtained using total RNA template levels in the range of 10 pg–1 µg per reaction, or mRNA template levels in the range of 1 pg–100 ng.

23. The AMV-RT should be inactivated to obtain high yields of amplification product when using thermophilic DNA polymerases such as Tfl DNA Polymerase *(35,36)*.

24. The most frequent cause of excessive enzyme levels is pipeting errors. Accurate dispensing of submicroliter volumes of enzyme solutions in 50% (v/v) glycerol is difficult. We recommend the use of reaction master mixes sufficient for the number of reactions being performed to obviate this problem. A master mix increases the volumes of pipeted reagents, reduces pipeting errors and greatly facilitates the reaction setup and decreases tube-to-tube variability of the reaction components. Use individual pipete tips for all additions, being careful not to cross-contaminate the samples.

25. The quality of the template influences the outcome of the PCR. For instance, large amounts of RNA in a DNA template can chelate Mg^{2+} and reduce the yield of the PCR. Also, impure templates may contain polymerase inhibitors that decrease the efficiency of the reaction. The integrity of the template is also important. Template DNA should be of high molecular weight. To check the size and quality of the DNA, run an aliquot on an agarose gel. When testing a new template, include a positive control with primers that amplify a product of known size and produce a good yield.

26. It is important to denature the template DNA completely. Initial heating of the PCR mixture at 94°–95°C for 2–4 min will completely denature complex genomic DNA so that the primers can anneal to the template as the reaction mix is cooled. If the template DNA is only partially denatured, it will tend to "snap-back" very quickly, preventing efficient primer annealing and extension, or leading to "self-priming", which can lead to false-positive results. Use the shortest time for complete denaturation of template DNA during the PCR step. Unnecessarily long denaturation times decrease the activity of *Taq* DNA Polymerase.

27. In an optimal reaction, less than 10 template molecules can be amplified in less than 40 cycles to a product that is easily detectable on a gel stained with ethidium bromide. Most transcripts can be detected using 25–35 cycles of amplification. If the target RNA is rare, or if only a small amount of starting material is available, it may be necessary to increase the number of cycles to 40–45. However, as cycle number increases, nonspecific products can also accumulate.

28. Denaturation at 94°–95°C for 20–30 s is sufficient, but this should be adapted for the thermal cycler and tubes being used (e.g., longer times are required for dena-

turation in 500 μl tubes than in 200 μl tubes). If the denaturation temperature is too low, the incompletely melted DNA snaps-back as described above, giving no access to the primers. Use a longer denaturation time or higher denaturing temperature for GC-rich template DNA.

29. For most purposes, primer annealing temperature has to be optimized empirically *(11)*. The choice of temperature is probably the most critical factor in designing a high specificity PCR. If the temperature is too high, no annealing occurs. If it is too low, nonspecific annealing will increase dramatically. Primer-dimers will form if the primers have one or more complementary bases so that base pairing between the 3' ends of the two primers can occur.

30. *Taq* DNA Polymerase can add approx 60 bases per second at 72°C. A 45-second extension is sufficient for fragments up to 1 kb. For extension of fragments up to 3 kb, allow about 45–60 s per kb. These times may need to be adjusted for specific templates. For improved yield, use the cycle extension feature of the thermal cycler. For instance, perform the first 10 cycles at a constant extension time (e.g., 45 s for a 1 kb product). Then, for the next 20 cycles, increase the extension time by 2–5 s per cycle (e.g., 50 s for cycle 11, 55 s for cycle 12, and so on.). Cycle extension allows the enzyme more time to do its job, because as PCR progresses, there is more template to amplify and less enzyme (owing to denaturation during the prolonged high PCR temperatures) to do the extension.

31. After the last cycle, a final 7 min extension at 72°C improves the quality of the final product by extending truncated product to full-length.

References

1. Saiki, R. K., Scharf. S., Faloona, F., Mullis, K. B., Horn, G. T., Erlich, H. A., and Arnheim, N. (1985) Enzymatic amplification of beta-globin genomic sequences and restriction site analysis for diagnosis of sickle cell anemia. *Science* **230,** 1350–1354.
2. Mullis, K., Faloona, F., Scharf, S., Saiki, R., Horn, G., and Erlich, H. (1986) Specific enzymatic amplification of DNA in vitro: the polymerase chain reaction. Cold Spring Harb. Symp. *Quant. Biol.* **51,** 263–273.
3. Bell, J. (1989) The polymerase chain reaction. *Immunol Today,* **10,** 351–355.
4. Gibbs, R. A. (1990) DNA amplification by the polymerase chain reaction. *Anal. Chem.* **62,** 1202–1214.
5. Mullis, K., Faloona, F., Scharf, S., Saiki, R., Horn, G., and Erlich, H. (1992) Specific enzymatic amplification of DNA in vitro: the polymerase chain reaction. 1986. *Biotechnology* **24,** 17–27.
6. Saiki, R. K., Gelfand, D. H., Stoffel, S., Scharf, S. J., Higuchi, R., Horn, G. T., et al. (1988) Primer-directed enzymatic amplification of DNA with a thermostable DNA polymerase. *Science* **239,** 487–491.
7. Templeton, N.S. (1992) The polymerase chain reaction. History, methods, and applications. *Diagn. Mol. Pathol.* **1,** 58–72.

8. Frohman, M. A. and Martin, G. R. (1989) Cut, paste and save: New approaches to altering specific genes in mice. *Cell* **56,** 145–147.

9. Dieffenbach, C. W. and Dveksler, G. S. (1993) Setting up a PCR laboratory. *PCR Methods Appl.* **3,** S2–S7.

10. Blumberg, D. D. (1987) Creating a ribonuclease-free environment. *Meth. Enzymol.* **152,** 20–24.

11. Rychlik, W., Spencer, W. J., and Rhoads, R. E. (1990) Optimization of the annealing temperature for DNA amplification in vitro. *Nucleic Acids Res.* **18,** 6409–6412.

12. Williams, J. F. (1989) Optimization strategies for the polymerase chain reaction. *Biotechniques* **7,** 762–769.

13. Wittwer, C. T. and Garling, D. J. (1991) Rapid cycle DNA amplification: time and temperature optimization. *Biotechniques* **10,** 76–83.

14. Harris, S. and Jones, D. B. (1997) Optimization of the polymerase chain reaction. *Br. J. Biomed. Sci.* **54,** 166–173.

15. Roux, K. H. (1995) Optimization and troubleshooting in PCR. *PCR Methods Appl.* **4,** S185–S194.

16. Sellner, L. N. and Turbett, G. R. (1998) Comparison of three RT-PCR methods. *Biotechniques* **25,** 230–234.

17. Sellner, L. N., Coelen R. J., and Mackenzie, J. S. (1992) A one-tube, one manipulation RT-PCR reaction for detection of Ross River virus. *J. Virol. Methods* **40,** 255–263.

18. Mallet, F., Oriol, G., Mary, C., Verrier, B., and Mandrand, B. (1995) Continuous RT-PCR using AMV-RT and Taq DNA polymerase: characterization and comparison to uncoupled procedures. *Biotechniques* **18,** 678–687

19. Birch, D.E. (1996) Simplified hot start PCR. *Nature* **381,** 445–446.

20. D'Aquila, R. T., Bechtel, L. J., Videler, J. A., Eron, J. J., Gorczyca, P., and Kaplan, J. C. (1991) Maximizing sensitivity and specificity of PCR by pre-amplification heating. *Nucleic Acids Res.* **19,** 3749.

21. Bassam, B. J., and Caetano-Anolles, G. (1993) Automated "hot start" PCR using mineral oil and paraffin wax. *Biotechniques* **14,** 30–34.

22. Sharkey, D. J., Scalice, E. R., Christy, K. G., Atwood, S. M., Daiss, J. L. (1994) Antibodies as thermolabile switches: high temperature triggering for the polymerase chain reaction. *Biotechnology* (NY) **12,** 506–509.

23. Kaijalainen, S., Karhunen, P. J., Lalu, K., Lindstrom, K. (1993) An alternative hot start technique for PCR in small volumes using beads of wax-embedded reaction components dried in trehalose. *Nucleic Acids Res.* **21,** 2959–2960.

24. Kwok, S., and Higuchi, R. (1989) Avoiding false positives with PCR. *Nature* (London) **339,** 237–238.

25. Victor, T., Jordaan, A., du Toit, R., Van Helden, P. D. (1993) Laboratory experience and guidelines for avoiding false positive polymerase chain reaction results. *Eur. J. Clin. Chem. Clin. Biochem.* **31,** 531–535.

26. Grillo, M., Margolis, F. L. (1990) Use of reverse transcriptase polymerase chain reaction to monitor expression of intronless genes. *Biotechniques* **9,** 266–268.

27. Huang, Z., Fasco, M. J., Kaminsky, L. S. (1996) Optimization of Dnase I removal of contaminating DNA from RNA for use in quantitative RNA-PCR. *Biotechniques* **20,** 1012–1014, 1016, 1018–1020.

28. Hengen, P. N. (1995) Fidelity of DNA polymerases for PCR. *Trends Biochem. Sci.* **20,** 324–325.

29. Longley, M. J., Bennett, S. E., and Mosbaugh, D. W. (1990) Characterization of the 5' to 3' exonuclease associated with Thermus aquaticus DNA polymerase. *Nucleic Acids Res.* **18,** 7317–7322.

30. Bell, D. A., DeMarini, D. M. (1991) Excessive cycling converts PCR products to random-length higher molecular weight fragments. *Nucleic Acids Res.* **19,** 5079.

31. Eckert, K. A., and Kunkel, T. A. (1990) High fidelity DNA synthesis by the Thermus aquaticus DNA polymerase. *Nucleic Acids Res.* **18,** 3739–3744.

32. Eckert, K. A., and Kunkel, T. A. (1991) DNA polymerase fidelity and the polymerase chain reaction. *PCR Methods Appl.* **1,** 17–24.

33. Ellsworth, D. L., Rittenhouse, K. D., Honeycutt, R. L. (1993) Artifactual variation in randomly amplified polymorphic DNA banding patterns. *Biotechniques* **14,** 214–217.

34. Baldino, F., Chesselet, M. F., Lewis, M. E. (1989) High resolution in situ hybridization histochemistry, *Methods Enzymol.* **168,** 761–777.

35. Sellner, L. N., Coelen, R. J., Mackenzie, J. S. (1992) Reverse transcriptase inhibits Taq polymerase activity. *Nucleic Acids Res.* **20,** 1487–1490.

36. Chumakov, K. M. (1994) Reverse transcriptase can inhibit PCR and stimulate primer-dimer formation. *PCR Meth. Appl.* **4,** 62–64.

20

Analysis of Gene Expression

Northern Blotting

Jonathan Rousell and El-Bdaoui Haddad

1. Introduction
1.1. RNA Expression and Detection

Messenger (m)RNAs represent the information-carrying intermediates for protein synthesis. Northern blotting gives a snapshot of the relative abundance of an RNA transcript at a set time point by measuring the steady-state levels of an RNA transcript. The steady-state level of a particular mRNA species is determined by its rate of production, degradation, and transport from the nucleus to cytoplasm. Northern blotting allows investigation and quantification of changes in gene expression.

It is important to determine the objectives of the proposed investigation before deciding on which methodology to use. For example Northern blotting requires relatively large amounts of RNA (10 µg) and is less sensitive than other methods. Where sample is scarce or RNA transcripts rare use of reverse transcriptase polymerase chain reaction (RT-PCR) is more appropriate (*see* Chapter 19). Equally, *in situ* hybridization and not Northern blotting is used to localize RNA distribution within tissue sections.

Northern blotting has a number of advantages over other methods used to detect and quantify mRNA transcripts, including:

1. It is readily quantifiable and, although less sensitive than solution hybridization assays, blots may be reprobed and screened for multiple RNA transcripts.
2. Once fixed to a solid support the RNA is relatively stable as long as RNases are not introduced. This allows easy handling of RNA and facilitates repeated probing of the RNA for various transcripts.

From: *Methods in Molecular Medicine, vol. 56:*
Human Airway Inflammation: Sampling Techniques and Analytical Protocols
Edited by: D. F. Rogers and L. E. Donnelly © Humana Press Inc., Totowa, NJ

3. Generation of an RNA probe (as in RNase protection assays or *in situ* hybridization) is not required, eliminating the need to clone the probe into in vitro transcription vectors. Instead the probe is easily manufactured from appropriate cDNA's, including PCR products.

RNA is readily degraded by RNases, which are robust proteins abundant on fingertips and breath. RNases are difficult to inactivate because they are heat stable, refold after denaturation, and do not require cofactors for activity. The key to success in RNA extraction is to mimimize the activity of RNases and we cannot stress enough the need to render equipment RNase-free, to wear gloves at all times, and to keep samples chilled (*see* **Notes 1** and **2**).

1.2. General Strategy

The strategy used in this chapter is summarized in **Fig. 1**. Disruption of cells in culture is relatively easy and is the principle protocol described in the present chapter. Although Northern blotting refers directly to the transfer of RNA to a solid support, such as a nitrocellulose membrane, this is only part of the process. Total cellular RNA is isolated according to the method of Chomczynski and Sacchi (**1**). For successful isolation of RNA, it is necessary to disrupt cells, denature RNA/protein complexes, and inactivate RNases within those cells. Finally, RNA is purified away from contaminating DNA and protein. Extracting polyA+ RNA (mRNA) may further purify RNA. The second portion of the chapter describes size fractionation of the RNA and transfer to a solid support via the Northern blot. The third section describes principles and protocols involved in probe generation and hybridization to the RNA transcript of choice. Finally, quantification of the signal is discussed, because the ultimate aim of the procedure is to detect the presence of an RNA transcript within a cell or tissue, and determine whether its expression is modulated in disease or in response to extracellular stimuli.

This chapter does not attempt to describe the many protocols and approaches available to the researcher for each of the procedures described. The protocols given are those we use routinely in our laboratories to isolate, detect, and quantify RNA transcripts from the airways of a number of species and from cultured cells.

2. Materials
2.1. Reagents

Unless otherwise stated, reagents are obtained from Sigma (Poole, Dorset, UK)

1. Saline: Hanks' balanced salt solution (HBSS) or phosphate-buffered saline (PBS) can be obtained commercially. PBS; for 1 liter dissolve 0.2g KCl, 8.0g NaCl, 0.2g KH_2PO_4, 1.15g Na_2HPO_4, and pH to 7.4 with NaOH.

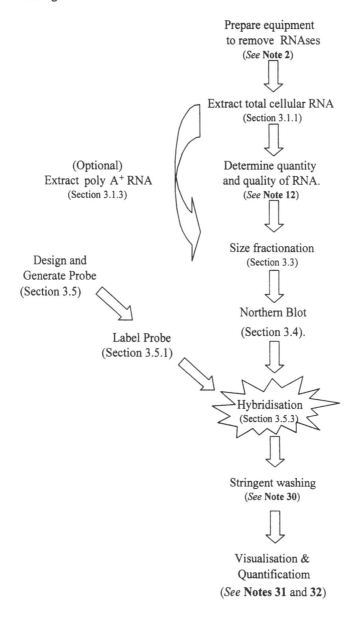

Fig. 1. Overview of Northern blotting. Northern blotting refers to the transfer of RNA to a solid support such as a nylon membrane. This, however, is only a small portion of the process described in this chapter. RNA is extracted, size fractionated, and transferred to a membrane where the RNA transcript of interest is probed for using a labeled DNA or RNA probe. This chapter describes general principles and detailed protocols used in our laboratory for each step of the chart.

2. Solution D: 4 *M* guanidinium thiocyanate, 1% (v/v) 2-mercaptoethanol, 0.5% (w/v) sodium sarcosyl (*see* **Note 3**). Solution D prepared without 2-mercaptoethanol is stable for several months at room temperature, but should be shielded from light. After addition of 2-mercaptoethanol, complete solution D is only stable for a few days.

3. Phenol/chloroform/isoamyl alcohol (50:49:1): Phenol (Rathburn Chemicals, Perthshire, UK) is extremely corrosive and standard safety precautions should be observed.

4. 4 *M* Sodium acetate (pH 4.0): pH to 4.0 with glacial acetic acid. A large volume (approx 50% vol) of acetic acid is required.

5. Isopropanol (BDH, Dorset, UK) and 75% (v/v) ethanol (BDH, Dorset, UK) are stored at –20°C for use in RNA extraction.

6. DEPC-treated water: 0.1% (v/v) diethyl pyrocarbonate (DEPC) in sterile water. To fully dissolve the DEPC it should be left at room temperature overnight (*see* **Note 4**). DEPC traces are removed by autoclaving. DEPC is a possible carcinogen.

7. Nuclease-free water (Promega or Ambion).

8. 10X MOPS: (3- [N-morpholino]-2-hydroxypropanesulfonic acid), pH 7.0. For 1 liter of 10X MOPS fully dissolve 83.72 g of MOPS (free acid) and 8.23g sodium acetate in 0.8 liters of DEPC-treated water. Add 20 mL of 0.5 *M* EDTA, pH 8.0 and pH to 7.0 with NaOH before making up to 1 liter. On autoclaving the solution will turn yellow. This will not affect its electrophoretic properties.

9. Agarose/formaldehyde gels: 1% (w/v) agarose gels containing 6.3% (v/v) formaldehyde, 20 m*M* MOPS (pH 7.0), 5 m*M* sodium acetate and 1 m*M* EDTA (*see* **Note 5**).

10. Ethidium Bromide (EtBr): Prepare as a 10mg/mL solution in DEPC-treated water (*see* **Note 6**).

11. 5X formaldehyde gel loading buffer: 0.1 *M* MOPS pH 7.0, 40 m*M* sodium acetate, 5 m*M* EDTA.

12. TE buffer: 10 m*M* Tris-HCl, pH 8.0, 1 m*M* EDTA.

13. Standard saline citrate (SSC): For 1 liter of 20X SSC, dissolve 173.3 g sodium chloride, 88.2 g sodium citrate in 800 mL distilled H_2O and pH to 7.0 with NaOH.

14. Nylon membranes: Magna+ nylon membranes (MSI, Westborough) or hybond N+ (Amersham/Pharmacia, Bucks, UK) are used as a solid support.

15. Formamide: available from a number of manufacturer's, although it varies in quality (*see* **Note 7**).

16. Labeling buffer: 250 m*M* Tris-HCl, pH 7.6, 25 m*M* $MgCl_2$, 10 m*M* dithiothreitol (DTT), 1 *M* HEPES, pH 6.6, 26 A_{260} units/mL of random hexadeoxyribonucleotides.

17. dNTP mixture, containing dATP, dGTP, and dTTP, 500 µ*M* each.

18. Denhardts solution: can be purchased as a 50X solution, but is prepared as follows: dissolve 1 g of Ficoll (Type 400; Amersham/Pharmacia), 1 g polyvinylpyrrolidine, 1g bovine serum albumin (BSA, Fraction V) in distilled H_2O. Make up to 100 mL, aliquot and store at –20°C.

19. Prehybridization/hybridization buffer: 50% (v/v) deionized formamide, 50 m*M* Tris-HCl (pH 7.5), 5X Denhardts solution, 0.1% (w/v) sodium dodecyl sulphate (SDS), 5 m*M* EDTA and 250 µg/mL denatured salmon sperm DNA.

20. Radiolabel: $[\alpha^{32}P]dCTP$ (specific activity >3000Ci/mmol, Amersham/Pharmacia, Bucks, UK).
21. Multiprime system nucleotide labeling kit (Amersham/Pharmacia, Bucks, UK).
22. Sephadex columns: Sephadex G50 is ideal for isolating probes ≈250bp. Spin columns are prepared in 2 mL syringes with glass wool pushed into the bottom. G50 Sephadex slurry (1:1 in TE from Amersham/Pharmacia) is pipeted into the column and centrifuged at 1000g for 5min.

2.2. Apparatus

1. Latex gloves (BDH, Dorset, UK) (*see* **Note 1**).
2. Tissue is homogenized with a single 30 s pulse (at ~14000 rpm) using a polytrontype homogenizer such as an Ultra Turrax Homogenizer.
3. Oakridge (thick-walled polypropylene tubes) and Corex glass tubing (suitable for use in a Sorval SS34 or equivalent rotor).
4. Agarose gel electrophoresis equipment (e.g., Submarine electrophoresis system from Bio-Rad).
5. UV crosslinkers such as the Stratalinker UV crosslinker from Stratagene or ultraviolet lamp/light box.
6. Hybridization ovens (e.g., Hybridizer HB1D from Techne): a shaking water bath is an acceptable alternative.
7. Kodak XAR film (or equivalent) and appropriate film cassettes.

3. Methods

3.1. Isolation of RNA

3.1.1. Isolation of RNA from Cells in Culture

This protocol is for isolation of RNA from a 175 cm^2 tissue culture flask containing approx 2–3 million cells, but may be scaled up or down as appropriate.

1. Wash cells twice with ice-cold HBSS to remove cell debris (*see* **Note 8**).
2. Add 10 mL solution D to flask or culture dish. Transfer into an Oakridge-style tube.
3. Isolate RNA by addition of 10 mL phenol:chloroform:isoamyl alcohol (at a ratio of 50:49:1).
4. Add 2 mL 4 M sodium acetate (pH 4.0).
5. Vigorously mix by shaking for 30 s. The solution should appear milky.
6. Stand on ice for 15 min.
7. Centrifuge at 10,000g for 15 min. The phenol/chloroform and aqueous phases should have separated.
8. Carefully remove the upper phase containing RNA and transfer to a 30 mL Corex tube. Extreme care should be taken to avoid removing or touching the protein at the phenol/water interface to prevent protein (and especially RNase) carry over. Protein should be visible as a white precipitate at the interface and smeared on the wall of the tube.

9. Precipitate RNA by addition of an equal volume of propan-2-ol. At 4°C this takes approx 15–30 minutes; however, 2–14 h at –20°C maximizes yield.
10. Pellet RNA by centrifugation at 12000*g* for 15 min at 4°C.
11. Carefully pour off the supernatant and resuspend RNA/salt pellet in 5 mL solution D and add a further 5 mL of isopropanol (*see* **Note 9**). RNA is precipitated for a minimum of 2 h at –20°C.
12. Pellet RNA by centrifugation at 12,000*g* for 15 min.
13. Residual salt is removed by washing in 70% (v/v) ethanol. The majority of the pellet is comprised of salt at this stage and may require an additional 70% (v/v) ethanol wash to remove it if the pellet is large.
14. Pellet RNA by centrifugation at 12000*g* for 15 min at 4°C.
15. Dry the RNA pellet in air or under vacuum at –20°C. It is important to remove residual ethanol, as this will prevent resuspension of the pellet (*see* **Note 10**).
16. Resuspend RNA pellet in 50–100µL of TE or nuclease free water (*see* **Notes 11** and **12**).

3.1.2. Isolation of RNA from Tissue Samples

See Chapter 22 for description of isolation of RNA from human lung tissue.

3.1.3. Isolation of Poly A⁺ RNA

It is possible to increase the sensitivity of Northern blotting by isolating the mRNA fraction of the RNA pool. Purification of mRNA makes use of the poly-adenylate tail found on the 3' end of mRNA. An oligonucleotide containing poly thymidine or poly uracil residues attached to a support matrix (such as cellulose) allows affinity purification of the mRNA (*2*).

1. Total RNA isolate (in column loading buffer such as 20 mM Tris-HCl, 1 mM EDTA, 0.1% w/v SDS) is heated and rapidly cooled to remove secondary structures within the RNA.
2. Oligo dT cellulose is added and the RNA is allowed to bind.
3. Once bound, the RNA is washed several times with column loading buffer before elution in 2–3 column volumes of elution buffer (such as 10 mM Tris-HCl, pH 7.6, 1 mM EDTA, 0.05% w/v SDS) or nuclease-free water (*see* **Note 13**).

3.2. Concentration of RNA before Size Fractionation

Once isolated it is necessary to concentrate the (m)RNA as only a small volume may be loaded onto the gel for size fractionation. Concentration of the RNA may be achieved by either alcohol precipitation or freeze-drying (for samples <0.5 mL). Lithium chloride may also be used to precipitate RNA. It has the advantage over precipitation in alcohol in that it does not coprecipitate carbohydrate, protein or DNA. A final LiCl concentration of 2–3 M is needed to precipitate RNA.

3.2.1. Freeze Drying

1. Snap-freeze RNA in liquid nitrogen.
2. Desiccate at –60°C under vacuum until the RNA appears as a white precipitate around the inside of the tube. This takes several hours.
3. Thoroughly resuspend the RNA in required volume of TE or nuclease-free water.

3.2.2. Precipitating with Alcohol

1. Add 0.1 vol of 3 M sodium acetate (pH 5.2) to the mRNA solution, then three volumes of ice-cold 100% ethanol (*see* **Note 14**).
2. After a minimum of 30 min on ice (we precipitate for 2 h to overnight at –20°C), centrifuge RNA at 12,000g at 4°C for 20 min.
3. Carefully pour off the supernatant and wash the pellet with 0.5–1 mL of 70% (v/v) EtOH.
4. Pellet the RNA by centrifugation at 12,000g at 4°C for 20 min.
5. Air-dry the pellet at room temperature (~15 min).
6. Resuspend in a small volume (to a concentration of 10 mg/mL) of TE or nuclease-free water.

3.3. Size Fractionation of RNA

The protocol given below is for a 150 mL gel, but may be scaled up or down as appropriate.

1. Dissolve 1.5 g agarose in 108 mL sterile water by heating in a microwave.
2. Allow the agarose solution to cool to approx 50°C.
3. Add 15 mL of 10X MOPS running buffer and 27 mL 35% (v/v) formaldehyde (*see* **Note 5**).
4. Pour the gel into an appropriate casting tray (containing "combs" for loading of the RNA) and allow the gel to set (*see* **Note 15**).
5. Once set, remove the combs and submerge the gel in 1X MOPS buffer, allowing buffer to just cover the gel. Prerun the gel for 10 min before loading the RNA.
6. Add RNA (10–20 µg) to 1X formaldehyde gel loading buffer and heat for 5 min at 65°C.
7. Cool on ice and add 2 µL EtBr (10 mg/mL) and 1 µL of tracking dye (such as 0.25% w/v bromophenol blue).
8. Load RNA/gel loading buffer into the pre-formed wells and apply current to the gel.
9. Electrophoresis is typically carried out at 150mA (*see* **Note 16**). The time of electrophoresis will depend on the equipment used.
10. Once electrophoresis is complete the RNA may be visualized under ultraviolet (UV) illumination (*see* **Note 17**) (*see* **Fig. 2** and **Note 18**).

3.4. Northern Blotting

Subsequent to size fractionation, RNA is transferred and fixed permanently to a solid support by Northern blotting. Transfer of the RNA is achieved using

A   **B**

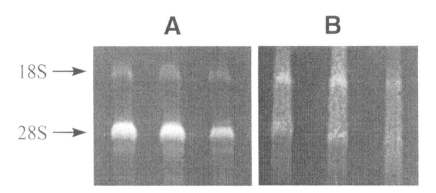

Fig. 2. Quality of RNA. Photographs of ethidium bromide-stained gels following RNA extraction and size fractionation on a 1% (w/v) agarose gel. **Panel A** shows good quality total RNA that has characteristic 28S and 18S bands in a ratio of approx 2:1. In contrast, the RNA in **panel B** has degraded showing typical smearing of the RNA along the lane.

capillary action, electrophoretic transfer, or vacuum transfer. Capillary action is slow, but does not require specialized equipment. We describe blotting by capillary action, as this is the method of transfer performed in our laboratory (*see* **Fig. 3**).

1. Place Whatman 3MM paper (three sheets) on a support larger and wider than the gel (*see* **Note 19**). The paper must make contact with the 20X SSC to allow wicking.
2. Roll the paper with a sterile pipet or glass rod to remove air bubbles.
3. Orientate the gel by cutting off the lower left-hand corner, and place onto the paper.
4. Label the nylon membrane (with pencil) and cut an appropriate corner to allow orientation after transfer. Briefly soak the membrane in 20X SSC and place on top of the gel (*see* **Notes 20** and **21**).
5. Roll the membrane (*see* **step 2** above) to remove air bubbles.
6. Surround the gel with cling film to prevent flow of SSC around the gel.
7. Place three sheets of 3MM paper onto the membrane and a pile of paper towels (~15 cm high) on top of the paper.
8. Place a glass plate on the pile and a 500 g weight (usually a bottle containing 500 mL water) on the top.
9. Allow transfer overnight. It may be necessary to replace soaked paper towels.
10. Remove membrane and fix the RNA by placing in an UV crosslinker using a 120μj burst for 30 s (*see* **Note 22**).
11. Wrap the membrane in Clingfilm and store at 4°C for several months or –20°C for longer.

3.5. Detection of Gene Expression

Detection of expression and quantification of the transcript of interest amongst other RNA transcripts expressed in the cell is the ultimate aim of

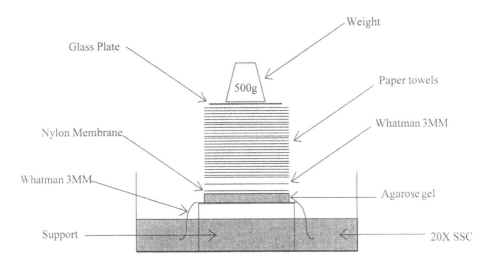

Fig. 3. Capillary blotting. Northern blots by capillary action are set up as shown in this figure. Buffer is drawn from the reservoir, through Whatmann paper, the agarose gel, the nylon membrane, and onto paper towels. RNA is drawn from the gel onto the nylon membrane by this action, where it is permanently fixed.

performing the Northern blot. It is beyond the scope of this chapter to detail the process of designing and generating probes for use in Northern blotting and the reader is referred to (*3*).

3.5.1. Labeling of Probes

There are two basic ways of labeling the DNA or RNA probes, namely end labeling and uniform labeling. The protocol below is optimized for labeling 25 ng of DNA template using the commercially available Multiprime system. We routinely label DNA generated by the PCR or from restriction enzyme digests from a plasmid (*see* **Note 23**).

1. Thaw all reagents on ice except the Klenow fragment of DNA polymerase (*see* **Note 24**).
2. Heat 25 ng DNA for 2–3 min at 95–100°C. Chill on ice.
3. Assemble the following components **in the order shown** in a microcentrifuge tube on ice:
   - a. Nuclease-free water (final volume of 50 µL)   x µL
   - b. Labeling 5X buffer   10 µL
   - c. dNTP mixture   2 µL
   - d. Denatured DNA template   25 ng
   - e. [α^{32}P]dCTP (specific activity 3000Ci/mmol) (*see* **Note 25**)   5 µL
   - f. DNA polymerase I, Large (Klenow) fragment   5 Y

4. Mix gently (with pipet tip) and incubate at room temperature for 1–2 h, or at 37°C for 30–60 min.
5. Add 200 µL TE and heat to 95–100°C to terminate the reaction.
6. Remove unincorporated radiolabel (*see* **Subheading 3.5.2.** below) (*see* **Note 26**).

3.5.2. Removal of Unincorporated Radiolabel using Size Exclusion Chromatography

1. Introduce 200 µL radiolabeled probe in TE buffer into the top of a Sephadex G50 spin column and centrifuge for 5 min at 1500*g*.
2. Transfer eluate to a fresh tube (dispose of spin column by appropriate route).
3. Remove 2 µL of probe and place in a scintillation vial. Count radioactivity in a β-scintillation counter (without scintillant).
4. The probe is now ready to hybridize to the filter containing the RNA, or may be stored (with shielding) at –20°C until required (*see* **Note 27**).

3.5.3. Hybridization and Washes

There are a number of methods for hybridization of probes to RNA or other nucleic acids attached to nitrocellulose or nylon membranes. It is beyond the scope of this chapter to detail these, and the reader is referred to (*3*). We use the following protocol:

1. Prehybridize the membrane in 5 mL hybridization buffer at 42°C for at least 4 h (*see* **Note 28**).
2. Add probe directly to the prehybrization mixture (*see* **Note 29**), and hybridize overnight (annealing of probe to RNA is slow in formamide).
3. Rinse filters in 2X SSC 0.1% (w/v) SDS at room temperature.
4. Further washes are performed in the hybridization chamber for 30 min per wash. The temperature is increased and the salt content decreased with each wash (*see* **Note 30**).
5. After washing, drain excess washing buffer from the membrane and wrap in cling film. Do not allow the membrane to dry out as probes may become irreversibly bound.
6. Expose the filter to X-ray film (Kodak XAR-2 or equivalent) overnight at –70°C, and develop film. Weak signals will require longer exposure times (up to 2 wk).
7. Quantification of the signal depends upon the equipment available (*see* **Note 31**). We use laser densitometry and image capture and quantification software (e.g., Quantity One Software, PDI, NY) (*see* **Note 32**).
8. If the autoradiographs exhibit high background, further washes at higher stringency may be performed. For more information readers are advised to refer to Meinkoth & Wahl (*4*).
9. If reprobing is to be performed (*see* **Note 33**), strip the filter by washing for 2–30 min in 50% (v/v) formamide, 1 mM NaHPO$_4$ at 70°C. The filter is then washed twice in SSC in readiness for reprobing.

4. Notes

1. We recommend that gloves be worn when handling reagents and reaction vessels. Gloves that have touched refrigerator handles, door handles, pipets and so on are not RNase-free and should be discarded.
2. A potential source of RNase contamination is the metal tip ejector mechanism on the side of pipets. Remove the metal ejector bar before using the pipet in any situation where the ejector could come into contact with the walls or contents of a vessel. Equipment such as gel tanks may be rendered RNase-free by soaking in 3% (v/v) hydrogen peroxide for several hours, followed by extensive rinsing in sterile or DEPC-treated water (DEPC inhibits RNases [5]). Solutions should be autoclaved to remove RNases. Glassware should be baked for at least 3 h at 180°C, except for Corex tubes which should be soaked in 0.05% DEPC-treated water overnight, followed by autoclaving to remove traces of the DEPC.
3. Solution D is an RNase inhibitor, eliminating the need for other inhibitors of RNAses.
4. DEPC has a half-life of approx 30 min in water and, at a concentration of 0.1%, solutions autoclaved for 15 min/liter can be assumed to be DEPC-free.
5. Formaldehyde should be added to the agarose/MOPS solution inside a fume cupboard after the solution has cooled below 60°C. Formaldehyde in the gel prevents secondary structures from forming in the RNA during electrophoresis that might affect its mobility through the gel. The formaldehyde also tends to make the gels more brittle, so care should be taken not to break the gel.
6. Ethidium Bromide is a known carcinogen and should be handled with care.
7. Formamide is often pure enough for use immediately in hybridization of Northern blots. A yellow tinge indicates the formamide is not deionized, but it is important to check the pH of the formamide to ensure this is the case regardless of the color. If it is not deionized, add Dowex XG8 mixed bed resin. Stir the solution for 60 min at room temperature before filtering twice through Whatmann #1 paper.
8. All extractions are carried out on ice as low temperatures inhibit RNAses (6).
9. RNA pellets are slimy, so care should be taken when pouring off the supernatant as the RNA can be dislodged.
10. The RNA should not be dried for too long. Under vacuum this typically takes 2–3 min. Excessive drying results in pellets that are difficult to resuspend and can damage the RNA.
11. RNA can be stored in a number of ways. For short-term storage, RNase-free H_2O or TE buffer can be used. RNA is stable at –80°C for up to a year without significant degradation. Magnesium and other metals catalyze nonspecific cleavages in RNA, and should be chelated by the addition of EDTA (RNase-free; older EDTA solutions may have microbial growth which could contaminate the RNA sample with nucleases). RNA solubilized in formamide may be stored at –20°C without degradation for at least 1 y (7). For long-term storage, RNA samples may also be stored at –20°C as ethanol precipitates.

12. Quantity of RNA is calculated by measuring absorbance (optical density, OD) at 260 and 280 nm wavelengths. Since an OD_{260} of 1 is equivalent to 40 µg/mL RNA, the concentration of RNA extracted can be determined. The ratio of OD_{260} to OD_{280} gives an indication of the quality of the RNA. The $OD_{260/280}$ for RNA is 2:1 (ratios of 1.7:1 to 2:1 are acceptable). $OD_{260/280}$ ratios >2.1 are due to contaminating protein, which may be removed by a phenol/chloroform/IAA extraction. This is not ideal, because up to 40% of the RNA may be lost during the reextraction procedure. $OD_{260/280}$ ratios <1.7 are usually caused by contaminating guanidine thiocyanate or 2-mecaptoethanol. These contaminants can be removed by EtOH precipitation of the RNA. However, it is difficult to measure the $OD_{260/280}$ when mRNA is isolated from small numbers of cells. The best way to determine the quality of the RNA is to visualize it after size fractionation by agarose gel electrophoresis.

13. A number of kits are available commercially to isolate mRNA. We use the PolyAtract system IV kit from Promega. Biotinylated oligo dT is bound to magnetic beads and allows rapid binding, washing, and elution of mRNA from 100µg–1mg of total RNA.

14. Precipitating RNA with alcohol (ethanol or isopropanol) requires monovalent cations (e.g., 0.2 M Na$^+$, K$^+$; 0.5 M NH$_4^+$) (*8*). Isopropanol is less efficient at precipitating RNA than ethanol, but in the presence of NH$_4^+$ it is better than ethanol at keeping free nucleotides in solution. RNA precipitation is faster and more complete at higher RNA concentrations. In general RNA concentrations of 10 µg/mL can be precipitated in several hours, but at lower concentrations a carrier nucleic acid or glycogen should be added to facilitate precipitation.

15. Pour gels as thin as possible, but thick enough to give a well depth sufficient to accommodate the sample volume. The thinner the gel, the faster and more efficient the transfer. Transfer is also impeded by agarose concentrations >1.2% (w/v).

16. Nucleic acids are negatively charged and move from the cathode to the anode, universally labeled black and red, respectively.

17. UV light is dangerous to skin and especially to eyes making it essential to wear a safety mask or goggles when visualizing RNA.

18. **Figure 2** shows RNA extractions that have produced either good or poor quality RNA. Total cellular RNA should have two prominent bands that represent the 28S and 18S rRNA and tRNA species, respectively (*see* **Fig. 2A**). These should be present in a ratio of approx 2:1. Extensive smearing in the lanes or a reversal in the 28S:18S intensity ratio is indicative of degradation of the RNA (*see* **Fig. 2B**). Poly A$^+$ RNA appears as a faint smear although it is often not possible to visualize this because of the small amounts of RNA extracted.

19. To limit evaporation of buffer, we use a sandwich box with two slits cut in the lid. A thin sponge is laid on the lid with the ends pushed through the slits to act as the wick.

20. Nitrocellulose or nylon membranes are the two basic types of membranes used in Northern blotting. Nitrocellulose membranes give low background noise, but suffer from two major problems:

1. the RNA is fixed to the nitrocellulose by baking, which makes the membrane extremely brittle.
2. The nucleic acid is not covalently bound to the nitrocellulose, which results in loss of the nucleic acid on washing, especially at high temperatures.

These two factors make it possible to probe nitrocellulose membranes only a few times. We prefer positively charged nylon membranes because they:

1. Bind nucleic acids irreversibly.
2. Are durable.
3. Give a more even signal than negatively charged membranes.
4. Are more sensitive than neutral membranes.

21. Use forceps when handling the membrane. Avoid touching the membrane, as this increases background noise and introduces RNases onto the membrane.
22. It is necessary to permanently fix the RNA to the membrane after transfer. Permanent attachment of the RNA to nylon membranes can be achieved by baking, but exposing the RNA to low levels of ultraviolet light (at 254 nm) is preferred *(9)*. UV crosslinking induces a cyclo-addition reaction between vicinal uridines or aromatic groups on the membrane resulting in covalent attachment of the RNA to the membrane. UV crosslinking is best achieved using a UV cross-linker such as the Stratalinker. An alternative is to use a UV light box or lamp, although we have found variation in UV output as the bulb ages seriously affects nonspecific binding of our probes. Using a hand-held lamp on the short wavelength setting results in crosslinking within 1–2 minutes.
23. It is important to remove any nonspecific DNA, such as that found in the plasmid vector, because it may significantly increase background.
24. Klenow is an enzyme stored in glycerol and does not need to be thawed. After use return immediately to –20°C.
25. It is not necessary to use [^{32}P]dCTP in the labeling reaction (e.g., [^{32}P]UTP is often used as a label for RNA probes). Other labels include ^{3}H, ^{35}S, or ^{125}I. Note local rules for handling and disposal of radioactivity.
26. Unincorporated radiolabel will significantly increase background noise if present during hybridization. Unincorporated radiolabel is removed either by selective precipitation of labeled DNA or by size exclusion chromatography. Selective precipitation relies on small (<20 bp) fragments of DNA not being precipitated in ethanol in the presence of ammonium acetate. In size exclusion chromatography, labeled probes are centrifuged through Sephadex G50 columns, which retain short (≤200 bp) oligomers. We prefer size exclusion chromatography because it is rapid.
27. The half-life of ^{32}P is approx 2 wk making it important to use the probe soon after labeling.
28. It is essential to include blocking agents such as Denhardt's solution and fragmented DNA when probing Northern blots, especially when probing for transcripts with low expression. Ideally, probing is carried out in a hybridization chamber inside a hybridization oven, although a sealed bag in a shaking water bath is an acceptable alternative.

29. The amount of probe added depends on the level of expression of the transcript of interest. Adding more than $5-10^6$ cpm/mL gives high background, and we use no more than $2-10^6$ cpm/mL. For abundant transcripts (e.g., glyceraldehyde-6 phosphate dehydrogenase, GAPDH), $0.25-10^6$ cpm/mL is sufficient to give a strong signal.

30. The stringency of washing depends on the melting temperature of the probe/RNA hybrid (this is usually determined empirically). We wash to a stringency of $55-65°C$ in $0.5-0.1$x SSC, depending on the probe.

31. For quantification of blots, differences in loading or efficiency of RNA transfer can be accounted for by probing the filter for expression of a gene which should remain constant. Enzymes involved in anerobic respiration (e.g., GAPDH) or structural components (e.g., β-actin) are often used, although there is now evidence that expression of these genes varies between tissues. An alternative is to monitor 18S or 28S ribosomal RNA levels, which are less susceptible to changes in levels of expression.

32. The method of detection depends upon the method of probe labeling. Common methods of detection are autoradiography or exposure of X-ray film to chemiluminescence. A more direct measurement of radioactivity after auto-radiography, is to cut out the appropriate area of blot and count using liquid scintillation counting, although this prevents reprobing of the blot. Alternative approaches include the Phosphorimager system (Molecular Dynamics Inc.) which detects ionizing radiation directly from the gel to generate an image and allow quantification of the signal.

33. One advantage of Northern blotting over techniques such as RNase protection assays or S1 nuclease assays is that the probe can be stripped from the filter and probed for other transcripts. This is useful for quantification of steady-state levels of RNA transcript. Reprobing with a "housekeeping" gene (e.g., GAPDH) allows variation in loading or transfer of the RNA to be assessed.

References

1. Chomczynski, P. and Sacchi, N. (1987) Single-step method of RNA isolation by guanidinium thiocyanate-chloroform extraction. *Anal. Biochem.* **162,** 156–159.
2. Aviv H. and Leder, P. (1972) Purification of biologically active globin messenger RNA by chromatography on oligothymidylic acid-cellulose. *Proc. Natl. Acad. Sci.* **69,** 1408–1412.
3. Sambrook, J., Fritsch, E. F., and Maniatis, T. (1992) *Molecular cloning. A laboratory manual.* 2nd ed. Cold Spring Harbour Laboratory, Cold Spring Harbour, NY.
4. Meinkoth, J. and Wahl, G. (1984) Hybridization of nucleic acids immobilized on solid supports. *Anal. Biochem.* **138,** 267–284.
5. Fedorcsak, I. and Ehrenberg, L. (1966) Effects of diethyl pyrocarbonate and methyl methanesulfonate on nucleic acids and nucleases. *Acta. Chem. Scand.* **20,** 107–112.
6. Han, J. H., Stratowa, C., and Rutter, W. J. (1987) Isolation of full-length putative rat lysophospholipase cDNA using improved methods for mRNA isolation and cDNA cloning. *Biochemistry.* **26,** 1617–1625.

7. Chomczynski, P. (1992) Solubilization in formamide protects RNA from degradation. *Nuc. Acids Res.* **20,** 3791–3792.
8. Wallace, D.M. (1987) Precipitation of Nucleic Acids. *Methods Enzymol.* **152,** 41–46.
9. Khandjian, I. (1987) Optimized hybridization of DNA blotted and fixed to nitrocellulose and nylon membranes. *Biotechnology* **5,** 165–170.

21

The Technique of *In Situ* Hybridization

Sun Ying and A. Barry Kay

1. Introduction

In situ hybridization (ISH) (also called "hybridization histochemistry" or "hybridization cytology") was first described in 1969 by Gall and Pardue who used the technique to localize ribosomal DNA in Xenopus oocytes *(1)*. In contrast to other techniques of hybridization (i.e., Northern or Southern blotting), ISH allows detection of specific DNA or RNA molecules in single cells, histological sections, or chromosomes. During the past decades, ISH has become a powerful tool in molecular biology and pathology, and has been widely applied to the localization of viral DNA, detection of expression of messenger RNA, and analysis of genes in chromosomes. This chapter describes the technique of ISH in some detail and also explains the pitfalls associated with its use.

1.1. Principle of ISH

The principle of ISH is based on the fact that the bases adenine (A) or cytidine (C) from DNA/or RNA sequences can pair specifically to the complementary bases thymine (T), guanine (G), or uridine (U) of other sequences of DNA/or RNA, by hydrogen bonds, respectively. Using a labeled nucleotide (probe), the DNA or RNA molecules in cells or sections of tissue can be localized. The hybridization signals are visualized through autoradiography or immunohistochemistry or fluorescence, depending on the methods of labeling the probe.

1.2. Types of Probes

Several types of labeled-probes can be used for ISH to detect DNA location or mRNA expression. These include:

From: *Methods in Molecular Medicine, vol. 56:*
Human Airway Inflammation: Sampling Techniques and Analytical Protocols
Edited by: D. F. Rogers and L. E. Donnelly © Humana Press Inc., Totowa, NJ

1. Double-stranded DNA probes. Usually, this probe can be labeled by methods of "random primer-labeling" *(2)* or "nick translation" *(3)*. However, since the amount of probes labeled by random primer is less than that of nick translation, the latter is often used for labeling of double-strand DNA for ISH.

2. Oligonucleotide probes. This probe is easily and commercially obtained by artificial DNA synthesis *(4,5)*. The 5' end extension (using T4 polynucleotide kinase) or 3' end extension (using terminal deoxyribonucleotidyl transferase) can be performed for labeling oligo probes. A major disadvantage of oligo probes is their relative insensitivity and nonspecific binding owing to their small sizes (in general 20–50 nucleotides of unique sequence).

3. Single-stranded DNA probes. Single-stranded DNA probe is produced by M13 phage and labeled by 3' or 5' end labeling. Becaues of difficulties in subcloning, it has been gradually replaced by asymmetrical polymerase chain reaction (PCR) to produce high specific single stranded DNA probes *(6,7)*.

4. Single-stranded RNA probes. This probe, also termed "riboprobe," was first described in 1984. Using this method, Cox and colleagues *(8)* had reported a sensitivity of 20 mRNA copies per cell. To generate RNA probes, a desired cDNA fragment must insert in downstream orientation from a RNA polymerase promoter *(9,10)*. When the RNA polymerase and nucleotides (UTP, GTP, ATP, and CTP, one of them is "labeled") are added, in vitro transcription is initiated. The "labeled" nucleotide is incorporated into the newly formed antisense probe (or cRNA, with complementary sequence to target mRNA) or sense probe (with identical sequence to target mRNA). The labeled antisense probes (cRNA probes) hybridize with target mRNA in the individual cells. In contrast, sense probes cannot hybridize to the target mRNA and can be used as a control **(Fig. 1)**.

   The advantages of RNA probes include:

   a. higher affinity and thermal stability of RNA:RNA hybrids than that of DNA:RNA hybrids.

   b. use of a constant defined probe size by direct or limited basic hydrolysis *(8)*.

   c. ability to generate the cRNA probe without vector sequences which may cause nonspecific binding.

   d. exclusion of competitive hybridization to the complementary strand, which may occur with double-stranded DNA probes.

   e. higher specificity than that of oligonucleotide probes.

After hybridization, RNase treatment can be relied upon to digest the unhybridized cRNA probe, which reduces background and provides strong specific signals. So far, several RNA expression vectors are commercially available, such as the pSp72 (Promega), pGEM (Promega), pT7/T3 (Gibco-BRL), and pBluscript (Northumbria Biologicals Ltd) systems. These vectors have two reverse orientation promoters of RNA polymerase (Sp6/T7 or T7/T3) and polylinkers between two promoters. Thus, the orientation of transcription will depend upon the RNA polymerase added **(Fig. 1)**. Because of the inconvenience of subcloning of desired cDNA fragments into RNA expression

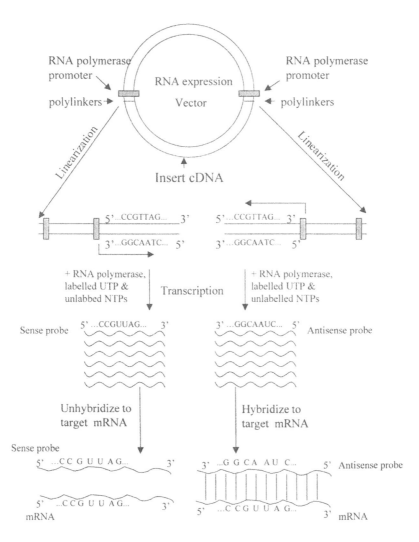

Fig. 1. The principle of *in situ* hybridization using riboprobes

vectors, some investigators have attempted to use PCR to generate cRNA probes *(11)*.

The types of probes and methods for labeling are summarized in **Table 1**.

1.3. Probe Labeling

Generally, there are two classes of labels for probes used in ISH, i.e., isotopic and nonisotopic labels. The former includes tritium (^{3}H), sulphur (^{35}S), phosphorus (^{32}P), and iodine (^{125}I). ^{3}H has the lowest energy emission and gives the finest resolution, and is therefore suitable for both cellular and sub-

Table 1
Methods for Labeling Probes

Probe	template	Method	Enzyme	Vector
DNA	dsDNA	Nick Translation	DNase I DNA polymerase I	Plasmid
DNA	dsDNA	Random Primer	Klenow polymerase I	Plasmid
DNA	ssDNA	3' end labeling	TdT	M13 phage
Oligo	—	5' end labeling	T4 polynucleotide kinase	no need
RNA	dsDNA	in vitro transcription	Sp6/T7/T3	RNA expression Vector

ds=double-strand; ss=single-strand; TdT: terminal deoxynucleotidal transferase

cellular localization of targets (i.e., chromosome mapping). However, the low energy emission needs longer exposure time, ranging usually from 6 wk to several months. ^{35}S is a popular label because of its short exposure time (7–14 d) although the background is somewhat higher than with ^{3}H, and the resolution is not as high. ^{32}P label can be used for rapid analysis because of its high sensitivity and very short exposure time (3–5 d) but with the risk of high background and poor resolution. ^{125}I provides a good resolution coupled with relatively short exposure time, allowing the demonstration of sequences of low density, but with higher background *(12)*. The characteristics of, and utilization of, labels are summarized in **Table 2**.

A number of nonisotopic labels have been used for ISH, such as biotin-, digoxigenin-, or fluorescence-labeled probes *(13)*. Potentially non-radioactive detection methods offer various advantages. The probes are stable, and obviate the need for long exposures used in autoradiography to visualize hybridization signals. Furthermore, excellent single-cell resolution can be obtained and special safety precautions associated with handling radioactive compounds are avoided. The major limitation of these probes is the relative reduced sensitivity compared with isotopic methods. Additionally, combining radio- and nonradio-labeled probes in which distinct labels are employed, multi-mRNAs can be detected in the same slide.

1.4. Fixation, Fixatives, and Hybridization Conditions

Successful ISH depends upon the retention of target nucleotide sequences (e.g., mRNA) and the preservation of tissue/cell morphology *(14)*. Optimal fixatives should have the following advantages: the preservation of the tis-

Table 2
Characteristics of Common Radio- and Nonradio-Labels Used in ISH

Label	Emission	Maximum energy (Mev)	Half life	Exposure time	Resolution
^{32}P	β	1.71	14.3 d	3–5 d	poor
^{35}S	β	0.167	87.4 d	7–14 d	moderate
^{3}H	β	0.018	12.35 y	mo (s)	excellent
Digoxiginin	—	—	N/A	—	excellent
Biotin	—	—	N/A	—	excellent

Note: The sensitivity of different labels: $^{32}P \geq {}^{35}S > {}^{3}H >$ or = nonradiolabels. The resolution of the labels: ^{3}H = nonradiolabels (biotin or digoxigenin) $> {}^{35}S > {}^{32}P$.

Table 3
Comparison of Fixatives for ISH

Fixative	Cell	Tissue	Fixation time (minutes) RNA Retention	Morphology
4% Paraformaldehyde	30	2–4 h	+++	+++
2% Glutarmaldehyde	30	2–4 h	+++	++++
Ethanol/acetic acid (95/5)	15	30	++	++
Methanol/ acetone (50/50)	4	20	+	++

sue integrity, retention of mRNA within the tissue and provision for efficient access of the probe to the target RNA. Generally, there are two types of fixatives, namely precipitating- and crosslinking. The former (e.g., combinations of methanol and acetone) provides the highest probe penetration and reasonable preservation of the tissue morphology, but relatively poor retention of RNA. The latter (e.g., glutaraldehyde) provides the best RNA retention but with poor probe penetration because of wide crosslinking of tissue. Another crosslinking fixative, buffered 4% paraformaldehyde appears to meet all three requirements *(15)*. Comparison of various fixatives is summarized in **Table 3**.

Compared with immunocytochemistry, an important advantage of ISH is that specificity of hybridization can be precisely controlled by changes in reaction conditions. The specificity of hybridization is based on the types of probes, temperature, pH, and the concentration of formamide and salt in the hybridization solutions. The extent to which mismatching base pairs are allowed is termed "stringency." Under high stringent conditions, the stable hybrids can be formed only when high homology sequences between probe and target RNA exist. In contrast, under low stringent conditions, the target sequences with 70–90% homology will also hybridize with the probe, causing nonspecific binding. Generally, the "stringency" can be increased by raising the temperature of the reaction and reducing the concentration of salt solution *(15)*. The optimal conditions of hybridization vary with different tissue, and type of probes used.

2. Materials

1. Phosphate buffered saline (PBS): 8 g/L NaCl, 0.2 g/L KCl, 1.44 g/L Na_2HPO_4, 0.24 g/L KH_2PO_4 in distilled H_2O , adjust pH to 7.4 with HCl.
2. 4% (w/v) paraformaldehyde (PAF): prewarm (56°C) PBS in a cupboard, add PAF, stir until completely dissolved, then keep the solution at 4°C until used. Fresh prepared PAF is always recommended for ISH.
3. 0.3% (v/v) Decon 90 (Decon Laboratories, UK): dilute Decon 90 in tap water.
4. Absolute ethanol and 70% (v/v), 95% (v/v) ethanol.
5. DEPC (diethyl pyrocarbonate, Sigma, UK) -treated H_2O: prepare distilled H_2O containing 0.1% (w/v) DEPC, leave the solution at 37°C overnight, autoclave it and keep at room temperature up to 6 mo.
6. 0.1% (w/v) solution of poly-L-lysine (PLL, MW > 150,000, Sigma): dissolve PLL in DEPC-treated H_2O, dispense the solution into aliquots, store at –20°C up to 6 mo to avoid frequent thawing and freezing.
7. Silicon treatment.
8. 15% (w/v) sucrose/PBS: sucrose (Sigma) in PBS, and keep at 4°C until used. To avoid any bacterial contamination, fresh prepared solution is always recommended.
9. Iso-Pentane, and OCT (Optimum Cutter Temperature compound).
10. RPMI 1640 medium (BRL, UK).
11. Normal human plasma.
12. Sodium azide (BDH, Dagenham, UK).
13. Transcription buffer (for radio-labeled riboprobes) (Promega, UK).
14. DTT (dithiothreitol) (Promega): dissolve DDT at 5 *M* concentration. Dispense the solution into aliquots, store at –20°C up to 12 mo to avoid frequent thawing and freezing.
15. RNasin (RNase inhibitor) (Promega).
16. Nucleotides (ATP, GTP, CTP, UTP, dATP, dCTP, dGTP, and dTTP) (Pharmacia Biotech, UK).
17. ^{35}S-UTP, ^{32}P-UTP, ^{32}P-dCTP, and ^{32}P-ATP (Amersham, UK).
18. RNA polymerases (Sp6, T7, and T3) (Promega).
19. RNase-free DNase (Promega).
20. Yeast tRNA (Sigma).
21. 4 *M* NaCl: 234 g/L NaCl in distilled H_2O.
22. Phenol and Chloroform (BRL, UK).
23. 7 *M* ammonium acetate: 539.56 g/L ammonium acetate in distilled H_2O and sterilize by filtration.
24. Transcription buffer (for digoxigenin-labeled riboprobes) (Boehringer Mannheim, Gemany).

25. RNA labeling Mix (containing CTP, GTP, ATP, and UTP-digoxigenin) (Boehringer Mannheim).
26. 0.5 *M* EDTA (disodium ethylenediaminetetraacetatic acid. $2H_2O$, Sigma): 186.1 g/L EDTA in distilled H_2O, adjust pH to 8.0, autoclave, and store at room temperature up to 6 mo.
27. 4 *M* LiCl: 16.95 g LiCl in 100 mL distilled H_2O, and sterilize by filtration.
28. Nick translation buffer (Promega)
29. Optimized enzyme mix (containing DNase I and DNA polymerase I) (Promega)
30. Calf intestinal alkaline phosphatase (CIAP) buffer and CIAP (Promega).
31. 1 *M* Tris- HCl (pH 7.4): 121.1 g /L Tris base in distilled H_2O, adjust pH with HCl to 7.4.
32. TE (Tris-EDTA) buffer (pH. 7.4): 10 m*M* Tris-HCl (pH. 7.4) and 1 m*M* EDTA (pH 8.0).
33. T4 polynucleotide kinase buffer and T4 polynucleotide kinase (Promega).
34. 0.1 *M* Glycine/PBS: 7.5 g/L Glycine (Sigma) in PBS.
35. 0.3% (v/v) Triton-X-100: dilute Triton-X-100 in PBS.
36. Proteinase K (Sigma) stock solution: 300 μg/mL Proteinase K in 20 m*M* Tris-HCl and 1 m*M* EDTA (pH 7.2), dispense the solution into aliquots (1 mL each), store at –20°C up to 6 mo. Working solution: take 1 mL of stock solution and put into 299 mL of prewarmed (37°C) 20 Tris-HCl, 1 mM EDTA, pH 7.2 before use.
37. 0.2 N HCl: 17.2 mL/L commercial HCl (11.6 N) in distilled H_2O.
38. Acetylation solution: 0.25% (w/v) acetic anhydride (Sigma) and 0.1 M triethanolamine (Sigma) in distilled H_2O. The solution should be freshly prepared.
39. Standard saline citrate (SSC): 1X: 0.1 5 *M* sodium chloride, 0.15 *M* sodium citrate, pH 7.0.
40. Prehybridization solution: 50% (v/v) formamide (Sigma) and 2X SSC.
41. Hybridization buffer: 50% (v/v) deionized formamide (Sigma), 5X SSC, 10% (w/v) dextran sulphate (Sigma), 5X Denhardts solution (Sigma), 0.5% (w/v) SDS (Sigma), 100 mg/mL denatured sperm DNA (Sigma), and 100 m*M* DTT. Dispense the buffer into aliquots, store at –20°C up to 6 mo.
42. 10% (w/v) SDS (sodium dodecyl sulfate): dissolve 100 g SDS (BDH) in 900 mL of distilled H_2O, adjust pH to 7.2 and add distilled H_2O to 1 liter.
43. RNase A, and RNase T1 (Sigma).
44. Graded ethanol: 70% (v/v), 95% (v/v) and 100% ethanol containing 0.3 *M* ammonium acetate.
45. Light-sensitive K-5 emulsion (Ilford, Moberley, UK): The new emulsion should be diluted in distilled H_2O as follows: warm the new bottle of emulsion in water bath (45°C) in darkroom for at least 1 h. Under safelight, pour the emulsion into a clean container, mix with one volume of distilled H_2O, and keep warm for further 30 min. Dispense the diluted emulsion into aliquots in dark bottles, seal with boxes and foil, store at 4°C up to 6 mo.
46. Developer (D-19) (Kodak, UK): dissolve the D-19 powder/can in 4000 mL prewarmed (38°C) tap water, adjust the water until 5000 mL. After filtration, dispense the solution into aliquots, covered with foil and store at room temperature up to 3 mo.

47. Working solution of fixer (Ilford Hypam) (Mobberley, UK): dilute fixer in distilled H_2O (1:5) before use.
48. Haematoxylin solution (BDH).
49. Graded ethanol 70% (v/v), 90% (v/v) and 100%.
50. Xylene and D.P.X mountant (BDH).
51. Tris buffered saline (TBS): 140 m*M* NaCl, 25 m*M* Tris-HCl buffer, pH 7.5.
52. Blocking solution: 1 g block reagent (Boehringer Mannheim) in 100 mL TBS, dispense the solution into aliquots and store at –20°C up to 6 mo.
53. Dig-AP-conjugate (sheep polyclonal antidigoxigenin antiserum conjugated with alkaline phosphatase).
54. TBT solution: TBS containing 0.1% (v/v) Tween-20.
55. Equalization buffer: 0.1 M Tris-HCl, 0.1 M NaCl, 50 mM $MgCl_2$, pH 9.5.
56. NBT/BCIP (Boehringer Mannheim) solution: 1.75 mg BCIP (X-phosphate-5-bromo-4-chloro-3-indoly-phosphate), 3.7 mg NBT (nitroblue tetrazolium salt) in 10 mL equalization buffer, 2 m*M* levamisole.
57. Glycergel (Dakopatts, High Wycombe, UK).

3. Methods
3.1. Preparation of Instruments and PLL-Coated Slides for ISH

1. Wash glassware and slides in 0.3% (v/v) Decon 90 for 2 h, rinse in tap water for 2 h, then in distilled water, and dip in 100% ethanol for 20 min (also *see* **Notes 1** and **4**).
2. Dry glassware and slides at room temperature, autoclave at 250°C for 4 h.
3. Coat the slides with 0.1% (w/v) PLL solution prior to applying sections or cytospins. The purpose of slide treatment is mainly to minimize nonspecific attachment of radiolabeled probes to slides and maximise section or bronchoalveolor lavage (BAL) cell retention on the slides throughout the various treatments involved in ISH procedures (also *see* **Note 1**).

3.2. Collection and Preparation of Tissues and Cells for ISH

In principle, any tissue or cells are suitable for ISH *(16–27)*. Ideally, the size of tissue is ~ 3 × 3 mm. Large tissue should be cut into small pieces by using RNase-free scalpel to minimize fixative penetration time. If tissues from animals are used for ISH, the fixation process can be initiated almost immediately by perfusion fixation. Fixed tissue can be frozen directly, or after washing with 15% (w/v) sucrose/PBS. Frozen tissue can be stored at –80°C at least 6 mo without significant loss of hybridization signals. Alternatively, fixed tissue can be embedded in paraffin for ISH. In our department, we prefer to use frozen tissue for ISH *(16–27)*. Thus, the protocol of ISH provided in this chapter bases on frozen sections and cytospins.

3.2.1. Tissue Preparation (Cryostat Sections)

1. Fix biopsies (3 × 3 mm) immediately in freshly prepared 4% (w/v) PAF/PBS for 2 (e.g., lung and nasal biopsies) or 4 (e.g., skin biopsies) hours (also *see* **Notes 1** and **4**).

2. Wash twice (1 h each) with 15% (w/v) sucrose/PBS, embed tissue with OCT, freeze in nitrogen-cooled isopentane, and store at −80°C until used.
3. Cut sections (6–10 μm thick) from the biopsies in a cryostat, mount on PLL-coated slides, and then air-dry overnight at 37°C. The slides should be immediately used for ISH or covered with foil and kept at −80°C up to 6 mo.

3.2.2. Preparation of Cytospins from Cells (e.g., BAL cells)

1. Pass the BAL (bronchoalveolar lavage) cells through sterile gauze **to remove any mucus.** Centrifuge BAL cells at 57.2*g*/min for 10 min at 4 °C. Wash the pellet twice in RPMI 1640 medium, and resuspend in 1.5 mL of RPMI 1640 with 5% (v/v) normal human plasma and 0.1% (w/v) sodium azide. After being counted on a Neubauer haemocytometer, resuspend BAL cells at a concentration of 0.5 to 1.0×10^6 cells/mL in RPMI 1640.
2. Prepare cytospins on PLL-slides with a Shandon 2 Cytospin (Shandon Southern Instruments, Runcorn, UK), air-dry for 10 min, fix in 4% (w/v) PAF/PBS for 30 min, and wash in 15% (w/v) sucrose/PBS for 1 hr each.
3. Incubate at 37°C overnight, then directly use for ISH or cover with foil and store at −80°C (also *see* **Notes 1** and **4**).

3.3. Labeling Probes (also see Note 2)

3.3.1. Labeling Riboprobes (RNA Transcription In Vitro) with Radio-Isotope (^{32}P or ^{35}S)

1. Add the following reagents in the order:

2 μL	5X Transcription Buffer
1 μL	100 m*M* DTT
0.5 μL	RNasin (RNase inhibitor, 25 u/μL)
2 μL	Mixture of ATP, GTP, CTP (2.5 m*M* each)
1 μL	linearized DNA template (1 μg/μL)
2.5 μL	^{35}S-UTP or ^{32}P-UTP (10 mCi/mL)
1 μL	T3, T7, or SP6 RNA polymerase (10 U/μL)

2. Incubate at 37°C for 30 min. Add another 1 μL RNA polymerase in and leave at 37°C for further 30 min.
3. Add 1 μL RNase-free DNase (1 μg/μL) into the reaction and leave at 37°C for 10 min to digest DNA template.
4. Add 1 μL Yeast tRNA (10 μg/μL), 5 μL 4*M* NaCl, and DEPC-treated disH$_2$O until to 200 μL.
5. Add 100 μL Phenol and 100 μL Chloroform (1:1), mix well, then centrifuge at 12,369*g* (approx 18,000 *g*) for 5 min.
6. Take the upper phase into a new tube, add 200 μL fresh chloroform, mix well, and centrifuge at 12,369*g* for 5 min.
7. Collect the upper phase into a new tube with 100 μL 7 *M* ammonium acetate and 750 μL 100% prechilled ethanol, mix well and then leave at −20°C overnight or −80°C for 2 h.

8. Centrifuge at 12,369g for 30 min, wash the pellet with 70% (v/v) pre-chilled ethanol twice, vacuum-dry for 15 min, and dissolve in 10 mL DEPC-treated H_2O.

Take one mL of probe for counting. Keep the rest at –80°C and use as soon as possible (also *see* **Notes 2, 3,** and **4**).

3.3.2. Labeling Riboprobes With Digoxigenin-UTP (Dig-UTP)

1. Add the following reagents in the order:
   2 μL   10X transcription buffer
   2 μL   1 *M* DTT
   1 μL   RNasin
   1 μL   linearized template DNA (1 μg/μL)
   2 μL   RNA labeling Mix
   disH₂O to total volume 18 μL
   2 μL   RNA polymerase (SP6 or T7 or T3, 20 U/μL)
2. Incubate for 2 h at 37°C.
3. Add RNase-free DNase (20 U) to the reaction and incubate at 37°C for 15 min to remove template DNA.
4. Add 2 μL 0.2 *M* EDTA (pH 8.0) to stop the reaction.
5. Add 2 μL 4*M* LiCl and 75 mL prechilled 100% ethanol and then leave at –70°C for 30 min or 2 h at –20°C to precipitate the transcripts.
6. Centrifuge at 12,369g for 15 min, wash the RNA pellet with 70% (v/v) cold ethanol, dry under vacuum and dissolve in DEPC-treated water. Usually, 4–10 mg Dig-labeled transcripts can be obtained from each reaction (1 mg DNA template).
7. Analyze the yield of transcripts by agarose-gel electrophoresis compared with a given concentration of control. The efficiency and specificity of Dig-labeled riboprobe can be detected by dot-blotting (following the instructions of manufacturer). The labeled Dig-riboprobes are stable at –20°C for no more than 6 mo.

3.3.3. Labeling DNA Probes (Nick Translation)

1. Mix the following reagents:
   5 μL   10X nick-translation buffer
   10 μL   dNTPs (dTTP, dATP, dGTP, each 20 m*M*)
   1 μg   sample DNA
   7 μL   [α-^{32}P]-dCTP (70 mCi at 400 Ci/mmole and 10 mCi/μL)
   5 μL   Optimized enzyme Mix (containing DNase I and DNA polymerase I)
   distilled H₂O until 50 μL
2. Incubate the mix for 60 min at 15°C, and then add 6 μL 0.5 M EDTA (pH 8.0) to stop the reaction.
3. Remove unincorporated dNTPs by chromatography or centrifuge using a small column of Sephadex G-50 (Sigma). The specific activity of labeled DNA can be calculated as the follows:

$$\frac{\text{cpm incorporated}}{\text{total cpm}} \times 100 = \% \text{ incorporation}$$

(The factor 33.3 is derived from using 3 mL of 1:100 dilution for counting.
The total volume is equivalent to 50 mL).

$$\frac{\text{cpm incorporated} \times 33.5 \times 50}{\text{mg input DNA}} = \text{cpm}/\mu g$$

3.3.4. Labeling of Oligo Probes (5'-end-labeling)

1. Remove the phosphate groups from 5' termini of linear molecule:
   5 μL   10X calf intestinal alkaline phosphatase (CIAP) buffer
   1 μL   substrate DNA (up to a total of 10 pM of 5' ends)
   0.5 U   CIAP (diluted in CIAP buffer)
   distilled H_2O to final volume 50 μL, 37°C 30 min
   Add another 0.1 U CIAP for further 30 min at 37°C
   Add 1 vol of TE-saturated phenol/chloroform, mix and spin at 12,369g) for 2
   min. Remove the aqueous phase into a fresh tube and repeat the extraction of
   phenol/chloroform. Collect the aqueous phase into a new tube and add 1/10 vol 2
   M NaCl. Add 2 vol of ethanol, mix well and leave at –80°C for at least 30 min.
   Spin (12,369g) for 5 min. Dry the pellet and resuspend the DNA in 34 μL 1 X T4
   polynucleotide kinase buffer.
2. Labeling
   Add the following reagents into the substrate DNA:
   15 μL   [g-^{32}P]-ATP (3,000 Ci/mM at 10 mCi/μL)
   1 μL   T4 polynucleotide kinase (8–10 U/μL)
   Incubate for 30 min at 37°C. Add 2 μL 0.5 M EDTA to stop the reaction. Add 1
   vol of TE–saturated phenol/chloroform, mix, and centrifuge (12,000 rpm) for 2
   min. Collect aqueous phase, add 0.5 vol of 7.5 M ammonium acetate, and 2 volumes of ethanol. Mix and leave at –80°C for at least 30 min. Spin (12,369g) for 5
   min. Redissolve the pellet in 50 μL TE buffer and take 1 μL labeled probe for
   counting. The rest of probe can be stored at –80°C and used as soon as possible
   (also *see* **Notes 2, 3,** and **4**).

3.4. In Situ Hybridization (ISH)

Although ISH has been widely used in many areas, there is still no standard protocol for this technique. Depending on different probes, targets and
specimens, some methodological modifications may be required. The readers may establish their own protocols for their own studies. In this section
we merely suggest the protocols for mRNA detection using riboprobes,
which have been used routinely in our department *(16–27)*.

3.4.1. ISH with Radio-Labeled Riboprobes

3.4.1.1. PREHYBRIDIZATION

All prehybridization and hybridization must be performed under RNase-free conditions (also *see* **Note 4**).

1. Rinse slide (frozen sections or cytospins) in PBS for 5 min.
2. Immerse slides in 0.1 *M* Glycine PBS for 5 min.
3. Place the slides in 0.3% (v/v) Triton X-100 in PBS for 10 min following by PBS supplemented with 0.1% (w/v) DEPC-H$_2$O for 5 min.
4. Permeabilize the samples with Proteinase K solution (1 μg/mL) for 30 min (sections) or 20 min (cytospins) at 37°C.
5. Rinse slides in PBS, fix in 4% (w/v) PAF/PBS for 5 min to terminate Proteinase K activity, then wash with PBS for 5 min.
6. Immerse slides in 0.2 *N* HCl for 20 min.
7. Rinse slides in 0.25% (w/v) acetic anhydride and 0.1 *M* of triethanolamine/L at 40°C for 10 min.
8. Prehybridize slides in prehybridization solution (50% (w/v) formamide and 2 x SSC) for 30 min at 40°C to reduce nonspecific binding.

3.4.1.2. HYBRIDIZATION

1. Wipe away the excess prehybridization solution and add 20 μL hybridization buffer containing 0.8 to 1.0×10^6 cpm ^{35}S- or ^{32}P-labeled riboprobe onto each slide.
2. Using fine forceps (RNase-free), gently place a cover slip coated with silicon treatment onto the section or cytospin.
3. Incubate slides in a sealed humid chamber containing 4X SSC at 42–50°C for 16 h (a different hybridization temperature might be needed for various probes according to their Tm (melting temperature).

3.4.1.3. WASHINGS POST HYBRIDIZATION

1. Remove the cover slips by immersing the slides in 4 x SSC/0.1% (w/v) SDS. The coverslips should float off after approx 1–2 min soaking.
2. Wash the slides in 2X SSC/0.1% (w/v) SDS at room temperature, 4×5 min.
3. Wash the slides in 0.1X SSC/0.1% (w/v) SDS at the same temperature used for hybridization shaking gently, 2×10 min (also *see* **Note 3**).
4. Wash the slides in 2X SSC twice (5 min for each) to remove any trace of SDS. Use the same container throughout, changing the solution quickly. Do not allow the slides to dry out in between any of the wash steps.
5. Incubate the slides with 20 μg/mL RNase A in 2X SSC (30 min at 37°C) to remove unhybridized RNA probe (which can increase background).
6. Wash the slides in 2X SSC and 0.1X SSC for 10 min each at the same temperature used for hybridization, rinse in distilled H$_2$O for 5 min at room temperature (also *see* **Notes 3** and **4**).

7. Dehydrate slides through graded alcohol (70% (v/v), 95% (v/v), and 100%) containing 0.3 M ammonium acetate, 5 min for each step.
8. Air-dry thoroughly before autoradiography.

3.4.1.4. Autoradiography

(The procedures (1–5) must be performed in darkroom)

1. Prewarm K-5 emulsion in water bath (45°C) in darkroom at least 1 h.
2. Put ~ 10 mL of the warmed emulsion (liquid) into a dipping chamber (Amersham International). Leave the chamber in water bath at 45°C for another 20 min. Dip a blank test slide (slowly and vertically) into the chamber to check that the emulsion is smooth and free from bubbles. Examine emulsion layer under the safelight. If free from streaks, lumps, bubbles, and so on, the emulsion is ready for dipping (also *see* **Note 3**).
3. Use thumb and forefinger to hold slide and dip slowly at an even speed. Make sure the slide is in the emulsion for 5 s. Absorb excess emulsion from bottom of the slide on blotting paper and place on drying rack. The slides must be kept vertical at all times. Try to dip all the slides to the same depth in emulsion. The thickness of the layer should be the same for all the slides.
4. Keep the slides on the rack in the darkroom for 4 h (or overnight). Ensure that the darkroom is really dark and switch off the safelight.
5. Collect the slides into light-tight autoradiography slide box with some silical gel. Seal the box with tape, label the dipping date and store at 4°C for 3–5 ds (for ^{32}P-labeled probes) or 2–3 wk (for ^{35}S-labeled probes).
6. Leave the slide box at room temperature for at least 1 h. In the meantime, prepare the solutions for developing: a) developer (D-19). b) distilled H_2O. c) fixer (1/5 dilution in disH_2O). Keep all solutions at 16–18°C. Sudden changes in temperature might damage the delicate emulsion layer.
7. Open the slide box in the darkroom (with the safelight on), put the slide rack into the developer for 3 min. Rinse in distilled H_2O for 30 s, and then fix in the fixer for 5 min.
8. The following procedures can be performed out of the darkroom. Rinse the slides thoroughly in running tap water for 20 min. Counterstain the slides with hematoxylin for 5 min, wash the slides with running tap water for 2 min.
9. Dehydrate in 70% (v/v), 90% (v/v) and 100% alcohol for 5 min each, immerse in xylene for 5 min, and then mount with D.P.X mountant.
10. Specific hybridization is recognized as clear dense deposits of silver grains in the photographic emulsion overlaying the tissue sections or cytospin preparations. Positive cells are identified as dense, discrete well-circumscribed areas of silver grains. When hybridizing positive cells are in close proximity, their numbers are determined by visualizing individual nuclei using dark field illumination *(16,20,21,23,25)* (**Fig. 2 A, B**).

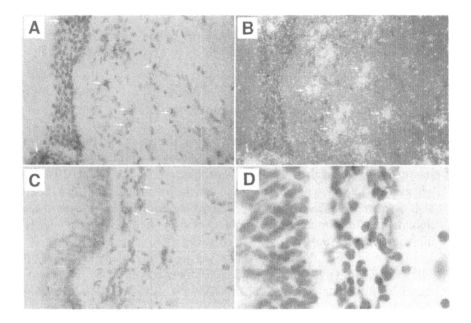

Fig. 2. *In situ* hybridization in bronchial biopsies. A depicts ISH with ^{35}S-labeled RANTES antisense riboprobe. B is the same section of A shown in darkfiled illumination. Some RANTES mRNA+ cells are indicated (arrows) (magnification × 400). C shows ISH with digoxigenin-labeled eotaxin antisense riboprobe (magnification × 200). D is the same section of C shown in high magnification (× 1000). Some eotaxin mRNA+ cells are indicated (arrows).

3.4.2. ISH with Digoxigenin (Dig)-Labeled Riboprobes

1. Immerse the slides in PBS for 5 min followed by treatment with 0.3% (v/v) Triton X-100 in PBS for 10 min.
2. Wash in PBS for 5 min, and then incubate with Proteinase K solution (1 µg/mL) for 30 min (tissue) or 20 min (cytospins) at 37°C.
3. Rinse in PBS, fix the slides in 4% (w/v) PAF/PBS for 5 min, rinse in PBS for 5 min.
4. Incubate the slides with prehybridization solution for 2 h at 40°C.
5. Wipe away the excess prehybridization solution, and add 20 to 30 µL of hybridization buffer contained 100 ng of Digoxigenin-labeled riboprobe onto each slide, cover with cover slips treated with silicon treatment and incubate overnight at 40°C in a humid chamber.
6. Wash the slides sequentially with 4X SSC at 42°C for 10 min twice, followed by incubation with 20 µg/mL RNase A in 2X SSC for 30 min at 37°C to remove unhybridized probe.
7. Wash in 2X SSC and 0.1X SSC for 10 min each at 42°C, then rinse in TBS for 2 min.
8. Incubate the slides with blocking solution at room temperature for 30 min to reduce nonspecific background.

9. Incubate the slides with 1:500 to 1:2000 dilutions of <Dig>-AP conjugate in TBT solution overnight at room temperature.
10. Wash in TBS 3 times (15 min for each), incubate the slides with equalization buffer for 5 min.
11. Develop with freshly prepared NBT/BCIP substrate solution for 20–40 min, at room temperature. Monitor the intensity of positive signals under microscope.
12. Stop the reaction by incubating in 10 mM Tris-HCl, pH 7.8, containing 10 mM EDTA.
13. Wash the slides in running in tap water, counterstain with hematoxylin for 5 s, and mount with glycergel (Dako).
14. The dark-blue deposits in cytoplasm are recognized as positive hybridization signals *(17–19,22,24)* (**Fig. 2 C** and **D**).

3.5. Controls for ISH

*3.5.1. Positive Controls (also see **Notes 3** and **4**)*

1. Tissue or cells (such as cell lines) known to contain the target nucleotide sequences of interest. This can be confirmed by Southern blot, Northern blot, or RT-PCR.
2. Using labeled probes specific for a housekeeping gene (e.g., β-actin) as a method control.

3.5.2. Negative Controls

1. Omit probe in hybridization buffer.
2. Pretreat sections or cytospins with nuclease (i.e., DNase or RNase) to remove the total DNA or RNA from the samples. For instance, pretreat the slides with RNase solution (RNase A 100 μg/mL, and RNase T1 10U/mL) before the prehybridization step with antisense probes.
3. Hybridize the slides with an irrelevant probe (i.e., labeled vector sequences).
4. Hybridize the slides with unlabeled probes.
5. Use the sense probes (having identical sequence to the target mRNA, therefore no hybridization occurs).
6. Omit primary antibody as a negative control for the nonradioactive ISH (i.e., omit anti-Dig antibody during Dig-ISH procedure).

3.6. Quantification of ISH Signals

Theoretically, the number of silver grains (in radio-ISH) is proportional to the number of hybrids formed which, at saturation, is equivalent to the number of mRNA sequences detected. In other words, counting the number of silver grains may reflect the number of mRNA copies. This provides the basis for quantitating the hybridization signals using computer assisted image analysis system *(28)*. However, it is a far from routine application because the results may be influenced by many factors, including the thickness of emulsion, the thickness of the sections, the amount of radioactivity of probes, exposure time, and so on. Thus, two other semiquantitative methods are often used. One method counts the numbers of ISH positive cells compared with background. The results are expressed as numbers of positive cells per unit of tissue section (i.e., per mm^2 of section) or per unit of total cells (i.e., per 500 or 1000 total cells) in cytospin preparations. This method has been used in our department for quantification of ISH with either radio- or nonradio-labeled probes *(16–27)*. Another method counts the number of silver grains presumably to represent the number of target mRNA copies *(29)*. Using ^{3}H-labeled probes, this semiquantitative method may be more reliable because of the high resolution of ^{3}H. However, long exposure time is the greatest disadvantage for this labeled probe.

Finally, the technique of ISH has become a powerful tool in molecular virology, molecular immunology, molecular pathology, and molecular oncology and is being gradually extended to a number of new fields such as molecular pharmacology and molecular physiology. The development of new nonisotopic labels is critical to the more extensive application of this technique.

4. Notes

1. Losing sections. This can occasionally happen before or after hybridization. If the numbers of sections lost are up to 30% (or more) of the total slides, the following steps should be considered: a) Slides may be not clean. PLL-coating requires completely grease-free slides (wearing gloves when handling slides) (also *see* **Methods**). b) After PLL-treatment, the slides must be completely dried. c) Once PLL-slides have been prepared, they should be used within 1 wk. d) After mounting sections on PLL-coated slides, the slides should be dried at 37°C for at least 4 h or overnight before using or storing for ISH. e) Overfixation also causes loss of sections because excessive crosslinking of tissue by fixatives may reduce potential binding of tissue to charged molecules in the coated slides *(30)*. Thus, the period of fixation is usually less than 4 h. f) 2% 3-aminopropyl-trethoxysilane in acetone prior to applying sections or cytospins may increase adhesion of sections or cells to the slides *(30)*.
2. Low incorporation of probe labeling. Any factors influencing the purity of DNA template, activity of enzymes and labels may lead to low incorporation of labeling. The following should be regularly checked prior to labeling: a) Purity of DNA templates. Lack of purity or incomplete linearization of DNA template may affect incorporation of labeled nucleotide into probes. The purity and degree of uncompleted linearization of the DNA template can be analyzed on the DNA gel. b) Activity of enzymes such as RNA polymerases (very sensitive to heat) and others. These enzymes must be always stored at –20°C or –70°C. Enzymes must always be placed on wet-ice when labeling is performed. After use, the enzymes must be returned to –20°C as soon as possible. Inactivity of enzymes is one of the common reasons for low incorporation of probe labeling. c) Activity of labels, particularly radioactive labels. These labels should be always used

within the half-life. d) Lost pellet of probe during washing procedures after pre-cipitation of labeled probes. Thus, particular attention should be taken during this procedure.

3. High background. Sometimes, positive signals can be observed not only at the sites of hybridization between probe and target, but also can appear at sites where there is some nonspecific binding, even where there are no cells or tissue. Strin-gency (low stringency, particularly on hybridization and washing procedures), concentration of probes, specificity of probes, repeated freezing and thawing of labels and emulsion, and prolonged exposure time of autoradiography are the common factors causing high background. The following solutions could give some help. a) The commonest nonspecific binding occurs between the probes and rRNA, which consists of >90% of total cellular RNA. High stringency wash-ing (such as high temperature and low concentration of salt) may help to reduce the nonspecific binding *(32)*. However, even under highly stringent conditions, nonspecific binding to some unrelated nucleotide sequences, owing to the high homology, may occur. In addition, in some circumstances, the antisense RNA might be expressed, which may lead to specific hybridization with sense probes *(33)*. Thus, the evaluation of each probe under a range of stringent conditions is strongly recommended. b) Avoid repeatedly freezing and thawing of labels and labeled probes, since this may increase nucleotide degradation and cause high background *(30)*. c) Proper concentrations of probes and exposure time is depen-dent on the abundance of target mRNA. Different tissues may have different abundance of various mRNA molecules. Thus, for each type of specimens and probes, proper concentration of probes and exposure time should be always opti-mized. d) Repeatedly using emulsion for the autoradiography is not recom-mended because melting and resolidifying several times may cause increased background counts. It is good practice to dispense a large amount of diluted emul-sion into small aliquots (e.g., 10 mL each). Each one can be used for a single experiment (up to 36 slides) only. In addition, emulsion can be used more eco-nomically if the tissue sections are mounted on the extreme end of the slides. e) ^{35}S-labeled riboprobes may be more "sticky" than DNA probes. Thus, for ^{35}S-labeled RNA probes, the slides should be treated in 10 mM iodoacetamide and 10 mM N-ethylmaleimide/PBS containing 10 mM DTT at 37°C for 30 minutes, then immersed in 0.5% acetic anhydride and 0.1 M triethanolamine at 37°C for 10 min (these procedures should be used before prehybridization) to reduce non-specific binding. f) Some difficulties are specific to the use of hapten-labeled probes and may lead to false positive signals even in the absence of nonradiolabeled probes. This is because of the endogenous hapten (such as biotin) or enzyme activity in tissue *(34)*. Using blocking reagents can much reduce the spurious positive signals.

4. No specific hybridization signals. RNase contamination, improper fixation, inap-propriate permeabilization of tissue sections or cells, or over-stringency of hybridization and washing posthybridization may result in false negative obser-vations. Common problems and solutions are as follows. a) Nuclease contamina-

tion. If the target nucleotide is mRNA, the collection and preparation of samples, as well as ISH procedures (prehybridization and hybridization), must be performed in RNase-free condition. RNA is much more sensitive to RNase than DNA is to DNase. On the other hand, RNase is quite resistant to physical and chemical factors. Thus, any contamination of RNase may destroy target mRNA in tissue, cell preparation, and sections, which may result in false negative observations. Although tissue should be directly frozen in liquid nitrogen-cooled isopentane, unfixed frozen tissue or cells are very sensitive to RNase during the process of cryostat sections, prefixation is recommended once the tissue is isolated. Additionally, the integrity of RNA can be influenced by many factors, including time delay between tissue acquisition and fixation, endogenous and exogenous RNase activity, the duration of tissue handling, and the integrity of tissue sample itself. Thus, fixation must be carried out as rapidly as possible (within 30 min). Gloves should always be worn throughout ISH procedures because of RNase contamination on fingers. Glassware and slides for ISH should be prepared in RNase-free conditions (*see* **Methods**). b) Tissue processing. Although tissue sections for ISH can be made from either frozen or paraffin-embedded tissue, cryostat sections require less tissue processing. Additionally, sensitive detection of nucleotide sequences is more readily attained on frozen sections than on paraffin sections. In contrast, high quality serial sections are more easily obtained from paraffin-embedded tissue than frozen tissue. For the fixatives, both PAF and glutaraldehyde give good RNA retention and morphology (*see* **Table 3**). However, PAF (4% in PBS) in particular is recommended for cells or cryostat sections. Because glutaraldehyde is a strong crosslinking fixative, it may reduce accessibility of probe to target sequences. Although using relatively high concentration of permeabilization reagent (e.g., protease) may overcome this, the overdigestion of samples may lead to poor morphology of tissue/cell. Thus, we prefer to use 4% PAF as a fixative in our studies (*16–27*). c) Overfixation of tissue or cells may also reduce positive signals, presumably by limiting accessibility of probes to the target sequences. d) A proper positive control (e.g. using a housekeeping gene as a probe) should be included to check the quality and retention of target sequences.

5. As described previously, ISH may be affected by many factors, including appropriate sample fixation, handling of tissue and slides, the labels, the quality and quantity of the probes, the reagents of permeabilization, hybridization conditions, stringency of posthybridization washings, and detection. All of these are vital to the ISH results. It is strongly recommended that investigators set up their own experimental conditions for each probe or target.

References

1. Gall, J. G. and Pardue, M. L. (1969) Formation and detection of RNA-DNA hybrid molecules in cytological preparations. *Proc. Natl. Acad. Sci. USA.* **63,** 378–381.
2. Feinberg, A. P. and Vogelstein, B. (1983) A technique for radiolabeling DNA restriction endonuclease fragments to high specific activity. *Anal. Biochem.* **132,** 6–13.

3. Rigby, P. W. J., Diekmann, M., Rhodes, C., and Berg, P. (1977) Labeling deoxyribonucleic acid to high specific activity in vitro by nick translation with DNA polymerase I. *J. Mol. Biol.* **113,** 237–251.

4. Stahl, W. L., Eakin, T. J., and Baskin, D. G. (1993) Selection of oligonucleotide probe for detection of mRNA isoforms. *J. Histochem. Cytochem.* **41,** 1735–1740.

5. Lathe, R. (1985) Synthetic oligonucleotide probes deduced from amino acid sequences data: theoretical and practical considerations. *J. Mol. Biol.* **183,** 1–12.

6. Gyllensten, U. B. and Erlin, H. A. (1988) Generation of single stranded DNA by the polymerase chain reaction and its application of direct sequencing of the HLA-DQA locus. *Proc. Natl. Acad. Sci. USA.* **83,** 7652–7656.

7. Cone, R. W. and Schlaepfer, E. (1998) Improved in situ hybridization to HIV with RNA probes derived from PCR products. *J. Histochem. Cytochem.* **45,** 721–727.

8. Cox, K. H., DeLeon, D. V., Angerer, L. M., and Angerer, R. C. (1984) Detection of mRNAs in Sea Urchin embryos by in situ hybridization using asymmetric RNA probes. *Develop Biol.* **101,** 485–502.

9. Melton, D. A., Krieg, P. A., and Rebagliati, M. R. (1984) Efficient in vitro synthesis of biologically active RNA and RNA hybridization probes from plasmids containing a bacteriophage SP6 promoter. *Nucleic Acid Res.* **12,** 7035–7041.

10. Schenborn, E. T. and Mierendorf, R. C. Jr. (1985) A novel transcription property of SP6 and T7 RNA polymerase: dependence on template structure. *Nucleic Acid Res.* **13,** 6226–6230.

11. Young, I. D., Ailles, L., Deugan, K., and Kisilevsky, R. (1991) Transcription of cRNA for in situ hybridization from polymerase chain reaction-amplified DNA. *Lab. Invest.* **64,** 709–712.

12. Allen, J. M., Sasek, C. A., Martin, J. B., and Heinrich, G. (1987) Use of complementary ^{125}I labeled RNA for single cell resolution by in situ hybridization. *Biotechniques* **5,** 774–777.

13. Bakkenist, C. J. and McGee J. O'D. (1998) The preparation of non-radioisotopic hybridization probes, in *In Situ Hybridization* (Polak, J. M. and McGee, J. O'D. eds) Oxford University Press, pp. 35–48.

14. Mcallister, H. A. and Rock, D. L. (1985) Comparative usefulness of tissue fixatives for in situ viral nucleic acid hybridization. *J. Histochem. Cytochem.* **33,** 1026–1032.

15. Bresser, J. and Evinger-Hodges, M. J. (1992) Comparison and optimization of in situ hybridization procedures yielding rapid sensitive mRNA detections. *Gene. Anal. Tech.* **4,** 89–104.

16. Ying, S., Robinson, D. S., Varney, V., Meng, Q., Tsicopoulos, A., Moqbel, R., et al. (1991) TNF-alpha mRNA expression in allergic Inflammation. *Clin. Exp. Allergy.* **21,** 745–750.

17. Ying, S., Durham, S. D., Barkans, J., Masuyama, K., Jacobson, M., Rak, S., Lowhagen, O., et al. (1993) T cells are the principal source of interleukin-5 mRNA in allergen-induced allergic rhinitis. *Am. J. Respir. Cell Mol. Biol.* **9,** 356–360.

18. Ying, S., Durham, S. D., Musuyama, K., Jacobson, M. R., Kay, A. B., and Hamid, Q. (1994) T cells are the principal source of interleukin-4 messenger RNA in the nasal mucosa in allergen-induced rhinitis. *Immunol.* **82,** 200–206.

19. Ying, S., Durham, S., Corrigan, C. J., Hamid, Q. and Kay, A. B. (1995) Phenotype of cells expressing mRNA for TH2-type (IL-4 and IL-5) and TH1-type (IL-2 and IFN-γ) cytokines in bronchoalveolar lavage and bronchial biopsies from atopic asthmatics and normal control subjects. *Am. J. Respir. Cell Mol. Biol.* **12,** 477–478.

20. Ying, S., Taborada-Barata, L., Meng, Q., Humbert, M., and Kay, A. B. (1995) The kinetics of allergen-induced transcription of messenger RNA for monocyte chemotactic protein-3 (MCP-3) and RANTES in the skin of human atopic subjects: Relationship to eosinophil, T cell, and macrophage recruitment. *J. Exp. Med.* **181,** 2153–2159.

21. Ying, S, Meng, Q., Barata, L. T., Corrigan, C. J., Barkans, J., Assoufi, B., et al. (1996) Human eosinophils express messenger RNA encoding RANTES and store and release biologically active RANTES protein. *Eur. J. Immunol.* **26,** 70–76

22. Ying, S., Robinson, D. S., Meng, Q., Rottman, J., Kennedy, R., Ringler, D. J., et al. (1997) Enhanced expression of eotaxin and CCR3 mRNA and protein in atopic asthma and their association with airway hyperresponsiveness and predominant co-localization of eotaxin mRNA to bronchial epithelial and endothelial cells. *Eur. J. Immunol.* **27,** 3507–3516.

23. Ying, S., Meng, Q., Barata, L. T., Robinson, D. S., Durham, S. R., and Kay. A. B. (1997) Associations between IL-13 and IL-4 (mRNA and protein), VCAM-1 expression and infiltration of eosinophils, macrophages and T cells in the allergen-induced late-phase cutaneous reactions in atopic subjects. *J. Immunol.* **158,** 5050–5057.

24. Ying, S., Humbert, M., Barkans, J., Corrigan, C. J., Pfister, R., Menz, G., et al. (1997) Expression of IL-4 and IL-5 mRNA and protein product by CD4+ and CD8+ T cells, eosinophils and mast cells in bronchial biopsies obtained from atopic and non-atopic (intrinsic) asthmatics. *J. Immunol.* **158,** 3539–3544.

25. Ying, S., Barata, L. T., Meng, Q., Grant, J. A., Barkans, J., Durham, S. R., and Kay, A. B. (1998) High affinity IgE receptor (FceRI)-bearing eosinophils, mast cells, macrophages and Langerhans cells in allergen-induced late-phase cutaneous reactions in atopic subjects. *Immunol.* **93,** 281–288.

26. Ying, S., Robinson, D. S, Meng, Q, Barata, L. T., McEuen, A. R., Buckley, M. G., et al. (1999) C-C chemokines in allergen-induced late-phase cutaneous responses in atopic subjects: Association of eotaxin with early 6-hour eosinophils, and eotaxin-2 and MCP-4 with the later 24-hour tissue eosinophilia, and relationship to basophils and other C-C chemokines (MCP-3 and RANTES). *J. Immunol.* **163,** 3976–3984.

27. Ying, S., Meng, Q., Zeibecoglou, K., Robinson, D. S., Macfarlane, A., Humbert, M., and Kay, A. B. (1999) Eosinophil chemotactic chemokines (eotaxin, eotaxin-2, RANTES, MCP-3, and MCP-4) and CCR3 expression in bronchial biopsies from atopic and non-atopic (intrinsic) asthma. *J. Immunol.* 1999

28. Nunez, D. J., Davenport, A. P., Emson, P. C., and Brown, M. J. (1989) A quantitative 'in-situ' hybridization method using computer-assisted image analysis. *Bioch. J.* **263,** 121–127.

29. Marfaing-Koka, A., Devergne, O., Gorgone, G., Schall, T. J., Galanaud, P., and Emilie, D. (1995) Regulation of the production of the RANTES chemokine by endothelial cells. Synergistic induction by IFN-gamma plus TNF-alpha and inhibition by IL-4 and IL-13. *J Immunol.* **154,** 1870–1878.

30. Wilcox, J. N. (1993) Fundamental principle of in situ hybridization. *J. Histochem. Cytochem.* **41,** 1725–1733.

31. Henderson, C. (1989) Aminoalkylisane: an inexpensive, simple preparation for slide adhesion. *J. Histochnol.* **12,** 123–124.

32. Hofler, H, Mueller, J., and Werner, M. (1998) Principle of in situ hybridization, in *In Situ Hybridization* (Ploak, J. M. and McGee, J. O'D. eds.) Oxford, University Press pp. 1–21.

33. Coghlam, J. P., Aldred, P., Haralambidis, J., Niall, H. D., Penschow, J. D., and Tregear, G. W. (1985) Hybridization histochemistry. *Anal. Biochem.* **149,** 1–28.

34. Potts, J. D., Vincent, E. B., Runyan, R. B., and Weeks, D. L. (1992) Sense and antisense TGF-β 3 mRNA levels correlate with cardiac valve induction. *Dev. Dynamics* **193,** 340–345.

22

Measurement of Airway Mucin Gene Expression

Kelly Pritchard, Alinka K. Smith, and Duncan F. Rogers

1. Introduction

Hypersecretion of airway mucus is characteristic of several severe lung diseases, particularly those involving chronic inflammation such as asthma, chronic obstructive pulmonary disease (COPD), and cystic fibrosis (CF) *(1)*. Mucins are the major macromolecular component of mucus and play a fundamental role in the pathophysiology of these diseases by determining the viscoelastic properties of mucus and its ability to interact with the cilia of the respiratory tract during mucociliary clearance.

Mucin structure and function has been difficult to study using traditional biochemical and immunological techniques, owing to the O-linked glycans which surround and tend to "mask" the core peptides. Research has begun to focus on the use of molecular biological methods to study the mucin (MUC) genes that encode the protein backbone of mucin *(2)*. Ten mucin genes are currently recognized: MUC1–4, MUC5AC, MUC5B, and MUC7–9. All except MUC9 (oviductin) are normally expressed to some extent as messenger RNA (mRNA) in adult respiratory epithelium *(3)*, in particular MUC1, MUC4, MUC5AC, and 5B *(2,4)*. The relative contribution of different MUC genes and their protein products in healthy and diseased airways has not been fully elucidated.

Some MUC gene expression has been demonstrated to be altered in certain diseases. For example, MUC2 is upregulated in the nasal mucosa of patients with CF *(5)*. MUC1, MUC3, and MUC4 expression has been shown to be upregulated in lung adenocarcinomas *(6)* and MUC1 is abundantly expressed and underglycosylated in many other human cancers *(7)*. Various inflammatory mediators also alter MUC gene expression, for example in human airways

From: *Methods in Molecular Medicine, vol. 56:*
Human Airway Inflammation: Sampling Techniques and Analytical Protocols
Edited by: D. F. Rogers and L. E. Donnelly © Humana Press Inc., Totowa, NJ

in vitro in response to TNFα *(8)*. Mucin mRNA from airway tissues may be examined using standard molecular techniques such as Northern blotting, but there are specific problems necessitating some technical modifications. The main difficulty is that MUC genes have large transcript sizes (2.4–40 kb) *(10)*. They are relatively sensitive to mechanical degradation and their large size can also lead to inefficient transfer during Northern blotting from the agarose gel to the nylon membrane prior to hybridization.

Many MUC genes (apart from MUC1 and MUC7) appear to have a high degree of polydispersity and are detected as smears or very wide bands rather than a distinct band of predicted size *(9)*. It was hypothesized that these smears were perhaps due to rapid turnover, several related genes producing varied transcript lengths, alternative splicing, or were simply artifacts. Debailleul et al. *(9)* developed a modified method of RNA purification, which reduces mechanical degradation. They concluded that the polydispersity was not an artifact but was due to allelic variations which are directly related to the variable number of tandem repeat (VNTR) polymorphisms seen at the DNA level.

The method described here for the study of airway mucin gene expression uses TRIzol following the manufacturer's instructions with some adaptations and also uses the modifications suggested by Debailleul et al. *(9)* for large transcript sizes (for general details of Northern analysis, *see* Chapter 20 of this volume). Total RNA is extracted from airway tissue using TRIzol Reagent, electrophoresed on a denaturing agarose gel to separate RNA according to molecular weight, then transferred by capillary action onto a nylon membrane. The RNA on the membrane is crosslinked by UV light to stabilize it and hybridized to a specific radiolabeled cDNA probe. The membrane is then exposed to X-ray film and the RNA under investigation appears as a dark band on the film.

Glyceraldehyde-3-phosphate dehydrogenase (GAPDH) is a common gene used as an internal standard to ascertain that the RNA has not degraded and is present in sufficient amounts on the membrane to be detected. Using densitometry, the RNA under investigation can be quantified in relation to the amount of GAPDH present.

2. Materials

2.1. RNA Isolation

1. Kreb's Henseleit solution made fresh from 20X stock (NaCl 118 mM, KCl 5.9 mM, MgSO$_4$ 1.2 mM, CaCl$_2$ 2.5 mM, NaHCO$_2$ 25.5 mM, glucose 5.05 mM).
2. TRIzol (Gibco-BRL Life Technologies, Paisley, Romfrewshire). Store at 4°C (*see* **Note 1**).
3. Diethyl pyrocarbonate (DEPC). Store at 4°C (*see* **Note 1**).
4. DEPC treated water (*see* **Note 2**).

5. Ethanol (75%) (BDH, Littleworth, Leics.) made up with DEPC water. Store at 4°C.
6. Isopropanol (BDH, Littleworth, Leics.). Store at 4°C.
7. Chloroform/isoamyl alcohol (49:1).
8. High salt buffer: 0.8 *M* sodium citrate with 1.2 *M* sodium chloride (*see* **Note 3**).
9. Nuclease-free water (Promega, Southampton).
10. Spectrophotometer.
11. Liquid nitrogen.
12. RNA*later* (Ambion, AMS Biotechnology, Abingdon, Oxon.).
13. Autoclaved Eppendorf tubes.

2.2. RNA Formaldehyde Gel Electrophoresis

1. RNAse-free agarose, 1% LE Analytical grade (Promega, Southampton).
2. 3-N-Morpholine-propanesulfonic acid (MOPS), 10X autoclaved. For 1 L: MOPS 41.845 g, sodium acetate 6.804 g, ethylenediaminetetraacetic acid (EDTA) 3.722 g, adjust to pH 7.0 with NaOH or HCl (*see* **Note 4**).
3. DEPC water (*see* **Note 2**).
4. Gel loading buffer: Deionized formamide (1 mL) (*see* **Note 5**), 25% formaldehyde (0.4 mL), 10X MOPS (0.2 mL), orange G in DEPC water (0.5 mL).
5. Ethidium bromide aqueous solution 10 mg/mL (Sigma Chemical, Poole). Use 0.4 mg/mL in DEPC water.
6. Formaldehyde: 37% solution.

2.3. Transfer of RNA from Agarose Gel to Nylon Membrane

1. Whatman chromatography paper, 3 MM (46×57 cm).
2. Blotting paper, 15×15 cm, extra thick (Sigma Chemical, Poole).
3. Nylon transfer membrane (MSI Magna, Genetic Research Instrumentation Ltd., Felsted Dunmow, Essex).
4. Plastic sandwich box and glass plates (approximately the same size as the gel).
5. Sponge.
6. UV Stratalinker-2400 (Stratagene, Cambridge).
7. UV transilluminator GDS 7500 (UVP Ultraviolet Products, Upland, CA.).
8. 20X Standard sodium citrate (SSC): 3 *M* NaCl, 0.3 *M* sodium citrate, pH 7.0, autoclaved.

2.4. Probes

Different researchers worldwide use their own selected probes for human MUC genes. Currently, MUC probes are not available commercially. We use probes designed by Dr. Yu-Chih Liu (*10*).

2.5. Hybridization

1. Prehybridization buffer (for 10 mL): deionized formamide (5 mL), RNAse-free water (1.05 mL), 20X SSC (2 mL), Tris-HCl, pH 7.5 (0.5 mL), 50X Denhardt's solution (1 mL; Sigma Chemical, Poole), EDTA 0.5 *M* (0.1 mL), salmon testes DNA stock 10.4 mg/mL (Sigma Chemical, Poole) (0.25 mL), 10% sodium dodecylsulfate (SDS) in DEPC water (0.1 mL).

2. [^{32}P]dCTP, specific activity >3000 Ci/mmol (Amersham Life Sciences Amersham, Bucks.).
3. Ready-to-Go labeling kits (Pharmacia, St. Albans, Herts.). Store at room temperature.
4. G50 Sephadex beads (Sigma Chemical, Poole).
5. Hybridization oven and chambers.
6. TE buffer: 10 mM Tris-HCl (pH 7.5), 1 mM EDTA (pH 8.0).
7. TES buffer: 10 mM Tris-HCl (pH 7.5), 1 mM EDTA (pH 8.0), and 0.1% SDS.

2.6. Post hybridization Washes

1. 20X SSC stock, autoclaved.
2. 10% SDS stock in DEPC water.

2.7. Detection of RNA

1. Cassettes.
2. X-Ograph XB-200 High Definition X-ray film, blue sensitive (X-Ograph Imaging Systems Ltd., Malmesbury).
3. Automatic film developer.

2.8. Stripping the Membrane

1. Stripping buffer: Formamide (50% v/v), Na$_2$HPO$_4$ (10 mM) in RNase free water.
2. 2X SSC/ 0.1% SDS in RNAse free water.

3. Methods
3.1. RNA Isolation

1. Obtain lung tissue segments (approximate size segmental bronchus 1.5 cm long × 0.3 cm outside diameter, parenchyma 3 × 2 cm) at surgery and immerse for several minutes in Kreb's solution on ice, aerated with 95% O$_2$: 5% CO$_2$.
2. Freeze the tissue (in small segments if possible) in liquid nitrogen and store at –70°C until required (*see* **Note 6**). Isolate total RNA from lung and other airway tissues using TRIzol Reagent, approx 100 mg tissue per 1 mL TRIzol Reagent. Wear gloves at all times to prevent RNAse contamination. Grind the tissue to a fine powder in liquid nitrogen using a pre-chilled pestle and mortar (*see* **Note 7**). Incubate at room temperature in TRIzol Reagent for 5 min in autoclaved Eppendorf tubes (*see* **Note 8**).
3. Centrifuge the tubes at 12,000g for 10 min and transfer the supernatant to fresh tubes.
4. Add chloroform (0.2 mL per mL of TRIzol Reagent) and shake the tubes by hand for 15 s.
5. Incubate at room temperature for 3 min. Transfer the upper colorless phase to fresh tubes.
6. Precipitate the RNA with 0.25 mL isopropanol and 0.25 mL high salt buffer per mL TRIzol Reagent at room temperature for 10 min (*see* **Note 9**). Centrifuge the samples at 12,000g for 10 min at 4°C. Carefully pour off the supernatant (*see*

Note 10). Wash the pellet once with 1 mL 75% ethanol and centrifuge at 7,500*g* for 5 min at 4°C. We have found that washing the pellet twice tends to reduce the amount of RNA retrieved.

7. Briefly freeze-dry the RNA in a vacuum dessicator (*see* **Note 11**). Carefully resuspend the pellet in 50 μL nuclease-free water and measure the absorption of UV light by an aliquot (4 μL in 96 μL distilled water) at 260 nm in a spectrophotometer to calculate yield in μg/μL, using the following equation:

$$[RNA] \ \mu g/mL = A260 \times 44.19 \times \text{dilution factor} \div 1000$$

$$\text{where } A_{260} = \text{absorbance at 260 nm}$$

$$\text{dilution factor} = 25 \text{ (in this case)}$$

$$44.19 = \text{extinction coefficient of RNA (\textit{see} \textbf{Note 12}).}$$

8. Store the RNA in aliquots in DEPC water at –70°C until required (*see* **Note 13**).

3.2. Total RNA Electrophoresis

1. To make a 0.8% agarose gel: Dissolve 1.2 g agarose in 110 mL DEPC water and 15 mL 10X MOPS by heating in a microwave for approx 2 min at a medium setting in a DEPC-treated glass bottle (*see* **Note 14**).
2. When the agarose has cooled to hand-hot, add 25 mL formaldehyde solution (*see* **Note 15**).
3. Seal the open edges of the gel casting tray with tape. Place the gel comb in the casting tray. Carefully pour the agarose into the center of the tray until it is approx 5 mm thick. Allow to set; this takes about 45 min (*see* **Note 16**).
4. Set up the electrophoresis tank: remove the tape from the gel. Cover the gel with 1X MOPS and carefully remove the comb (*see* **Note 17**).
5. Prepare the RNA samples: Aliquot the appropriate volume of DEPC water containing 15 μg RNA (*see* **Note 18**).
6. Add 2 vol of gel-loading buffer and 1 μL of 400 μg mL^{-1} ethidium bromide.
7. Heat at 65°C in a waterbath for 5 min, then chill on ice for 5 min.
8. Pulse spin in microcentrifuge.
9. Load the RNA samples carefully into the wells using sterile pipet tips (*see* **Note 19**).
10. Electrophorese the samples at a maximum of 5 V per cm of gel length (*see* **Note 20**).
11. After approx 1.5 h, or when the samples have moved approximately half the length of the gel, turn off the voltage and examine the gel in its casting tray on a UV transilluminator. At this point it is possible to see if the RNA has been degraded. Photograph if required (*see* **Fig. 1**) (*see* **Note 21**).
12. If the RNA is satisfactory (i.e., does not appear as a smear) (*see* **Fig. 2**), return the gel to the electrophoresis tank and continue until the orange dye runs off the edge of the bottom of the gel (*see* **Note 22**).
13. Soak the gel for 20 min in 0.05 *M* NaOH, then rinse with DEPC water for 2 min.

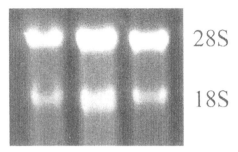

Fig. 1. Total RNA from human lung. Parenchymal tissue was collected at surgery and 15 μg RNA per lane electrophoresed on agarose gel (visualized with ethidium bromide). Note the clear 28S and 18S bands, demonstrating that the RNA has not degraded (compare with **Fig. 2**, and *see* **Notes 6** and **21**).

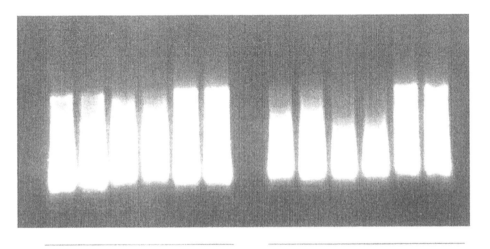

Fig. 2. Total RNA from human lung. Parenchymal tissue was collected at autopsy from three normal subjects and three asthmatic patients and 15 μg RNA per lane in duplicate electrophoresed on agarose gel (visualized with ethidium bromide). The smeared bands demonstrate that the RNA has degraded.

3.3. Transfer of RNA from Agarose Gel to Nylon Membrane

1. Fill a sandwich box with 20X SSC. Cut 2 slits in the lid and slot the sponge through the 2 slits so that it acts as a wick in the SSC.
2. Cut 2 pieces of chromatography paper the same size as the gel, soak them in 20X SSC and lay on top of the sponge. Roll flat with a sterile pipet to avoid air bubbles.
3. Place the gel upside down on the chromatography paper. Cut a corner off the gel with a sterile scalpel for future orientation.

4. Cut a piece of nylon membrane the same size as the gel (*see* **Note 23**). Write the date on the corner in pencil and cut off the corner corresponding with the gel. Place on top of the gel and roll flat as before.
5. Soak two more pieces of chromatography paper in 20X SSC and place on top of the nylon membrane. Roll flat.
6. Place approximately six sheets of thick blotting paper evenly on top of the chromatography paper.
7. Place a pile of paper towels approx 5 cm thick on the pile.
8. Place a flat glass plate on top of the paper towels and then a heavy weight on top of the plate.
9. Allow to blot overnight.
10. Wash the nylon membrane in 5X SSC.
11. Wrap in Saran wrap to prevent the membrane drying out.
12. Covalently crosslink the membrane under UV light.
13. Look at the membrane under UV to check that the RNA transferred properly and mark in pencil on the side of the membrane the level of the 28 S and 18 S bands.
14. Keep the membrane wrapped in Saran wrap at 4°C until required.

3.4. Preparation of Probes

Human mucin cDNAs and glyceraldehyde-3-phosphate dehydrogenase (GAPDH) were cloned by Liu *(10)*.

3.5. Hybridization

1. Prehybridize the nylon membranes (2–3 per chamber) in a cylindrical glass hybridization chamber with 6 mL prehybridization buffer comprising 50% deionized formamide, 2X SSC, 50 mM Tris-HCL (pH 7.5), 5X Denhardt's solution, 0.1% SDS, 5 mM EDTA and 250 µg/mL denatured salmon sperm DNA, for a minimum of 4 h at 42°C in a hybridization oven.
2. Label 30–50 ng of all cDNA probes with [^{32}P]dCTP utilizing a commercial random-primed labeling kit (Easy-to-go; Pharmacia Biotech, St. Albans), according to the manufacturer's instructions (*see* **Note 24**).
3. Purify the radiolabeled probes: first break off the tip of a glass Pasteur pipet. Put some glass wool in the top and push down to the tip. Sterilize by washing with ethanol.
4. Fill the pipet with G50 Sephadex beads in TE buffer (pH 7.5) (*see* **Note 25**).
5. Wash the column twice with 200 µL TES buffer (Tris, pH 7.5 – EDTA, pH 8.0, 0.1% SDS).
6. Add TES buffer (200 µL) to the labeled cDNA and then add all of the reaction mix to the top of the column and allow to drip through into an Eppendorf tube.
7. Continually add TES buffer (200 µL) to the column and collect 7–10 fractions in separate Eppendorf tubes (*see* **Note 26**).
8. Count a sample (1 µL) of each fraction in a beta-counter and select the fraction with the highest counts (*see* **Note 27**).
9. Add the labeled probes to the chamber at a concentration of 1.0×10^6 cpm per mL of prehybridization buffer (2×10^6 cpm / chamber for GAPDH) and leave to hybridize overnight at 42°C.

3.6. Post hybridization Washes

Post hybridization washes are performed to remove nonspecific binding of the cDNA probes. Carry out washes as follows:

1. Wash 1. 2X SSC/0.1% SDS   room temperature   10 min
2. Wash 2. 2X SSC/0.1% SDS   45°C   15 min
3. Wash 3. 1X SSC/0.1% SDS   50°C   15 min
4. Wash 4. 0.5X SSC/0.1% SDS   55°C   30 min
5. Wash 5. 0.1X SSC/0.1% SDS   60°C   30 min

3.7. Detection of RNA

1. Wrap the membranes in Saran wrap and place in autoradiography cassettes.
2. Expose the membranes to X-ray film for appropriate time periods (*see* **Note 28**).
3. Quantitate the autoradiographs by densitometry (GelWorks ID Intermediate, Cambridge, Cambridgeshire, UK) with the relative amounts of RNA calculated as a ratio of GAPDH.

3.8. Stripping the Membrane

1. Strip the membranes before re-probing in a chamber containing 50 mL stripping buffer comprising 50% formamide (v/v) and 10 mM Na_2HPO_4 in RNase free water.
2. Leave the filters in the hybridization chamber for at least 1 h at 65–70°C.
3. Rinse twice with 2X SSC and 0.1% SDS in DEPC water at 25°C for 10 min.

4. Notes

1. Highly toxic, use in a fume hood.
2. Add 0.1% (v/v) DEPC to distilled water and make sure they are thoroughly mixed. Incubate at 37°C for 12 h and then autoclave to break down the DEPC.
3. For 50 mL use 2 M sodium chloride (30 mL) and 2 M sodium citrate (20 mL).
4. Turns yellow when autoclaved and is light sensitive, so store wrapped in foil.
5. Formamide is deionized by placing on a magnetic stirrer with mixed bed resin for approx 30 min. Adjust to pH 7 with either resin or formamide. Filter through Whatman filter paper. Store in aliquots at –20°C.
6. It is important that the tissue is frozen as quickly as possible to reduce RNA breakdown by Rnases (*see* **Fig. 1**). RNA*later* is a useful solution to put the tissue in straight away and can be stored at room temperature for 1 wk and 4°C for 1 mo or longer.
7. The tissue must not be allowed to thaw so repeatedly pour on liquid nitrogen.
8. Avoid homogenization, vigorous shaking and vortexing to limit mechanical degradation of large transcripts (*9*).
9. This removes proteoglycan and polysaccharide contamination from the isolated RNA.
10. The RNA does not stick avidly to the side of the tube, so ensure it is not discarded with the supernatant.
11. Do not over-dry the RNA as it is difficult to redissolve.
12. In the presence of excess salt or proteins the absorbance can be skewed, so use A_{260}/A_{280} ratio to give an indication of the quality of the RNA. A pure sample of RNA has an A_{260}/A_{280} ratio of 2 ± 0.05 (*11*).

13. Avoid repeated freezing and thawing.
14. Loosen the lid of the bottle.
15. Swirl the bottle gently to keep the agarose warm and in solution when adding the formaldehyde. Use a fume hood.
16. The gel can be covered in Saran wrap and kept at 4°C until required.
17. Adding buffer before the removal of the comb reduces the vacuum formed by the comb when it is pulled out and is less likely to damage the gel.
18. Use a maximum of 20 μg RNA per lane to prevent loss of resolution.
19. Load slowly to avoid the force of the pipet blowing the sample out of the well. If possible, avoid using the outer lanes, as the RNA does not transfer optimally onto the nylon membrane.
20. Our gel is 11 cm long and we find 75 V to be optimal. A lower voltage allows for better separation but takes too long (>4 h) whereas a higher voltage may overheat the gel. RNA runs from negative to positive.
21. Ribosomal RNA, 28 S and 18 S, should be visible as two distinct bands. The intensity of the 28 S rRNA is about twice that of the 18 S rRNA (*see* **Fig. 1**) Do not expose to UV for longer than necessary to reduce RNA degradation.
22. The large mucin mRNA should be between the 18 S band and the wells of the gel so it is better to run the gel for as long as possible for maximum separation of these larger molecules.
23. It is convenient to use a clean gel casting tray to mark the size required.
24. Probe with GAPDH first then repeat the hybridization for the MUC gene under investigation.
25. It is important not to allow the column to dry out.
26. Each fraction takes approx 3–5 min to drip through the column.
27. This is generally fraction 6, although it may be worth keeping fractions 5 and 7 to use or combine for further experiments.
28. GAPDH is more strongly expressed than MUC genes and generally needs approx 4 d exposure, depending on the strength of the radioactivity on the membrane. MUC probes are used separately and the film exposed for up to 10 d.

References

1. Rogers, D. F. (1994) Influence of Respiratory Tract Fluid on Airway Calibre in *Airways Smooth Muscle: Regulation of Contractility* (Raeburn, D. and Giembycz, M.A., eds.) Birkhäuser Verlag, Basel, p. 375–409.
2. Rose, M.C. and Gendler, S.J. (1997) Airway Mucin Genes and Gene Products in Airway Mucus: Basic Mechanisms and Perspectives (Rogers, D. F. and Lethem, M. I.,eds.). Birkhäuser Verlag, Basel, p. 41–66.
3. Berger, J.T., Voynow, J.A., Peters, K.W., and Rose, M.C. (1999) Respiratory carcinoma cell lines: MUC genes and glycoconjugates. *Am. J. Resp. Cell Mol. Biol.* **20**, 500–510.
4. Reid, C.J., Gould, S., and Harris, A. (1997) Developmental expression of mucin genes in the human respiratory tract. *Am. J. Respir. Cell Mol. Biol.* **17**, 592–598.
5. Li, D., Wang, D., Majumdar, S., Jany, B., Durham, S.R., Cottrell, J., Caplen, N., Geddes, D.M., Alton, E.W., and Jeffery, P.K. (1997) Localization and up-regula-

tion of mucin (MUC2) gene expression in human nasal biopsies of patients with cystic fibrosis. *J. Pathol.* **181**, 305–310

6. Nguyen, P.L., Niehans, G.A., Cherwitz, D.L., Kim, Y.S., and Ho, S.B. (1996) Membrane-bound (MUC1) and secretory (MUC2, MUC3 and MUC4) mucin gene expression in human lung cancer. *Tumour Biol.* **17**, 176–192.

7. Agrawal, B., Krantz, M.J., Reddish, M.A., and Longenecker, B.M. (1998) Cancer-associated MUC1 mucin inhibits human T-cell proliferation, which is reversible by IL-2. *Nat. Med.* **4**, 43–49.

8. Levine, S.J., Larivee, P., Logun, C., Angus, C.W., Ognibene, F.P., and Shelhamer, J.H. (1995) Tumor necrosis factor-alpha induces mucin hypersecretion and MUC-2 gene expression by human airway epithelial cells. *Am. J. Respir. Cell Mol. Biol.* **12**, 196–204.

9. Debailleul, V., Laine, A., Huet, G., Mathon, P., Collyn d'Hooghe, M., Aubert, J.P., and Porchet, N. (1998) Human mucin genes MUC2, MUC3, MUC4, MUC5AC, MUC5B, and MUC6 express stable and extremely large mRNAs and exhibit a variable length polymorphism. *J. Biol. Chem.* **273**, 881–890.

10. Farrell, R.E. (1993) RNA Methodologies: A laboratory guide for isolation and characterization. Academic Press, U.S.A.

11. Liu, Y-C. (1999) Airway mucus secretion: control mechanisms, pharmacological regulation and mucin gene expression. PhD Thesis, University of London.

23

Transcription Factors
and Inflammatory Gene Regulation

Strategic Approaches

Robert Newton and Karl J. Staples

1. Introduction

In chronic inflammatory diseases, the expression of multiple genes, including those for cytokines, chemokines, adhesion molecules, receptors, and
inflammatory enzymes, is often upregulated. The problem for many academic
or industrial scientists is to elucidate the mechanisms behind this upregulation
to further the understanding of inflammation or to explore possible means of
therapeutic intervention. Common research problems faced by investigators
would be to analyze the regulation of a novel gene in response to various
inflammatory stimuli or alternatively to investigate the mechanisms of induction of an established gene in response to novel stimuli. Whereas the induction
of many inflammatory genes is thought to occur, at least partly, at the level of
increased transcription, it is important to address the possible role of posttranscriptional, translational, or even posttranslational control. For example, release
or synthesis of the protein of interest from suitably stimulated cells could be
examined in the presence or absence of transcriptional inhibitors, such as actinomycin D, or translational inhibitors, such as cycloheximide. Thus, a dependence on *de novo* transcription and/or translation may be demonstrated.
Therefore, whether the protein of interest is simply released from preformed
cellular stores or is synthesized from preformed mRNA can be elucidated.
Northern blot analysis, reverse transcription polymerase chain reaction (RT-PCR),
or ribonuclease protection assays can be used to examine steady-state mRNA
levels, which if elevated gives rise to a presumption of transcriptional control.

From: *Methods in Molecular Medicine, vol. 56:*
Human Airway Inflammation: Sampling Techniques and Analytical Protocols
Edited by: D. F. Rogers and L. E. Donnelly © Humana Press Inc., Totowa, NJ

However, before undertaking any of the methods listed below, investigators should ensure that changes in steady-state mRNA are in fact because of changes in transcription rate as opposed to posttranscriptional changes in mRNA half-life. To this end, mRNA half-life studies using actinomycin D, and nuclear run on analysis, to assess the actual transcription rate, should be performed. Assuming that a transcriptional mechanism is implicated, it would then be appropriate to commence analysis of promoter regions and factors that bind to promoter elements.

Typical problems would include identification of candidate promoter regions and their corresponding binding factors. One approach is simply to scan the putative promoter region for consensus transcription factor binding sites (*see* **Note 1**). However, as the binding sites for most transcription factors are highly degenerate, this results in the identification of vastly more potential binding sites than are functionally relevant. To some extent, investigators may limit these numbers by virtue of knowledge of either the type of gene or the nature of the stimulus used. For example, proinflammatory stimuli such as interleukin (IL)-1β or tumor necrosis factor (TNF)-α are potent inducers of factors such as nuclear factor (NF)-κB, activator protein (AP)-1, cyclic AMP response element binding protein (CREB) and CAAT/enhancer binding proteins (C/EBP). Thus, a novel promoter region can be searched for binding sites that have been previously shown to confer responsiveness on other genes given a particular stimulus. Another useful approach, where homologous genes have been cloned from different organisms, is to perform a sequence comparison of the promoter regions (*see* **Note 1**). Because regions of DNA that are functionally constrained will evolve at a slower rate than regions where no selective pressure is operating, important regions are often conserved between species. Although such an approach may help identify important functional regions, whether these regions are involved in any particular responses can only be determined experimentally.

In this chapter we shall describe, using examples that are relevant to gene regulation in inflammatory conditions, some of the methodologies used to examine the mechanisms of gene activation.

2. Materials

2.1. Electrophoretic Mobility Shift Assay (EMSA)

All reagents are from Sigma Chemical Co., Poole, Dorset, UK unless otherwise stated.

1. Buffer A: 10 mM HEPES pH 7.9, 1.5 mM MgCl$_2$, 10 mM KCl, 0.5 mM dithiothreitol (DTT), 0.1% (v/v) Nonidet P40 (NP-40).
2. Buffer C: 20 mM HEPES pH 7.9, 25% (v/v) glycerol, 0.42 M NaCl, 1.5 mM MgCl$_2$, 0.2 mM EDTA pH 8.0, 0.5 mM PMSF, 0.5 mM DTT.
3. Buffer D: 20 mM HEPES pH 7.9, 20% (v/v) glycerol, 50 mM KCl, 0.2 mM EDTA pH 8.0, 0.5 mM phenylmethylsulfonylfluoride (PMSF), 0.5 mM DTT.

4. Bradford Reagent (Bio-rad, Hemel Hempstead, Herts., UK).
5. NF-κB consensus (underlined) double-stranded oligonucleotide 5´ - AGT TGA <u>GGG GAC TTT CCC</u> AGG - 3´ (sense strand) (Promega, Southampton, UK). AP-1, Sp-1 and Oct 1 consensus probes (Promega).
6. T4 polynucleotide kinase and 10X kinase buffer (Promega).
7. TE buffer: 10 mM Tris-HCl pH 7.5, 1 mM ethylenediaminetetraacetic acid (EDTA) pH 8.0.
8. Sterile G-25 sephadex (Amersham Pharmacia Biotech, Little Chalfont, Bucks., UK) in 1X TE.
9. 5X EMSA buffer: 20% (v/v) glycerol, 5 mM MgCl$_2$, 2.5 mM EDTA, 250 NaCl, 50 mM Tris-HCl pH 7.5, 0.4 mg/mL denatured salmon sperm DNA, 2.5 mM DTT.
10. 10X Gel loading buffer: 50% (v/v) glycerol, 0.05% (w/v) bromophenol blue.
11. 10X TBE: 108 g Tris base, 55 g boric acid, 20 mL EDTA (pH 8.0), H$_2$O to 1 L.
12. 40% (w/v) acrylamide / 2.105% (w/v) *bis*-acrylamide solution (Scotlab, Cotbridge, Strathclyde), N',N',N',N'-tetramethylethylenediamine (TEMED), ammonium persulphate (APS) (*see* **Note 2**).
13. Hyperfilm MP (Amersham-Pharmacia Biotech).

2.2. Transfection of Promoter Constructs into Lymphocytes/Monocytes

1. Biorad Gene Pulser II electroporator (Biorad, Hemel Hempstead, Herts).
2. 0.4 cm cuvets (Biorad).
3. 5X Reporter lysis buffer (Promega).
4. Luciferase assay reagent (Promega).
5. TD 20/20 Luminometer (Turner Designs, Steptech, Stevenage, UK).

2.3. Western Blotting for Phosphorylated Transcription Factors

2.3.1. Polyacrylamide Gel Electrophoresis

1. 40% (w/v) acrylamide (38% (w/v) acrylamide/2% *bis*-acrylamide 19:1) (Anachem, Luton, Beds); 1 M Tris (pH 8.8); 1 M Tris (pH 6.8); 10% (w/v) sodium dodecyl sulphate (SDS); 10% (w/v) APS, TEMED.
2. 2X Laemmli Buffer: 125 mM Tris-HCl, pH 6.8, 1% (w/v) SDS, 10% (v/v) glycerol, 0.1% (w/v) bromophenol blue, 2% (v/v) 2-mercaptoethanol.
3. Rainbow Markers (Amersham Pharmacia).

2.3.2. Transfer of Protein to Membranes (Blotting)

1. 10X Gel running buffer: 30.3 g Tris base, 144 g glycine, 10 g SDS, H$_2$O to 1 L.
2. 10X Blotting buffer: 30.3 g Tris base, 145.8 g glycine, H$_2$O to 1 L.
3. 1X Blotting buffer: 100 mL 10 X Blotting buffer, 700 mL H$_2$O, 200 mL methanol (BDH, Lutterworth, UK).
4. India Red: 500 mg Ponceau S, 500 mL H$_2$O, 25 mL glacial acetic acid (BDH).
5. Hybond-enhanced chemiluminescence (ECL) membrane (Amersham Pharmacia).

2.3.3. Immunodetection

1. 10X TBS (Tris buffered saline)/Tween: 24.2 g Tris Base, 80 g NaCl, make up to 1 L with H_2O then adjust pH to 7.6 with HCl then add 10 mL Tween-20.
2. Nonfat powdered milk (*see* **Note 3**).
3. Bovine serum albumin (BSA).
4. α-phospho-CREB, α-CREB and α-rabbit antibodies (New England BioLabs, Hitchin, Herts, UK).
5. LumiGLO™ reagents (New England BioLabs).
6. 15 mL stripping buffer: 3 mL 10% (w/v) SDS, 0.9375 mL 1M Tris (pH 6.8), 115 µL 2-mercaptoethanol, 9.475 mL H_2O.
7. Hyperfilm-ECL™ (Amersham Pharmacia).

2.4. Pull Down Kinase Assay

2.4.1. Immunoprecipitation

1. Buffer A: (*see* **Subheading 2.1.**) supplemented with 25 µg/mL aprotinin, 10 µg/mL leupeptin, 0.5 mM Na_3VO_4, 1 mM sodium pyrophosphate, 50 mM NaF and 5 µg/mL N-tosyl-L-phenylalanine-chloromethyl (TPCK).
2. Protein A agarose (Santa Cruz Antibodies, Santa Cruz, CA).
3. α-IKKα (H744) and α-IKKβ antibodies (Santa Cruz).
4. Normal rabbit IgG (Santa Cruz)

2.4.2. Kinase Assay

1. Kinase assay buffer: 20 mM HEPES pH 7.9, 2 mM $MgCl_2$, 2 mM $MnCl_2$, 10µM adenosine triphosphate (ATP), 10 mM β-glycerophosphate, 10 mM NaF, 10 mM 4-nitrophenyl phosphate, 0.5 mM Na_3VO_4; 1 mM benzamidine; 0.5 mM PMSF; aprotinin at 25 µg/mL; leupeptin at 10 µg/mL; pepstatin at 2 µg/mL and 1 mM DTT.
2. $[\gamma^{-32}P]$ATP 10 mCi/mL, >5000 Ci/mmol (Amersham Pharmacia Biotech).
3. Substrate: GST-IκBα (1–54) or mutant GST-IκBα (1–54; S32A, S36A) (*see* **Note 4**).

2.5. Metabolic Labeling of Proteins

1. Phosphate-free media (usually RPMI or Dulbeccos modified eagles medium (DMEM).
2. $[^{32}P]$ Orthophosphate 10mCi/mL (Cat No. PBS13) (Amersham Pharmacia Biotech).
3. 1X radio immunoprecipitation (RIPA) buffer: 1X phosphate buffered saline (PBS) (8 g NaCl, 1.16 g Na_2HPO_4, 0.2 KCl, 0.2 KH_2PO_4, H_2O to 1 L), 1% NP-40, 0.5% sodium deoxycholate, 0.1% SDS.
4. α-p65 Antibody-agarose conjugate (SC-109AC) (Santa Cruz).
5. α-p65 (C-20) antibody (Santa Cruz).

3. Methods

3.1. Electrophoretic Mobility Shift Assay

The fact that many transcriptional activators, including NF-κB, AP-1, and CREB, bind DNA in a sequence specific manner allows investigators to assay

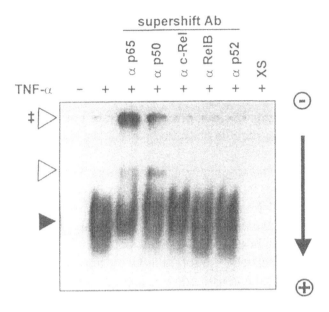

Fig. 1. EMSA and supershift analysis of NF-κB activation in U937 monocytic cells. Cells were either unstimulated (–) or treated (+) with TNF-α (10 ng/mL) as indicated. After 1 h, cells were harvested and nuclear proteins prepared. EMSA was performed using a probe containing the consensus NF-κB recognition site (underlined) (5' - AGT TGA <u>GGG GAC TTT CCC</u> AGG - 3'). Specific DNA binding complexes are indicated with a solid arrow. XS indicates EMSA performed with nuclear extracts from TNF-α treated cells but incubated with a 100-fold excess of consensus unlabeled probe. Antibodies directed against the Rel proteins; p65, p50, c-Rel, RelB and p52 were incubated with nuclear extracts as indicated. Supershifted complexes are indicated by open arrows and the position of the wells is indicated with a ‡. The direction of migration is indicated and free probe migrating to the bottom of the gel is not shown. Data are taken from *(3)*.

for the presence of particular DNA binding activities by means of an EMSA. Briefly, nuclear extracts are prepared from and then incubated with a double-stranded radiolabeled DNA probe containing the relevant consensus recognition sequence. Binding of factors to the probe is analyzed by nondenaturing polyacrylamide gel electrophoresis (PAGE). Free probe migrates rapidly through the gel whereas bound probe is retarded due to binding of the protein. Thus, the presence of a particular DNA binding activity can be detected, for example between different cell types or following treatment with drugs or stimuli (*see* **Fig. 1**) (*see* **Note 5**) *(1)*. Alternatively, this technique can be used to determine whether uncharacterized DNA elements are capable of binding proteins from test extracts *(2)*. In each case, the composition of DNA binding complexes may be further examined by supershift analysis (*see* **Fig. 1**) *(2,3)*. This technique involves setting up binding reactions as before, and including antisera directed to proteins that the investigator wishes to test for. Binding of antibody to a protein in a DNA/protein complex increases the size of the complex and leads to a greater mobility shift (hence supershift). Alternatively, the antibody may interfere with DNA binding and will cause reduced, or loss of, DNA binding. In either instance supershift or reduced binding, the investigator may infer that the particular protein is a component of the complex (*see* **Note 6**).

The use of EMSA and supershift analysis allows investigators to test for the presence of particular DNA-binding activities in cells of interest and test the effect of various stimuli and drugs. Thus, the relationship between transcription factor binding (and composition) and the kinetics of putative response genes can be analyzed. In addition inhibitor studies can be performed to further test the relationship between transcription factor binding and gene induction (*see* **Note 7**). Finally, the construction of appropriate probes can be used to address whether putative sites from a "real" gene are able to bind particular factors *(2)*.

3.1.1. Preparation of Nuclear Extracts

The protocol for the preparation of nuclear extracts is one modified from Dignam et al. *(4)*. This procedure uses soft lysis to rupture the plasma membrane, following which nuclei are spun out and a high salt concentration is used to extract the soluble nuclear proteins.

1. Pellet cells in suspension at 14,000*g*, 4°C, 2 min in a bench-top centrifuge and remove medium (*see* **Note 8**).
2. Lyse cells by resuspension in 200 µL of Buffer A. Vortex briefly and incubate on ice for 5–15 min (*see* **Note 9**).
3. Pellet nuclei at 14,000*g*, 4°C, 5 min and discard supernatant (*see* **Note 10**).
4. Retain nuclear pellet and resuspend pellet in 15 µL Buffer C (*see* **Note 11**). Leave on ice for 20–60 min with occasional agitation.
5. Pellet nuclear debris at 14,000*g*, 4°C, 15 min and carefully remove all the supernatant to a fresh tube containing 75 µL Buffer D.
6. Measure protein concentrations using the Bradford assay (*see* **Note 12**). Generation of standard curves using BSA and measurement of optical density (OD) at 600 nm allows protein concentrations to be determined.

3.1.2. Preparation of Radiolabeled Probe

Radiolabeled DNA probes can be generated by numerous end-fill and strand replacement processes involving various DNA polymerase activities *(5)*. However, one convenient method for radiolabeling oligonucleotides is the 5' end labeling of DNA using T4 polynucleotide kinase. Often investigators will not be able to use commercially available probes, for instance when analyzing binding of proteins to putative sites in an uncharacterized promoter or to allow the incorporation of mutations in order to characterize the binding specificity. In such cases the appropriate oligonucleotides should be synthesized and annealed prior to end labeling (*see* **Note 13**).

1. Add: 2 μL consensus double-stranded oligonucleotide (1.75 pmol/μL), 2 μL 10X kinase buffer, 13 μL H_2O, 2 μL [$\gamma_{32}P$] ATP (3,000 Ci/mmol at 10 mCi/mL), 1 μL T4 polynucleotide kinase (5–10 U/μL).
2. Incubate at 37 °C, 30 min.
3. Prepare G-25 Sephadex spin column by removing the plunger of a 1-mL syringe. Plug the tip end with a pinch of glass fiber or polymer wool. Pack column with G-25/TE slurry. Allow slurry to settle, topping up as necessary. Spin at 800–1000 g, 5 min in a swing-out bucket rotor.
4. Add 180 μL TE to the labeling reaction and apply the mix to the G-25 column. Respin at 800–1000g, 5 min.
5. Collect sample from the column (unincorporated nucleotide remains on the column) and monitor to ensure probe has been labeled. Probe can be stored at 4°C for at least one half-life and usually two for most applications.

3.1.3. Binding Reactions

In EMSA, it is essential to ensure that excess radiolabeled probe is present in the binding reactions otherwise the intensity of the shifted signal observed on a gel will not reflect the amount of DNA binding activity in a sample. In such cases, less nuclear extract or more probe is required. Binding of proteins to the probe may either be specific or nonspecific. Nonspecific binding can be identified by incubation of extracts with excess cold (competitor) probe. Specific complexes will be readily competed out whereas nonspecific complexes will remain (*see* **Fig. 1**). Such an approach also allows the sequence specificity of binding complexes to be determined by the addition of excess competitor probes harboring various point mutations in the putative binding site. Mutations that are not involved in DNA binding will not affect the ability to compete out the signal whereas mutations that affect DNA binding will result in an impaired ability to compete against the native sequence *(2)*.

1. Binding reactions are set up on ice (*see* **Note 14**). Add: Sufficient H_2O to give a final vol of 20 μL, 4 μL 5X EMSA buffer, 1–10 μg nuclear proteins and 1 μL radiolabeled probe. Normally probe is added 5 min after the nuclear proteins. For competition experiments, unlabeled probe, usually a 100-fold excess over the labeled probe, is added 15 min prior to addition of labeled probe. In the case of supershift analysis, 1–2 μL of supershift antibody (1–2 mg/mL) is added to the

binding reaction and incubated on ice for 2 h prior to the addition of probe (*see* **Note 15**).
2. Incubate on ice for 90 min.
3. Add 2 μL 10X gel loading buffer.

3.1.4. Nondenaturing Polyacrylamide Gel Electrophoresis

Nondenaturing PAGE is used for separation of free probe from the slower migrating DNA/protein complexes. As DNA/protein interactions are often weak and are easily disrupted, low ionic strength electrophoresis buffers are used and rapid running of gels is not recommended.

1. Assemble gel plates in gel casting stand (*see* **Note 16**).
2. Prepare 50 mL of a 6% acrylamide gel mix (but can use from 4–8%) (sufficient for 2 gels): 7.5 mL 40% acrylamide, 41 mL H_2O, 1.25 mL 10X TBE, 0.6 mL 10% (w/v) APS, 0.06 mL TEMED. After addition of APS and TEMED, quickly pour the gels and insert combs ensuring that no bubbles become trapped. Gels will usually set within 15 min. However, it is normal to leave at least 1 h prior to use.
3. When required, remove the combs carefully and flush out the wells with 0.25X TBE to remove unpolymerized acrylamide. Add fresh 0.25X TBE to wells.
4. Load samples to the bottom of the each well using an extended tip.
5. Run gels in 0.25X TBE at 200 V until the bromophenol blue loading dye reaches the bottom of the gel.
6. At the end of the run, separate the gel plates, adhere wet gel to 3MM Whatman paper and cover with Saran wrap.
7. Place on slab gel drier at 80°C for 1 h with vacuum.
8. Autoradiograph dried gels with intensifying screens as required.

3.2. Transfection of Lymphocytes and Monocytes

One important caveat to EMSA is that the DNA binding activity of transcription factors does not necessarily correlate with transcriptional activity. Many transcription factors, for example AP-1 and CREB, are constitutively present in the nucleus (*6*). In the case of AP-1 and related factors, signal transduction processes involving mitogen activated protein (MAP) kinase cascades result in active kinases that translocate to the nucleus to phosphorylate specific transcription factors and cause transcriptional activation (*6*). Thus, considerable DNA binding activity may be detected independently of stimulus and only minor changes (if any) observed following cell stimulation.

To address the issue of transcriptional activation of such factors appropriate transcriptional reporters are required. In essence these consist of conventional cloning plasmids in which a reporter gene, chloramphenicol acetyl transferase (CAT) or more recently firefly luciferase, is placed downstream of a multiple cloning region. Investigators may then clone putative promoter regions upstream of the reporter gene to allow assessment of promoter activity. A com-

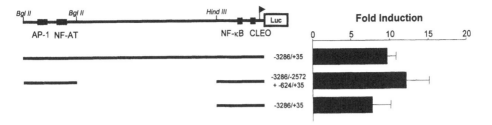

Fig. 2. Transient transfection analysis of GM-CSF promoter constructs in Jurkat T-cells. Cells were transfected with the GM-CSF promoter constructs depicted *(11)* (EMBL Accession No. HSA224149). Following transfection, cells were stimulated with $5 \times 10^{-8}\ M$ PMA + 5 µg/mL phytohemagglutinin (PHA) and harvested after 12 h for luciferase assay and protein determination. Data (n = 3) are shown as luciferase units normalized to protein and expressed as fold induction of stimulated to untreated.

mon strategy to analyze a promoter of interest is to generate a series of reporter constructs containing the transcription start site (+1) and usually 10–80 bases downstream along with progressively larger regions of 5' or upstream regions of the putative promoter. Transfection of such constructs into cells of interest may allow determination of the promoter regions required for transcriptional activation (*see* **Fig. 2**). Specific transcription factor binding sites, for example as identified by sequence comparison and/or EMSA, may be mutated by site-directed mutagenesis to verify a role in transcriptional activation (*see* **Note 17**) *(7)*. In addition, particular elements may be cloned upstream of a minimal promoter, for example containing a TATA box plus transcription start driving an appropriate reporter gene, to address the ability of particular elements to produce a transcriptional response.

3.2.1. Electroporation of Cells in Suspension Culture

Transfection refers to the introduction of essentially naked DNA into a cell. A number of processes, including electroporation, calcium phosphate coprecipitation, and liposome-mediated transfer or lipofection, have been developed for this purpose. Of these, calcium phosphate coprecipitation and lipofection are most readily applicable to cells cultured as mono-layers and their use is discussed elsewhere *(7)*. Electroporation is most suitable for transfection of cells in suspension culture and is described herein. We have successfully used this approach for transfection of T-cell lines, such as Jurkat and HUT78 cells, primary human T cells, and monocytic cell lines such as U937 cells.

1. Harvest cells and resuspend at 2×10^7 cells/mL (*see* **Note 18**).
2. To a 0.4 cm electroporation cuvet, add 10 µg of plasmid DNA and 250 µL of cells (i.e., 5.0×10^6 cells) (*see* **Note 19**). Leave for 5 min.

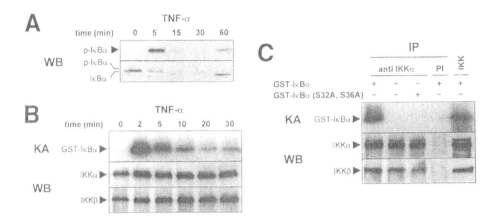

Fig. 3. Analysis of IκBα protein and IKK kinase activity following TNF-α treatment of U937 monocytic cells. Cells were treated with TNF-α (10 ng/mL) for the times indicated. (A) Cytoplasmic extracts were prepared and Western blotting (WB) performed for the Ser-32 phosphorylated form of IκBα (p-IκBα) (upper panel). Membranes were stripped and reprobed with a pan-IκBα antibody (IκBα) (lower panel). (B) IKK complexes were immunoprecipitated using an IKKα (H744). Immunoprecipitates were divided into halves and one-half subjected to IKK kinase assay (KA) using GST- IκBα (1–54) as a substrate. The second half was subject to Western blot analysis for IKKα (middle panel) and IKKβ (lower panel). (C) Immunoprecipates from cells treated with TNF-α for 2 min were subject to IKK kinase assay (KA) using either wild type GST-IκBα (1–54), or mutant GST- IκBα (1-54: S32A, S36A) or no substrate. In addition kinase assay on immunoprecipitates using rabbit preimmune antisera (PI) and biochemically purified IKK complex from HeLa cells (IKK) was performed as indicated.

3. Electroporate cells at 260 V, 975 μF in a Bio-Rad Gene Pulser II.
4. Immediately add cells to 3 mL RPMI, 10% FCS (for cell lines, use 10 mL media).
5. Incubate at 37°C for 30 min.
6. Pellet cells and resuspend in 350 μL serum free media. (2×10^6 cells/mL for cell lines).
7. Add 100 μL per well to a 96-well plate (*see* **Note 20**). Treat as required and harvest after 12 h for luciferase assay.

3.2.2. Luciferase Assay

1. Harvest cells by centrifugation at 14,000*g* for 1 min at 4°C.
2. Resuspend cell pellet in 100–200 mL 1X reporter lysis buffer (Promega).
3. Vortex vigorously and subject to one freeze/thaw cycle.
4. Spin down debris at 14,000*g* for 1 min at room temperature.
5. To 20 μL cell lysate add 40 μL luciferase assay reagent (Promega).
6. Immediately measure luminescence on a luminometer.
7. Determine protein concentration of sample using the Bradford assay.
8. Normalize luciferase readings to total protein (*see* **Note 21**).

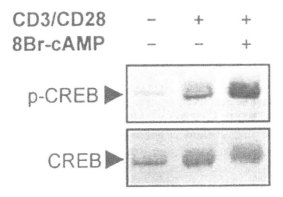

Fig. 4. Analysis of phospho-CREB in human peripheral blood mononuclear cells. Cells were stimulated with anti-CD3 (500 ng/mL) and anti-CD28 (500 ng/mL) alone or with 1 mM 8-Br-cAMP for 30 min in a 37°C incubator, with 95% air, 5% CO_2 and constant humidity. Cells were then resuspended in Buffer A supplemented with protease inhibitors. Proteins, 20 µg, were loaded on a 10% acrylamide gel and run for approx 1 hour before being transferred to a nitrocellulose membrane and probed with α-phospho-CREB antibody (New England Biolabs) (p-CREB) (upper panel). After stripping, the same membranes were reprobed with the antipan-CREB antibody (CREB) (lower panel).

3.3. Western Blotting for Phosphorylated Transcription Factors

In the preceding sections, we have noted that DNA binding of many transcription factors does not necessarily provide a guide to transcriptional activity. Phosphorylation of transcription factors such as CREB, c-*jun*, and c-*fos* has been shown to activate these factors at a transcriptional level *(6)*. To monitor protein phosphorylation, it is often possible to detect a mobility shift on SDS-PAGE (*see* **Fig. 3A**). In addition, a number of other approaches are available. One approach involves metabolic labeling of proteins followed by immunoprecipitation of the protein of interest and autoradiography to detect incorporation of ^{32}P labeled phosphate. However, a number of signal transduction pathways have now been characterized in sufficient detail to allow the elucidation of specific phosphorylation sites on various transcription factors and upstream kinases. For example, in the case of CREB, phosphorylation of Ser-133 is linked to activation and can therefore be used as a marker for transcription factor activation. The development of commercially available antibodies that are capable of specifically recognising these phosphorylated proteins allows the activation status to be addressed using conventional Western blot analysis (*see* **Note 22**). In each case Western blot analysis is also performed for the total (phosphorylated and nonphosphorylated) to allow normalization and control for loading or expression effects. Analysis of Ser-133 phosphorylated CREB is described below (*see* **Fig. 4**).

3.3.1. SDS-PAGE

1. Prepare 20 mL, sufficient for 4 mini-gels (using 1.0 mm spacers), of 8% denaturing-polyacrylamide gel mix by adding: 7.5 mL H_2O, 5.0 mL 40% acrylamide, 7.5 mL 1 *M* Tris-Cl (pH 8.8), 200 μL 10% SDS, 200 μL 10% w/v APS, 20 μL TEMED. Immediately following addition of the APS and TEMED mix by inversion and pour 4.5 mL/mini-gel (*see* **Note 23**).
2. Add 200 μL water-saturated butan-1-ol to the top of each gel and allow the acrylamide mix to set at room temperature for 1 h.
3. Wash off any unpolymerized acrylamide and butan-1-ol using H_2O and dry using Whatman 3MM paper.
4. Prepare 10 mL 5% stacking gel mix by adding: 7.28 mL H_2O, 1.26 mL 40% acrylamide, 1.26 mL 1 *M* Tris-Cl pH6.8, 100 μL 10% SDS, 100 μL 10% APS, 10 μL TEMED. Immediately following the addition of APS and TEMED, mix by inversion and fill gels to the top. Insert combs ensuring that no air bubbles are introduced.
5. Once stacking gel is set, assemble the gel tanks and fill with 1X running buffer.
6. Remove combs and flush wells with buffer to remove unpolymerized acrylamide.
7. Prepare samples (*see* **Note 24**) using 10–20 μg protein with an equal volume of 2 X Laemmli Buffer and boil for 3 min. Centrifuge to pellet debris and load samples and Rainbow markers (7.5 μL) to gel using a Hamilton syringe or extended gel loading tip.
8. Run gels at 200 V for 45–60 min until bromophenol blue reaches the bottom of gel.

3.3.2. Electroblotting

1. Cut 4 pieces of Whatman paper (10 cm × 8 cm) per gel and 1 Hybond-ECL nitrocellulose membrane (9 cm × 6.5 cm) per gel and soak in 1X blotting buffer.
2. Carefully separate glass plates and discard stacking gel. Trim gel to remove any unwanted regions.
3. Assemble blotting sandwich in the transfer cassette in the following order: two sheets of Whatman paper, nitrocellulose membrane, gel, two sheets of Whatman paper. Remove air bubbles at each stage using a plastic pipet as a rolling pin.
4. Place in blotting apparatus ensuring that the nitrocellulose layer is on the positive side of the gel (*see* **Note 25**).
5. Load cassette into blotting tank and insert icebox. Fill tank with 1X blotting buffer.
6. Run at 400 mA for 1 h (voltage should start at approx 150 V and reduce over time).
7. After running, check transfer of proteins by staining with India Red for 30 s and washing off excess stain with H_2O.

3.3.3. Immunodetection

1. Block membrane at room temperature in 10 mL 1X TBS/Tween, 5% nonfat milk for approx 1 h with shaking.
2. Wash 3 times for 5 min in 1X TBS/Tween with shaking.
3. Incubate membrane with rabbit α-phopsho-CREB antibody (New England BioLabs), diluted 1:1000 in 5% BSA 1X TBS/Tween overnight at 4°C (*see* **Notes 26** and **27**)
4. Wash 3 times for 5 min in 1X TBS/Tween.
5. Incubate membrane with α-rabbit IgG-HRP conjugated antibody diluted 1:2000 in 5% nonfat milk, 1X TBS/Tween for 1 h at room temp.
6. Wash 3 times for 5 min in 1X TBS/Tween, dry membrane against Whatman 3MM paper.
7. Incubate membrane for 1 min with 2 mL 1X LumiGLO™ (0.5 mL 20x LumiGLO, 0.5 mL Peroxide mix, 9 mL H_2O).
8. Drain and remove excess LumiGLO™ with Whatman paper prior to wrapping membrane in Saran wrap.
9. Place membrane next to film in cassette (using appropriate safety lighting) and expose for between 1–5 min, as necessary, prior to developing.
10. Density of bands of interest can be quantified using image analysis.
11. To probe for the pan-CREB, heat 15 mL stripping buffer per filter to 80°C. Then incubate with the membrane with shaking in a fume hood for 2 min.
12. Wash 3 times for 5 min in 1X TBS/Tween.
13. Repeat **steps 1–9** using the pan-CREB as the primary antibody.
14. Data should be shown or expressed as a ratio of phospho-CREB/pan-CREB.

3.4. Kinase Assay

In the preceding sections, it has been noted that kinase cascades result in the phosphorylation of target transcription factors and cause activation. In the context of examining the relationship between various stimuli and transcriptional activation, it is often desirable to assay for kinase activity. The two main approaches are the in gel kinase assay and the pull down kinase assay.

With the "in gel" approach, protein samples are size separated by SDS-PAGE using gels in which the substrate for the kinase of interest is covalently linked to the gel matrix. Following electrophoresis, gels are washed to remove SDS. After a gradual renaturation process, many proteins will adopt their natural conformation and enzymatic activity is restored. Addition of radiolabeled ATP will result in phosphorylation of the substrate linked in to the gel matrix, which after extensive washing to remove excess radiolabel can be visualised by autoradiography. This technique suffers from being a lengthy process, requires large (mg) quantities of substrate and identifies kinase activities based on size and substrate selectivity, which may confound identification of the specific kinase concerned. Conversely, the "in tube" assay requires small (μg) quantities of substrate and will identify specific kinase activities. However, the "in tube" approach can only be used where suitable antibodies are available to immunoprecipitate the relevant kinase. In such cases, or where the kinase is uncharacterized, the "in gel" approach is the method of choice. Here, we describe the "in tube" type kinase assay to assay for IκBα kinase (IKK) activity (*see* **Fig. 3B, C**). These kinases are responsible for the Ser-32 and Ser-36 phosphorylation of the NF-κB inhibitory molecule IκBα. These phosphorylation events lead to the degradation of IκBα and subsequent activation of NF-κB.

3.4.1. Immunoprecipitation of Proteins

1. Appropriate numbers of cell are harvested on ice into 100 µL Buffer A supplemented with 25 µg/mL aprotinin, 10 µg/mL leupeptin, 0.5 mM Na$_3$VO$_4$, 1 mM sodium pyrophosphate, 50 mM NaF, 0.5 mM PMSF and 5 µg/mL N-tosyl-L-phenylalanine chloromethyl ketone (*see* **Note 28**).
2. Subject lysate to one freeze/thaw cycle before spinning down debris at 14000g, 4°C, 5 min. Remove supernatants to new tube and perform Bradford protein assay. Each immunoprecipitation routinely requires 200 µg protein.
3. Mix normal rabbit IgG, 1 µg/200 µg protein, with Protein A-agarose beads, 20 µL/200 µg protein, and add to 200 µg cellular lysate.
4. Allow to preclear for 1 h at 4°C on a rotating wheel, prior to centrifugation to remove agarose beads.
5. Transfer supernatants to a new tube and incubate with 1 µg IKKα antibody (H744) (Santa Cruz) for 30 min at 4°C on a rotating wheel. Add 20 µL Protein A-agarose and mix for a further 90 min at 4°C.
6. Taking care not to remove agarose beads, wash four times with Buffer A supplemented with inhibitors and 0.05% Tween-20. Samples should be used immediately or stored at –70°C until required.

3.4.2. IKK Kinase Reaction

1. Resuspend one half of each immunoprecipitate in 25 µL kinase buffer, supplemented with 1 µg GST-IκBα substrate and 2 µCi [γ-^{32}P]ATP, and incubate at 20°C for 1 h on a rotating wheel. In addition, controls to test for specificity of the pull-down assay should be included (*see* **Fig. 3C**, lanes 1–4). As an alternative to using preimmune antiserum, immunoprecipitates can be carried out in the presence of specific blocking peptide.
2. Spin briefly to collect sample at bottom of tube and add 5 µL 6 X Laemmli buffer to stop reaction.
3. Run samples on a 10% SDS-PAGE for 1 h (conditions as above in **Subheading 3.3.1.**).
4. Dry gel on a slab vacuum dryer for 2 h.
5. Transfer gel to film cassette and autoradiograph at –70°C overnight.
6. The remaining half of each immunoprecipitation should be analyzed by SDS-PAGE and Western blotting (*see* **Subheading 3.3**) performed for IKKα (IKKβ) to confirm loading and check immunoprecipitation of the IKK complex.

3.5. Metabolic Labeling of Proteins

Detection of phosphorylated proteins by metabolic labeling involves incubation of cells in phosphate-free media and direct detection of radiolabeled proteins. Addition of radiolabeled inorganic phosphate to the media results in incorporation of radiolabel into the cellular ATP pool. When cells are subsequently stimulated immunoprecipitation and autoradiography can detect incorporation of radiolabel into specific proteins. This type of methodology is useful where the actual phosphorylation sites are not fully characterized and can be used as the first step toward mapping phospho-acceptor sites by phospho-amino acid analysis or peptide mapping (not discussed here). Herein we describe a protocol that has been successfully used to study the phosphorylation status of the p65 subunit of NF-κB (*3*).

3.5.1. Detection of ^{32}P-Labeled Proteins

1. Incubate cells in phosphate-free media for 2 h prior to the addition of [^{32}P] ortho-phosphate (Amersham Pharmacia Biotech) at 0.2 mCi/mL (*see* **Note 29**).
2. Incubate cells for 4 h and stimulate as normal. At the desired time, harvest cells in 200 μL 1 X RIPA buffer supplemented with 0.5 mM PMSF, 2 mM Na$_3$VO$_4$, 10 μg/mL leupeptin.
3. Immunoprecipitate p65 protein using 5 μL α-p65 antibody-agarose conjugate (SC-109AC) (Santa Cruz) according to the protocol above.
4. Split the immunoprecipitates into two halves and subject each to SDS-PAGE on separate gels. Vacuum dry one gel, using a slab drier, and autoradiograph to detect ^{32}P labeled proteins. On the second gel perform western analysis for p65, using the anti C-20 antibody (Santa Cruz).
5. Normalize data to total p65 present to obtain the relative level of phosphorylation.

4. Notes

1. Nucleotide sequence databases are found at www.ncbi.nlm.nih.gov and these may be searched using the BLAST program. Sequence comparisons may also be performed using BLAST. Lists of such consensus sequences, and tools designed to find transcription factor binding sites in DNA sequences, are found at http://transfac.gbf.de and http://pdap1.trc.rwcp.or.jp/research/db/TFSEARCH. html.
2. Unpolymerized acrylamide is a potent and irreversible neurotoxin. Appropriate precautions should be taken when using acrylamide solutions.
3. In our hands, brand name dried nonfat milk powder such as Marvel work well.
4. The recombinant GST-IκBα fusion protein used in this assay consists of an IκBα peptide corresponding to the first 54 amino acids and, therefore, containing the two phospho-acceptor sites Ser-32 and Ser-36, cloned in-frame and downstream of a GST tag. The construct is driven by a bacterial promoter to allow overexpression and purification from bacterial cells. Appropriate fusion proteins can be generated using substrate sites for other kinases.

5. It should be noted that EMSA is essentially a qualitative technique and is best suited to the detection of large changes (for example activation of NF-κB by TNFα) or simply the presence/absence of particular binding activities. This notwithstanding, EMSA can be successfully used in a semiquantitative manner, for example comparison of patient groups *(8)*. In this instance prior planning is essential, as samples prepared and analyzed separately cannot be readily compared. We have found that paired samples (e.g., group 1 vs group 2) which are processed and analyzed simultaneously may yield meaningful data. However, the best option is to prepare and analyze all samples in a study simultaneously to allow direct comparison of data.

6. The absence of a supershift or no reduction in DNA binding following incubation with excess antibody does not necessarily exclude the presence of a factor from the complex. To reach this conclusion appropriate positive controls would be required.

7. The inhibition of gene expression, but not DNA binding of a particular transcription factor does not necessarily exclude the involvement of that factor in gene induction. It is possible that either transcriptional activity is modulated by phosphorylation and not solely by changes in DNA binding or the inhibitor is acting downstream of DNA binding on other processes necessary for activated transcription *(9)*.

8. The optimal number of cells to be harvested needs to be determined empirically and will depend on the yield of nuclear proteins. For monocytic cells lines, such as U937, we have used 5×10^5 cells per sample. For adherent cells, such as blood-derived monocytes, we find that 3×10^6 cells, or confluent epithelial cells in 6-well plates works well. These are usually scraped in media on ice prior to pelleting and resuspension in Buffer A.

9. The appropriate incubation time varies considerably depending on the cell type or cell line. This should be determined empirically by adding buffer A and examining cells by light microscopy using a stain such as Kimura (add: 11 mL Toluidine Blue (0.05%,), 0.8 mL Light Green (0.03%), 0.5 mL Saponin (saturated), 5 mL phosphate buffered saline), which stains the nuclei. The appropriate time is that required to lyse the plasma membrane but leave the nuclear membrane intact in most cells. In addition, we commonly use Gough I buffer (10 mM Tris-Cl pH 7.5, 0.15 M NaCl, 1.5 mM MgCl$_2$, 0.65% NP-40) in place of buffer A, which contains a higher NP-40 level and when supplemented with 20–40 U RNasin (Promega), allows preparation of cytoplasmic RNA *(10)*.

10. These cytoplasmic lysates may be used for simultaneous western analysis of cytoplasmic proteins or alternatively can be used to obtain cytoplasmic RNA for RT-PCR or northern analysis *(10)* (*see* **Note 9**).

11. We find this step to be critical to the successful isolation of nuclear proteins. The nuclear pellet is usually small and compact. This can usually be dispersed with the end of the yellow tip prior to or simultaneously with resuspension. Vigorous agitation is essential to release nuclear proteins successfully. Vortexing is <u>not</u> sufficient. We drag our tubes up and down an empty Eppendorf rack to generate a violent flicking action. This is repeated at intervals during the incubation.

12. In addition to standardization of the amount of protein to be added, we routinely perform EMSA on a noninducible transcription factor, for example Oct 1, in parallel with the factor to be tested. This allows easy identification of loading or processing artefacts and, in many instances, normalization to the constitutive factor will improve the rigor of experimental data.

13. Double-stranded oligonucleotide probes are generated by mixing forward and reverse oligonucleotides (usually 20–25 mers) at a concentration of 100 pmol/μL in TE buffer. This mix is then heated to 100°C for 2 min and allowed to cool to ~30°C. Annealed probe can be diluted to a working concentration of 2 pmol/μL for radiolabeling.

14. Sheared and denatured salmon sperm works well for NF-κB EMSA. However, for CRE, NFIL6, or GRE EMSA, we often use an identical buffer except that the 0.4 mg/mL salmon sperm DNA is replaced with 0.25 mg/mL poly dI/dC (Pharmacia). Binding reactions may also be performed at room temperature, 30°C or even 37°C. The optimum will depend on the transcription factor to be analyzed and in each case should be determined empirically. Where higher incubation temperatures are used, the incubation time may also be reduced.

15. A number of commercial suppliers produce high concentration (1–2 mg/mL) antibodies (for example Santa Cruz) that are suitable for use in supershift analysis.

16. We routinely use a Hoefer SE 600 vertical electrophoresis system for 14×16 cm slab gels. Typically gels are run with 20-well combs and spacers of 1.0 mm thickness.

17. Numerous methods now exist for site-directed mutagenesis. We find the QuickChange site-directed mutagenesis kit (Stratagene, CA) to work efficiently.

18. Preparation of human T cells using MACS™ pan T cell magnetic selection (Milteny Biotech Ltd, Bergisch Gladbach, Germany) routinely results in around 93% of cells being CD3$^+$ as measured by fluorescent assisted cell sorting (FACS). Incubation of cells in RPMI supplemented with 10% fetal calf serum (FCS) and IL-2 (10 ng/mL) for 3 d results in a cell population that is 97% CD3$^+$ and can be successfully used for electroporation.

19. We have successfully used 1×10^7 U937 and Jurkat T cells per electroporation. In each case appropriate cell densities were obtained empirically using a luciferase reporter, pGL3control (Promega) that gives rise to constitutively high levels of luciferase expression.

20. After electroporation of cell lines, cells are resuspended in 10 mL of RPMI, 10% FCS and incubated at 37°C for 30 min. Cells are then resuspended in 2 mL serum-free media and 500 μL aliquots used for analysis.

21. Because of the variable nature of transient transfection, it is common for investigators to cotransfect a reporter plasmid that gives rise to constitutively high levels of β-galactosidase expression. This can be measured in cell extracts harvested as below and used to normalize the luciferase reading. However, variations in β-galactosidase expression as a result of stimulation, drugs or overexpression of signalling molecules are often observed. Consequently, normalization to protein concentration to control for variations in cell number may also be acceptable.

However, this does not control for transfection efficiency and such variations will therefore show up as an experimental error.

22. Probably the widest range of phospho-specific antibodies is available from New England Biolabs which, in addition to CREB, includes phospho-specific antibodies for transcription factors such as: c-Jun, ATF-2, Elk-1, c-Myc, Stat3, and Stat1. In addition, the phosphorylated form of the NF-κB inhibitor, IκBα, and kinases such as ERK1/2, JNK1/2, p38 MAP kinase, MEK1/2, SEK1, and MKK3 are also available.

23. We routinely use the Bio-Rad mini-protean II electrophoresis and blotting system.

24. Cells are routinely harvested in Buffer A (*see* **Subheading 2.1**) supplemented with 25 μg/mL aprotinin, 10 μg/mL leupeptin, 0.5 mM Na$_3$VO$_4$, 1 mM sodium pyrophosphate, 50 mM NaF, 0.5 mM PMSF and 0.5 mM DTT.

25. SDS coated proteins are negatively charged and therefore migrate away from the negative electrode (cathode) toward the positive electrode (anode).

26. We recommend incubation of membranes with primary antibody in sealed plastic bags, which can be placed on a rotary shaker. This allows total incubation volumes to be reduced to only 2–3 mL.

27. Incubation in primary antibody may also be for 1 h in 5% milk 5% BSA powder at room temperature.

28. As an alternative cells may be harvested in 1X RIPA buffer: RIPA buffer: 1X PBS, 1% NP-40, 0.5% sodium deoxycholate, 0.1% SDS. This is a higher stringency buffer, which will reduce protein-protein interactions and reduce nonspecific bands.

29. The exact phosphate-free media (RPMI, DMEM, and so on) will depend on the cell line being studied.

References

1. Newton, R., Adcock, I.M., and Barnes, P.J. (1996) Superinduction of NF-kappa B by actinomycin D and cycloheximide in epithelial cells. *Biochem. Biophys. Res. Commun.* **218,** 518–523.

2. Newton, R., Kuitert, L.M., Bergmann, M., Adcock, I.M., and Barnes, P.J. (1997) Evidence for involvement of NF-kappa B in the transcriptional control of COX-2 gene expression by IL-1β. *Biochem. Biophys. Res. Commun.* **237,** 28–32.

3. Nasuhara, Y., Adcock, I.M., Catley, M., Barnes, P.J., and Newton, R. (1999) Differential IKK activation and IkappaBalpha degradation by interleukin-1beta and tumor necrosis factor-alpha in human U937 monocytic cells: Evidence for additional regulatory steps in kappaB-dependent transcription. *J. Biol. Chem.* **274,** 19,965–19,972.

4. Dignam, J.D., Lebovitz, R.M., and Roeder, R.G. (1983) Accurate transcription initiation by RNA polymerase II in a soluble extract from isolated mammalian nuclei. *Nucleic. Acids. Res.* **11,** 1475–1489.

5. Sambrook, J., Fritsch, E.F., and Maniatis, T. (1989), Molecular Cloning — *A Laboratory Manual.* Cold Spring Harbor Laboratory Press, New York.

6. Karin, M. (1995) The regulation of AP-1 activity by mitogen-activated protein kinases. *J. Biol. Chem.* **270,** 16,483–16,486.

7. Newton, R. and Adcock, I.M. (2000) Analysis of transcription factor activation: NF-kappaB as regulator of inflammatory genes in epithelial cells, in: *Asthma; Methods and Protocols.* Chung, K.F. and Adcock, I.M., eds. Humana Press Inc., pp. 143–159.

8. Hart, L.A., Krishnan, V.L., Adcock, I.M., Barnes, P.J., and Chung, K.F. (1998) Activation and localization of transcription factor, nuclear factor- kappaB, in asthma. *Am. J. Respir. Crit. Care Med.* **158,** 1585–1592.

9. Bergmann, M., Hart, L., Lindsay, M., Barnes, P.J., and Newton, R. (1998) IkappaBalpha degradation and nuclear factor-kappaB DNA binding are insufficient for interleukin-1beta and tumor necrosis factor-alpha induced kappaB-dependent transcription: Requirement for an additional activation pathway. *J. Biol. Chem.* **273,** 6607–6610.

10. Gough, N.M. (1988) Rapid and quantitative preparation of cytoplasmic RNA from small numbers of cells. *Anal. Biochem.* **173,** 93–95.

11. Bergmann, M., Barnes, P.J., and Newton, R. (2000) Molecular regulation of granulocyte-macrophage colony-stimulating factor in human lung epithelial cells by IL-1, IL-4 and IL-13 involves both transcriptional and posttranscriptional mechanisms. *Am. J. Respir. Cell Mol. Biol.* **22,** 582–589.

V

MEDIATORS

EXPRESSION AND FUNCTION

24

Inflammatory Mediators
in Spontaneously Produced Sputum

Adam Hill, Simon Gompertz, Darren Bayley, and Robert Stockley

1. Introduction

Airway inflammation is currently the subject of intense research interest concerning both the nature of the inflammatory cells, proteins, and cytokines present. These data are being used to define and assess the severity, cause, prognosis, and response to treatment of airway inflammatory disease. Spontaneous sputum is a useful method for studying inflammation in the larger airways, in diseases such as asthma, bronchitis, and bronchiectasis.

Although many assays are readily available, it is absolutely critical to validate them within the biological sample to be studied. For instance, monoclonal antibodies by definition are epitope specific but in biological fluids such as sputum the presence of proteolytic activity or protein-protein complex formation may lead to the loss or "masking" of the specific epitope identified by the monoclonal antibody. This may lead to the false assumption that the antigen is reduced or not present. In addition, many proteins bind to the mucopolysaccharide component of sputum and may be excluded from the sol phase, whereas they may be released if chemicals such as dithiothreitol (DTT) break down the mucopolysaccharides. However, this approach also has its problems in that the mucopolysaccharides may not be completely broken down and DTT itself may interfere with protein measurements. Methodologies should therefore clearly be validated before being applied to sputum and this should involve the "spiking" of sputum samples with the pure protein or cytokine to determine recovery.

The neutrophil and, in particular, the serine proteinase neutrophil elastase, released from activated neutrophils, has been implicated in the pathogenesis of chronic lung diseases e.g., chronic obstructive pulmonary disease (COPD) and

From: *Methods in Molecular Medicine, vol. 56:*
Human Airway Inflammation: Sampling Techniques and Analytical Protocols
Edited by: D. F. Rogers and L. E. Donnelly © Humana Press Inc., Totowa, NJ

bronchiectasis. This chapter discusses the methods of sputum collection, processing, and assay validation. A variety of methods are available for measuring neutrophil elastase and its inhibitors, and the following will be described:

1. Total neutrophil elastase concentration.
2. Free elastase activity.
3. Elastase inhibitory capacity.
4. Sodium dodecyl sulfate-polyacrylamide gel electrophoresis (SDS-PAGE) with immunoblotting (to confirm the identity and relative molecular mass of the protease inhibitors).
5. Direct measurement of inhibitors.
6. Measurement of neutrophil chemotaxis, including inhibition studies to determine the contribution of individual cytokines, and the direct measurement of chemoattractant concentrations.
7. Measurement of myeloperoxidase as a surrogate marker of neutrophil influx are described.

2. Materials (*see* Note 1)

2.1. Reagents

All reagents from Sigma Chemical Co., Poole, Dorset, UK unless stated otherwise.

2.1.1. Neutrophil Elastase ELISA

1. Acid washed immunoplate II (Nunc, Inc., Newbury Park, CA).
2. Neutrophil elastase (−70°C).
3. 10 mM Phosphate, 0.6 M NaCl (pH 7.4).
4. 1% (w/v) Ovalbumin (4°C).
5. 0.1% (v/v) Tween-20.
6. 1% (w/v) Bovine serum albumin (BSA) (4°C).
7. Sheep antineutrophil elastase IgG (4°C) (Cappel, Malvern, PA).
8. Polypropylene RIA vials (Sarstedt, Princeton, NJ).
9. Peroxidase conjugated rabbit antisheep IgG (4°C).
10. O-phenylenediamine (4°C).
11. Citrate buffer.

2.1.2. Neutrophil Elastase Activity

1. Microtiter plate.
2. Neutrophil elastase (−70°C).
3. N-Methoxysuccinyl-ala-ala-pro-val-paranitroanilide (4°C).
4. Neutrophil elastase buffer: 0.01 M Tris-HCl, 0.5 M NaCl, 0.1% (v/v) Triton X 100 (pH 8.6).
5. Acetic acid.

Table 1
SDS-PAGE Gel Composition

Reagent	Running gel	Stacking gel	Vol
% Acrylamide (final concentration in gel)	12.5	5	
Distilled water	5.55	3.6	mL
Running Buffer (1.875 M Tris/HCl pH 8.8)	3.0		mL
Stacking Buffer (1.25 M Tris/HCl pH 6.8)		0.5	mL
Acrylamide (29.1% (w/v) acrylamide and 0.9% (w/v) bis-acrylamide)	6.25	0.8	mL
SDS (w/v) (10%)	150	50	μL
Ammonium persulphate (w/v) (10%)	50	17	μL
N,N,N',N'-Tetramethylethylenediamine (TEMED)	7.5	5.0	μL

2.1.3. Elastase Inhibitory Capacity

1. Microtiter plate.
2. Neutrophil elastase (–70°C).
3. Neutrophil elastase buffer: 0.01 *M* Tris-HCl, 0.5 *M* NaCl, 0.1% (v/v) Triton X 100 (pH 8.6).
4. N-succinyl ala-ala-ala p-nitroanilide (4°C).

2.1.4. SDS-PAGE Gel Electrophoresis

1. Tall mighty small multiple gel caster SE 200 (Hoefer Scientific Instruments, San Francisco, CA).
2. Tall mighty small vertical slab gel unit SE 280 (Hoefer Scientific Instruments).
3. Well comb (Hoefer Scientific Instruments, San Francisco, USA).
4. Power supply (Pharmacia Biotech Electrophoresis power supply EPS 600).
5. Running and stacking gel (*see* **Table 1**).
6. Methanol.
7. Electrode buffer (25 m*M* Tris, 192 m*M* glycine, and 0.1% (w/v) SDS) (4°C).
8. Sample buffer store at –20°C [0.125 *M* Tris/HCl pH 6.8 (2.5 mL stacking buffer), 4% (w/v) SDS, 20% (v/v) glycerol, 10% (v/v) β-2-mercaptoethanol (1 mL), 0.2 mg Bromophenol blue].

2.1.4.1. Fast Staining

1. Fast stain (ZOION Biotech, Newton).
2. Destain (5 parts water, 5 parts methanol, and 1 part glacial acetic acid).
3. 10% (v/v) acetic acid.
4. 1.5% (v/v) glycerol.
5. Easy Breeze gel drier (Hoefer Scientific Instruments).

2.1.4.2. SILVER STAINING

1. Silver staining kit (Sigma-Aldrich).
2. Fixing solution [made up to 200 mL in ultra pure water (10 mL "silver fixing solution", 100 mL methanol, and 20 mL glacial acetic acid)] (4°C).
3. Prepare staining and developing solution immediately before use adding each solution sequentially while stirring (35 mL ultra pure water, 5 mL provided components 1 to 3, and 50 mL provided component 4).
4. Stop solution (10 mL glacial acetic acid made up to 200 mL in ultra pure water).
5. 1.5% (v/v) glycerol.
6. Easy Breeze gel drier (Hoefer Scientific Instruments).

2.1.5. Immunoblotting

1. Nitro-cellulose sheet (Bio-Rad Laboratories).
2. Filter paper (Whatman No. 1).
3. Destaining chamber (Conalco Ltd.).
4. Transfer buffer [25 mM Tris/HCl (pH 8.3), 192 mM glycine/20% (v/v) methanol] (4°C).
5. Phosphate-buffered saline (PBS) (NaCl 4.5 g/L, $NaH_2PO_4.2H_2O$ 2.8 g/L, Na_2HPO_4 anhydrous 8.0 g/L).
6. NaCl/PBS/10% (v/v) colloidal gelatin (Hemaccel)/Tween 20 [Hemaccel stored at −70°C].
7. Mouse monoclonal antibody against human alpha-1-antitrypsin (4°C).
8. Peroxidase-conjugated donkey anti-mouse IgG (4°C).
9. 3-amino-9-ethylcarbazole (4°C).
10. H_2O_2 (4°C)

2.1.6. Alpha-1-Antitrypsin

1. MAXISORP (Nunc) microtiter plate.
2. Goat antihuman α_1-antitrypsin antibody (4°C) (The Binding Site Limited, Birmingham, UK).
3. 0.05 M Sodium carbonate/bicarbonate pH 9.6 (4°C).
4. PBS containing 1% (v/v) Tween 20.
5. Goat antihuman α_1-antitrypsin antibody conjugated with horseradish peroxidase (4°C) (The Binding Site Limited).
6. O-phenylamine dihydrochloride (4°C).
7. O-phenylamine dihydrochloride buffer (0.01% (v/v) H_2O_2 in 1 vol 0.1 M Citric acid/2 vol 0.1 M Na_2HPO_4, pH 5).
8. Citric acid.

2.1.7. Chemotaxis

2.1.7.1. AGAROSE CHEMOTAXIS

1. 0.5 g Agarose.
2. RPMI (4°C) supplemented with gelatin (0.82 g RPMI-1640 medium, 0.25 g gelatin).

3. 50 mm diameter vented tissue culture petridishes (Greiner).
4. RPMI assay medium [0.41 g RPMI-1640 medium with HEPES modification in 25mL sterile distilled water] (4°C).
5. Freshly harvested peripheral blood neutrophils from healthy volunteers.
6. Chemoattractant or sputum sol phase (–70°C).
7. Glutaraldehyde 2.5% (v/v) in PBS.
8. Diff-Quick (Gamidor Ltd, Oxford).

2.1.7.2. BOYDEN CHEMOTAXIS

1. Boyden chamber (Neuro Probe 48-well chemotaxis chamber, Neuro Probe Inc., Cabin John, MD).
2. PVP-free Nucleopore polycarbonate filter with 2 µM pores (Costar, High Wycombe, UK).
3. 10% (v/v) 7X-PF detergent solution (ICN Biomedicals Ltd, Irvine, Scotland).
4. Freshly harvested neutrophils.
5. RPMI 1640 medium containing 0.2% (w/v) bovine serum albumin (4°C).
6. Chemoattractant or sputum sol phase (–70°C).
7. Diff-Quik.

2.1.7.3. ENDOTHELIAL TRANSMIGATION ASSAY

1. Human pulmonary artery endothelial cells.
2. Transwell polycarbonate membrane filter [6.5 mm diameter, 3.0 µM pore size (Corning Costar Corp., Cambridge, MA) previously coated with human type 4 collagen].
3. 24-well culture plates.
4. Scanning electron microscope.
5. Hanks balanced salt solution (4°C).
6. Chemoattractant or sputum sol phase (–70°C).
7. Freshly harvested neutrophils.
8. Hanks balanced salt solution containing (HBSS) 0.25% (w/v) Brij-35 (4°C).

2.1.7.4. ASSESSING CONTRIBUTION OF INDIVIDUAL CHEMOATTRACTANTS TO CHEMOTAXIS

The following uses assessment of interleukin (IL)-8 as an example.

1. Monoclonal antihuman IL8 antibody (4°C) (R & D Systems, Abingdon, UK).
2. 10 nM pure leukotriene (LT)-B$_4$ (–70°C).
3. 10 nM pure IL8 (-70°C) (R & D Systems).
4. RPMI solution containing 0.2% (w/v) BSA (4°C).

2.1.8. IL-8 ELISA

1. IL-8 Quantikine kit (4°C) (R&D Systems Europe Ltd, Abingdon, UK).
2. Assay diluent RD1-8 (4°C).
3. IL8 standard (–70°C).
4. RD5P Calibrator diluent (4°C).

5. IL8 conjugate (4°C).
6. Wash buffer.
7. Substrate solution (1 vol of color reagent A to 1 vol of color reagent B) (4°C).
8. 1 *M* sulfuric acid.

2.1.9. Myeloperoxidase

1. O-dianisidine dihydrochloride (4°C).
2. 30% (v/v) H_2O_2 (4°C).
3. 50 m*M* K_2HPO_4.
4. 0.5% (w/v) hexadecyl trimethyl ammonium bromide pH 6.

2.2. Apparatus

1. Microplate reader: Dynatech MR 5000 (Dynatech Corporation, Burlington, VT).

3. Methods

3.1. Sputum Collection and Processing

1. Collect sputum samples into a sterile container over a fixed period (often 4 h) following rising from bed.
2. Process sputum sample within 4 h of sputum collection.
3. Ultracentrifuge sputum sample at 50,000*g* for 90 min at 4°C.
4. Remove the sol phase by pipet and store at –70°C until analyzed (*see* **Note 2**).

3.1.2. Assay Validation

1. Obtain a standard curve using a pure preparation.
2. Assay sputum sol phase from a pooled sample (*n* = 6) of mucoid and mucopurulent phlegm (to ensure the assay is valid for the range of samples that may be tested).
3. Assay each pooled sample at different dilutions (4 to 6 times for each dilution) (*see* **Notes 3** and **4**).
4. Assay again after a known quantity of the pure mediator has been added to the sample (*see* **Fig. 1**).
5. Compare optical density to the standard curve and derive the result for the new value by interpolation.
6. To obtain the amount of spike recovered, subtract the original sample amount (step 3) from the latter result (step 5), and divide the result by the amount of spike added (expressed as %) (*see* **Note 5**).
7. Finally to study the effect of active neutrophil elastase (which may interfere with the assay), add increasing concentrations of active neutrophil elastase to a known amount of the mediator (*see* **Note 6**). Assay the mixture to determine whether there is any change in the value obtained.
8. To ensure the assay is reproducible, aim for an interassay coefficient of variation <10% (add a known concentration of mediator to serial assays). This process should be carried out for every assay.

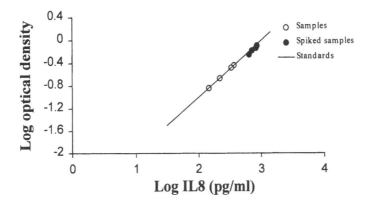

Fig. 1. The optical density of the ELISA reaction (vertical axis) is plotted against the IL-8 concentration (horizontal axis). The open circles are four sample results and the closed circles are spiked with known amounts of IL-8. Results lie close to the line of the standard curve indicating good recovery of the sample spike (>85%) (reproduced with permission *Eur. Respir. J.* 2000: 15; 778–781).

3.2. Elastase ELISA (1)

1. Coat acid washed immunoplate II with 1 µg neutrophil elastase in 10 mM phosphate, 0.6 M NaCl (pH 7.4) and incubate overnight at 4°C.
2. Wash the plates repeatedly with 10 mM phosphate, 0.6 M NaCl (pH 7.4) to remove unbound protein.
3. To block additional protein binding sites, block overnight with 200 µL of 1% (w/v) ovalbumin in 10 mM phosphate, 0.6 M NaCl, 0.1% (v/v) Tween-20 (pH 7.4) at 4°C.
4. Dilute standards or samples in 10 mM phosphate, 0.6 M NaCl, 1% (w/v) BSA (pH 7.4) and incubate overnight at 4°C with 5 µg/mL monospecific sheep anti-NE IgG in polypropylene RIA vials in a total volume of 130 µL.
5. Transfer 100 µL of the standard or samples into each well of the neutrophil elastase coated plate and incubate overnight at 4°C.
6. Wash the plate repeatedly with 10 mM phosphate, 0.6 M NaCl (pH 7.4).
7. Add 200 µL peroxidase conjugated rabbit antisheep IgG and incubate for 90 min at 37°C.
8. Develop the assay using 1 mg/mL o-phenylenediamine in 50 mM citrate buffer (pH 4.5).
9. Read the plate at 450 nm using a microtiter plate reader and calculate the amount of neutrophil elastase in the samples by interpolation from the standard curve.

3.3. Neutrophil Elastase Activity

1. Purify neutrophil elastase standard from empyema pus according to the method of Baugh and Travis (2).

2. Determine the activity of the elastase standard by active site titration using published kinetic constants *(3)*.

3. Measure neutrophil elastase activity in the samples and standards spectrophotometrically using the synthetic substrate *N*-methoxysuccinyl-ala-ala-pro-val-paranitroanilide (MeOSAAPVpNa).

4. Add 20 µL of standard or sample to wells of a microtitre plate (*see* **Note 7**).

5. Add 150 µL MeOSAAPVpNa (0.3 m*M*) in neutrophil elastase buffer.

6. Allow the reaction to continue for 1 h at 37°C.

7. Stop by adding 200 µL of 1 *N* acetic acid.

8. Read the absorbance at 410 n*M* and calculate the elastolytic activity from the standard curve by interpolation.

3.4. Elastase Inhibitory Capacity

1. Neutrophil elastase of known concentration is made up to 2.5 µ*M* in neutrophil elastase assay buffer (*see* **Note 8**).

2. Place 10 µL in triplicate across 11 columns of a 96-well flat-bottomed microtiter plate.

3. Insert 10 µL of assay buffer into column 12 (blank wells).

4. Into the first set of wells, add 1 µL undiluted sputum sol phase.

5. Into the second set, add 2 µL undiluted sputum sol phase.

6. Into the third set, add 3 µL undiluted sputum sol phase and so on until the eleventh set which provides the control activity.

7. Add assay buffer to each well to give a final volume of 110 µL and then gently mix by tapping on side of the plate with a finger.

8. Wrap the plate in cling film and incubate at 37°C for 20 min.

9. After incubation, add 150 µL N-succinyl-ala-ala-ala p-nitroanilide (1 mg/mL) into each well and then gently mix.

10. Incubate plate for 45 min at 37°C.

11. Read plate at 410 nm on the microplate reader.

12. Subtract the blanks from each result and then plot the percentage of zero inhibition against the volume of sol added.

13. The amount of elastase inhibitory capacity of the sample is then calculated from the x axis intercept (*see* **Fig. 2** and **Note 9**).

3.5. SDS-PAGE

1. Prepare 12.5% running gel (*see* **Table 1**) and pour carefully using a syringe into the tall mighty small multiple gel caster SE 200 [combine 6.25 mL 29.1% (w/v) acrylamide/ 0.9% (w/v) *bis*-acrylamide with 3 mL running buffer (1.875 *M* Tris/HCl; pH 8.8), 150 µL 10% (w/v) SDS, 5.55 mL distilled H_2O, 50 µL 10% (w/v) ammonium persulphate and 7.5 µL *N,N,N',N'*-tetramethylethylenediamine (TEMED)].

2. Top up to approx 2 cm below the top of the back plate once the gel becomes level.

3. Pour methanol carefully on top of the gel to create a level interface between the running and stacking gels.

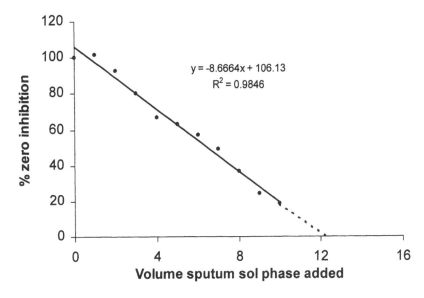

Fig. 2. Elastase inhibitory capacity calculated from x axis intercept.

4. Allow the gel to set for 1 h and then pour the methanol off.
5. Prepare the stacking gel [combine 800 µL acrylamide/*bis*-acrylamide with 500 µL stacking buffer (1.25 M Tris/HCl; pH 6.8), 50 µL 10% (w/v) SDS, 3.6 mL H₂O, 17 µL 10% (w/v) ammonium persulphate and 5 µL TEMED] and pour on top of the running gel (*see* **Table 1**).
6. Insert a well comb into the apparatus, and leave the gel to set.
7. Remove the well comb and flush the wells with distilled water using a Hamilton syringe.
8. Remove the gel and place in a tall mighty small vertical slab gel unit SE 280.
9. Fill the upper and lower tanks with electrode buffer.
10. Prepare gel filtration fractions by combining 40 µL sample with 20 µL sample buffer.
11. Denature the protein by placing in a boiling water bath for 3 min (100°C) and then transfer to ice for 1 min.
12. Use a Hamilton syringe to dispense 5 µL of a wide range molecular weight markers into the outer well and 10–15 µL sample is loaded into the remaining wells.
13. Connect the gel to a high voltage power supply.
14. Perform electrophoresis through the stacking gel at 50 V and through the running gel at 150 V.
15. On completion, the gel is removed and protein bands visualized by fast or silver stain.

3.5.1. Fast Staining (see **Note 10**)

1. After electrophoresis, remove the gel carefully from the assembly, place in a tray of Destain, and place on a rotary shaker for 20 min.
2. Repeat with another wash of Destain.

3. Stain the gel then with fast stain for 20 min.
4. Several washes with 10% (v/v) acetic acid to ensure removal of background staining.
5. Immerse in destain containing 1.5% (v/v) glycerol.
6. Dry the gel between sheets of cellophane in an Easy Breeze gel drier for a minimum of 2 h.

3.5.2. Silver Staining

1. After electrophoresis, remove the gel carefully from the assembly, immerse in 200 mL fixing solution, and place on a rotary shaker for 20 min.
2. Wash for 10 min in ultra pure water, repeating the wash step once more.
3. The gel is then incubated with gentle shaking in 100 mL staining and developing solution until the required staining intensity has been reached (typically 1 h).
4. The staining reaction is then stopped by transferring the gel into 200 mL of the stop solution for 20 min.
5. Incubate the gel overnight in a 1.5% (v/v) glycerol solution.
6. Dry the gel between sheets of cellophane in an Easy Breeze gel drier.
7. Amend as appropriate according to manufacturer's instructions.

3.6. Immunoblotting (4)

3.6.1. Transfer of Protein from SDS-PAGE to Nitro-Cellulose Sheet (Electroblotting)

1. The SDS gel is put onto a dampened filter paper and overlaid with a nitro-cellulose sheet soaked in transfer buffer.
2. Cover the nitro-cellulose with a further layer of filter paper.
3. Electroblotting is then carried out by electrophoresis in a modified destaining chamber with the nitro-cellulose sheet facing the anode.
4. Protein transfer is completed overnight at 40 mA in transfer buffer.

3.6.2. Immunological Detection of Proteins on Nitro-Cellulose (see **Fig. 3**)

1. The nitro-cellulose membrane is soaked for 30 min in NaCl/PBS/10% (v/v) colloidal gelatin (Hemaccel)/Tween 20.
2. Wash thoroughly in NaCl/PBS buffer; 3 × 10 min (*see* **Note 11**).
3. The membrane is then incubated for a further 2 h with a primary mouse monoclonal antibody against human alpha-1-antitrypsin.
4. Wash thoroughly in NaCl/PBS buffer; 3 × 10 min.
5. To allow subsequent visualization of specific alpha-1-antitrypsin bands, incubate with a peroxidase-conjugated donkey antimouse IgG for 2 h.
6. Wash again in NaCl/PBS buffer (3 × 10 min).
7. Add the substrate 3-amino-9-ethylcarbazole for 20 min (may require less time) followed by H_2O_2.

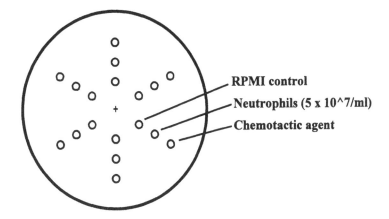

Fig. 3. Schematic representation of immunoblots for native α_1 antitrypsin, complexed and proteolysed forms (the latter two after the addition of elastase). **Lane 1** illustrates specific antibody staining of native α_1 antitrypsin (N) alone. **Lanes 2** and **3** show samples which contain complexed (C) and proteolyzed α_1 antitrypsin (P). The sample in **Lane 2** also contains some native α_1 antitrypsin.

3.7. Direct Measurement of Inhibitor (e.g., α_1-antitrypsin by ELISA)

1. Add 200 µL goat antihuman α_1-antitrypsin antibody in 0.05 M sodium carbonate/ bicarbonate pH 9.6 to a microtiter plate and incubate overnight (4°C).
2. Wash the plate three times with PBS containing 1% (v/v) Tween 20 and 1% (v/v) Haemaccel.
3. Add 200 µL standard or sample (*see* **Note 12**) to the plate followed by a 60 min incubation at 37°C.
4. Wash the plate three times with PBS containing 1% (v/v) Tween 20 and 1% (v/v) Hemaccel.
5. Add 200 µL goat antihuman α_1-antitrypsin antibody peroxidase conjugate in PBS containing 1% (v/v) Tween 20 to each well.
6. Incubate the plate for 60 min at 37°C.
7. Wash each well three times with PBS containing 1% (v/v) Tween 20 and 1% (v/v) Hemaccel.
8. Add 200 µL of 1 mg/mL O-phenylamine dihydrochloride in O-phenylamine dihydrochloride buffer to each well followed by an incubation for 10 min at 25°C.
9. Stop the reaction with 50 µL of 0.5 *M* citric acid.
10. Read the plate at 450 nm and the α_1-antitrypsin concentration is calculated from the standard curve by interpolation.

3.8. Neutrophil Chemotaxis

3.8.1. Agarose

1. Boil 0.5 g agarose in 25 mL sterile distilled water (100°C).
2. Dissolve RPMI/gelatin in 25 mL sterile distilled water for 20 min at 56°C.

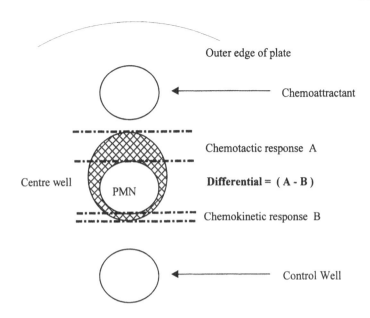

Fig. 4. A template for the preparation of agarose chemotaxis plates

3. Allow agarose to cool to 56°C in water bath.
4. The agarose and RPMI/gelatin are mixed and kept at 56°C. 6 mL is then pipeted into each agar plate. The plates are left to set at room temperature for 20 min and then placed at 4°C for 10 min. Wells are then cut into the agar with a punch (diameter 3.2 mm) using the following template (*see* **Fig. 4** and **Note 13**).
5. Freshly harvested neutrophils are resuspended at 5×10^7 cells/mL in RPMI.
6. 10 μL RPMI are placed into each of the inner wells, 10 μL suspended neutrophils into each of the center wells, and 10 μL chemoattractant (10^{-7} *M* *N*-formyl-methionyl leucyl phenylalanine, fMLP, in RPMI) or sputum sol phase (pure) into each of the outer wells (*see* **Notes 14** and **15**).
7. Incubate plates at 37°C (5% CO_2) for 2 h and then flood with glutaraldehyde for overnight fixation of the cells.
8. Carefully remove gel and wash plates under a slow running tap water.
9. Stain plates with Diff-Quik and leave to dry.
10. For each well the chemotactic and chemokinetic responses are read using an eye piece graticule.
11. The overall response to the chemoattractant (chemotactic differential) is calculated by subtracting the chemokinetic from the chemotactic response (*see* **Fig. 5**).

3.8.2. Boyden Chamber Chemotaxis

1. The chemotaxis chamber consists of a top and bottom acrylic plate, a silicone gasket, and assembly hardware.
2. The lower plate has 48 wells, each of 27 μL vol.

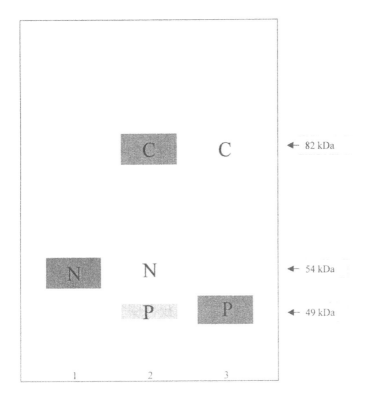

Fig. 5. The overall response to the chemoattractant (chemotactic gradient) in the agarose assay is calculated by subtracting the chemokinetic from the chemotactic distance moved by the neutrophils (PMN).

3. Corresponding holes in the top plate form the upper wells of 50 µL.
4. The membrane used to separate the two portions is a PVP-free (polyvinylpyrrolidone) Nucleopore polycarbonate filter with 2 µm pores.
5. Prepare the chambers by soaking overnight in 10% (v/v) 7X-PF detergent solution.
6. Wash the components thoroughly under running tap water and then with distilled water (*see* **Note 16**).
7. Shake thoroughly dry and place in an incubator at 37°C to complete the drying process.
8. Resuspend harvested neutrophils at 1.5×10^6 cells/mL in RPMI 1640 medium (0.2% (w/v) BSA).
9. To the lower wells add 27.5 µL (to ensure a raised meniscus) of chemoattractant or sputum sol phase (*see* **Note 17**) in RPMI containing 0.2% (w/v) BSA.
10. Carefully place membrane with matt side lowermost over the wells.
11. Place the silicone gasket on top of the membrane followed by the upper plate.
12. 50 µL of resuspended neutrophils is then carefully pipeted into the upper wells (*see* **Note 18**).

13. Incubate chamber for 20 min at 37°C.
14. After incubation the chamber is carefully disassembled and the membrane removed.
15. Cells that have migrated are adherent to the matt side of the membrane, whereas cells that have not migrated are removed by floating the membrane on the PBS, shiny side down and wiping this side three times on a wiper blade.
16. Air-dry membrane for 1 h and then stain with Diff-Quik.
17. Count neutrophils under × 400 magnification.
18. For each well the total number of cells wholly contained within five random equal size fields are counted and the mean is taken.
19. Perform each test in triplicate.

3.8.3. Endothelial Transmigration Assay (5)

1. Human pulmonary artery endothelial cells are cultured at 1.5×10^5 cells/transwell filter insert for 4 days.
2. Transfer cultured human pulmonary artery endothelial cells (after 4 d) on the transwell filter inserts to a fresh 24-well tissue culture plate.
3. For each migration assay, retain one filter and process for scanning electron microscopy to confirm the presence of an intact continuous cell layer covering the filter.
4. Remove the culture medium carefully from the other filter inserts.
5. Gently rinse the cells with 100 μL HBSS (prewarmed to 37°C).
6. Replace medium with 100 μL HBSS.
7. Preincubate cells for 45 min at 37°C.
8. Add 600 μL of either the chemoattractant (e.g., fMLP 0.1–100 nM) in HBSS, or HBSS alone, to the lower compartments of the Transwell system (in place of the chemoattractant sputum sol phase can be used).
9. Initiate the migration assay by the addition of 1×10^6 neutrophils in 100 μL HBSS to all upper compartments.
10. Add an additional 200 μL of either fMLP or HBSS to the bottom compartment to equalize the liquid levels in the top and bottom compartments of the Transwells.
11. Incubate the plates at 37°C in 100% humidity and 5% CO_2 for 3 h.
12. Place the plate on ice.
13. Separate non-migrated and migrated neutrophils populations by lifting the filter inserts from the upper compartment out of the well from the lower compartment in which they had been suspended.
14. Rinse any loosely attached migrated neutrophils from the filter undersurface into the population of migrated neutrophils in the lower compartment of the transwell.
15. Collect the nonadherent neutrophils that have not migrated (remaining in the volume contained in the filter insert in the upper compartment of the transwell system) by gently washing with HBSS.
16. Centrifuge both neutrophil populations and their respective supernatants at 300g for 10 min.
17. Lyse the neutrophils by suspending in HBSS containing 0.25% (w/v) Brij-35.
18. Remove the human pulmonary artery endothelial cells monolayer with associ-

ated neutrophils by carefully cutting the filter membrane out of the insert and lyse by suspending in HBSS containing 0.25% (w/v) Brij-35.

19. For each experiment, prepare a range of neutrophil concentrations and incubate in either fMLP or HBSS for 3 h at 37°C.

20. After this time collect the neutrophils by centrifuging at 300g for 10 min.

21. Resuspend in HBSS containing 0.25% (w/v) Brij-35 and lyse concurrently with migration assay samples.

22. Assay all neutrophil isolates for Myeloperoxidase activity (*see* **Subheading 3.10.**).

23. Construct a standard curve of the numbers of neutrophils vs Myeloperoxidase activity, and the numbers of non adherent, adherent, and migrated neutrophils are quantified by extrapolation from the myeloperoxidase activity present in upper, monolayer, and lower compartments respectively.

3.8.4. Assessing Contribution of Individual Chemoattractants to Chemotaxis

The following uses interleukin (IL-8) as an example to assess whether chemotactic activity can be suppressed by a monoclonal antibody to IL-8.

1. Add increasing concentrations of the IL8 antibody (10^{-9} to 10^{-1} mg/mL) to study the effect on the chemotactic response to optimal concentrations of pure IL-8 (10 nM).

2. Each concentration of IL8 antibody is preincubated with 10 nM pure IL-8 suspended in RPMI solution containing 2 mg/mL BSA at 37°C for 1 h prior to performing the chemotaxis assay.

3. Repeat the experiments to determine whether the chemotactic responses can be abrogated in the same way in a mixture of chemoattractants (e.g., IL-8 and LTB$_4$ as might be found in airway secretions).

4. Using dose responses to varying dilutions of sputum sol phase, obtain the maximal neutrophil chemotaxis (*see* **Note 17**).

5. At this dilution, incubate with IL-8 antibody (10^{-9} to 10^{-1} mg/mL) to determine the contribution of IL-8.

3.9. Interleukin 8

1. IL-8 is measured by enzyme-linked immunosorbent assay (ELISA) using a commercially available kit.

2. Add 100-μL assay diluent RD1-8 to each well.

3. Add 50-μL standard or sample (dissolved in calibrator diluent RD5P) (*see* **Note 19**).

4. Add 100-μL IL8 conjugate to each well.

5. Cover the wells with an adhesive strip and incubate the plate for 2.5 h at 25°C.

6. Dissolve 20 mL wash buffer concentrate in 480 mL distilled water to produce 500 mL wash buffer.

7. Wash each well six times with wash buffer.

8. Add 200 μL substrate solution (equal volumes of colour reagents A and B) to each well.

9. Incubate the plate for 30 min at 25°C.
10. Stop the reaction by using 50 μL of 1 M sulphuric acid.
11. Measure the absorbance at 450 nm with a 570 nm correction using a Dynatech MR 5000 microplate reader.
12. Calculate the IL8 concentration by interpolation from the standard curve.

3.10. Myeloperoxidase

Myeloperoxidase activity in sputum sol phase is measured by chromogenic substrate assay relative to a preparation of lysed neutrophils (*see* **Note 20**).

1. Add 10 μL standard or sample to the wells of a microtiter plate (*see* **Note 21**).
2. Add 150 μL 1 mg/mL (w/v) O-dianisidine dihydrochloride, 0.01% (v/v) 30% H_2O_2 in 50 mM K_2HPO_4 and 0.5% (w/v) hexadecyl trimethyl ammonium bromide (pH 6).
3. Incubate the plate for 15 min at 25°C.
4. Measure the absorbance at 450 nm.
5. Obtain the myeloperoxidase concentration by interpolation from the standard curve and express as arbitrary units/mL or absolute amounts if a commercially available pure standard is used.

4. Notes

1. Materials stored at room temperature unless otherwise indicated.
2. Pipet sol phase into approx 5 aliquots into cryovials (this avoids repeat freeze thaw cycles).
3. Coefficient of variation (%) = standard deviation/mean *100. Aim for intra-assay coefficient of variation <10%.
4. The aim is to provide a working range for the assay using dilutions that have an intra-assay coefficient of variation <10% and providing similar concentrations (error <10%) after correction for dilution within the working range of the assay (coefficient of variation <10%).
5. Use assays that give results after spiking close to the standard curve (aim for ⊕ 85% recovery) *(6)*.
6. 10^{-9} to 10^{-6} M usually spans the range of active neutrophil elastase found in sputum sol.
7. The standards range from 0.8 nM to 0.1 μM. Sample dilutions vary from pure sample to 1 in 100. The lower limit of detection of the assay is 0.8 nM and the interassay coefficient of variation is less than 1%.
8. To determine the contribution of secretory leukoprotease inhibitor (SLPI), repeat the assay using 1 μM porcine pancreatic elastase (Type 4, Sigma) (SLPI inhibits neutrophil elastase but not porcine pancreatic elastase and, therefore, the difference in activity reflects the contribution by SLPI).
9. Elastase inhibitory capacity = (10/ χ intercept) × elastase concentration.
10. Fast as opposed to silver staining is quicker but is less sensitive (50 ng protein/ mm^2 vs 1 ng/mm^2 of gel).

11. Ensure thorough washes at each stage to remove background staining.
12. The standards range from 0.001 to 1.08 nM. Sample dilutions vary from 1 in 500 to 1 in 100,000. The lower limit of detection of the assay is 1.68 nM and the inter-assay coefficient of variation is less than 10%.
13. Use sterile needle to remove punch inserts.
14. For all the chemotaxis assays described, reverse pipette to avoid bubbles.
15. Add RPMI, then the chemoattractant/sputum sol phase, and finally the neutro-phils to avoid diffusion of the chemoattractant prior to the start of the assay.
16. To ensure thorough cleaning use a toothbrush.
17. To assess chemotaxis, dilute 1 in 6 for mucopurulent and purulent samples and 1 in 8 for mucoid sputum *(7)*.
18. Reverse pipet with tip, very gently touching the membrane without piercing it. If higher then there is a tendency for air bubbles that will interfere with the chemo-taxis assay.
19. For IL-8, the standards range from 0.004 to 0.25 n*M*. Sample dilutions vary from 1 in 20 to 1 in 500. The lower limit of detection of the assay is 0.008 n*M*, the interassay coefficient of variation is less than 10%, and samples spiked with pure sample result in greater than 85% recovery.
20. Studies have shown that the myeloperoxidase ELISA using the commercial immune assay (R&D systems, Abingdon, UK) gives poor recovery in "spiking" experiments using sputum sol, and is dependent on the degree of sample dilution and elastase content *(6)*. The chromogenic assay, on the other hand, gives good recovery in spiking experiments and is therefore described herein.
21. The standards range from 0.0976 to 50 U/mL. Sample dilutions vary from 1 in 5 to 1 in 500. The lower limit of detection of the assay is 0.1 U/mL and the interassay coefficient of variation is less than 10%.

References

1. Campbell, E. J., Silverman, E. K., and Campbell, M. A. (1989) Elastase and Cathepsin G of human monocytes. *J. Immunol.* **143,** 2961–2968.
2. Baugh, R. J. and Travis, J. (1976) Human leukocyte granule elastase: rapid isolation and characterization. *Biochem.* **15,** 836–841.
3. Nakajima, K., Powers, J. C., Ashe, B. M., and Zimmerman, M. (1979) Mapping the extended substrate binding site of cathepsin G and human leukocyte elastase. Studies with peptide substrates related to the alpha 1-protease inhibitor reactive site. *J. Biol. Chem.* **254,** 4027–4032.
4. Afford, S. C., Burnett, D., Campbell, E. J., Cury, J. D., and Stockley, R. A. (1988) The assessment of α-1-proteinase inhibitor form and function in lung lavage fluid from healthy subjects. *Biol. Chem. Hoppe-Seyler.* **369,** 1065–1074.
5. Mackarel, A. J., Cottell, D. C., Russell, K. J., Fitzgerald, M. X., and O'Connor, C. M. (1999) Migration of neutrophils across human pulmonary endothelial cells is not blocked by matrix metalloproteinase or serine protease inhibitors. *Am. J. Respir.Cell Mol. Biol.* **20,** 1209–1219.

6. Stockley, R. A. and Bayley, D. (2000) Validation of assays for inflammatory mediators in sputum. *Eur. Respir. J.* **15,** 778–781.
7. Mikami, M., Llewellyn-Jones, C., Bayley, D., Hill, S. L., and Stockley, R. A. (1998) The chemotactic activity of sputum from patients with bronchiectasis. *Am. J. Respir. Crit. Care Med.* **157,** 723–728.

25

Flow Cytometry

Measurement of Leukocyte Receptor Expression and Function

Adele Hartnell

1. Introduction

Flow cytometry is an invaluable tool for the analysis of leukocyte populations in inflammation. Flow cytometers, particularly those designed purely for analysis rather than cell sorting, have now become user-friendly machines and are commonplace in many laboratories. Any cell type can be analyzed, as long as a single-cell suspension can be prepared, and small numbers of cells can be used, often without the need for purification, thus making measurements rapid and less susceptible to artifacts associated with lengthy cell separation procedures.

Once introduced into the flow cytometer, cells are accelerated past a beam of light one at a time. At least four parameters can be measured for each cell by means of separate light detectors, two for reflected light and two or more for emitted fluorescent light of different wavelengths. Light scattered by cells at small angles to the incident beam (forward scatter, FSC) and at 90° to the incident beam (side scatter, SSC) is proportional to their size and granularity, respectively. Therefore, a two-dimensional plot of FSC vs SSC is distinctive for different cell types, and lymphocytes, monocytes, and neutrophils can be distinguished from each other on this basis. However, eosinophils and neutrophils have overlapping FSC vs SSC profiles, as do large lymphocytes, basophils, and small monocytes. Therefore, in many cases individual leukocyte types in a mixed cell population, such whole blood, mixed mononuclear cells or granulocytes, or bronchoalveolar lavage (BAL) fluid, have to be distinguished by specific surface markers. For T cells this is usually CD3, CD4, or

From: *Methods in Molecular Medicine, vol. 56:*
Human Airway Inflammation: Sampling Techniques and Analytical Protocols
Edited by: D. F. Rogers and L. E. Donnelly © Humana Press Inc., Totowa, NJ

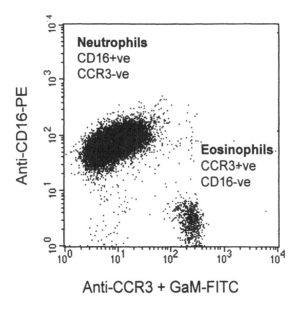

Anti-CCR3 + GaM-FITC

Fig. 1. Immunostaining of mixed granulocytes (eosinophils and neutrophils), separated from peripheral blood, for CC chemokine receptor 3 (CCR3) expression. Cells were stained with an anti-CCR3 mAb (7B11) followed by FITC-conjugated F(ab')$_2$ goat antimouse Ig and then PE-conjugated anti-CD16 to distinguish the neutrophils from the eosinophils. The CD16-ve eosinophils express high levels of CCR3, whereas the CD16+ve neutrophils do not express this chemokine receptor (7).

CD8. Monocytes are generally identified as CD14 positive cells. Where neutrophils and eosinophils have to be distinguished from each other, the neutrophils can be stained with anti-CD16 (*see* **Fig. 1**) (*1*) or the eosinophils with anti-CD9 or anti-VLA-4 (CD49d). As more monoclonal antibodies to surface receptors and fluorescent dyes become available the number of possible applications continues to increase.

The most common application of flow cytometry is to analyze immunofluorescence staining of cells for surface receptor expression. T-cell subset analysis has progressed from simple CD4 and CD8 ratios to defining states of activation (*2*), memory T cells (*3*), and Th1 and Th2 subsets. Leukocytes can be examined for markers of activation or phenotypic changes associated with migration into sites of inflammation, such as the lung (*4*). The expression patterns of chemokine receptors, adhesion molecules, and Fc receptors are particularly relevant to the processes of leukocyte transendothelial migration and then activation in the tissues. A comparison of leukocytes in the blood and those recovered from the lungs by BAL provides valuable information in inflammatory diseases, revealing selective recruitment of subpopulations of leukocytes or activation of cells in the lung.

As well as surface receptor expression, flow cytometry can be used with fluorescent dyes or particles to study many functional responses of phagocytes, including calcium flux, adhesion, phagocytosis, and respiratory burst. Intracellular cytokines can also be measured in combination with cell surface markers to dissect functional characteristics of T cells.

Herein, a detailed method for immunofluorescence staining is described, with protocols for single staining, as well as for staining with combinations of two or three antibodies. These protocols can be applied to any cells in suspension. In addition, a flow cytometric assay of respiratory burst activity is outlined.

2. Materials

2.1. Reagents for Immunofluorescence Staining of Cell Surface Receptors

2.1.1. Direct Immunofluorescence

All reagents are from Sigma-Aldrich (Poole, Dorset, UK), unless otherwise stated.

1. Phosphate buffered saline (PBS), pH 7.2-7.4: make 10X stock solution (68g NaCl, 14.5g Na_2HPO_4, 4.3g KH_2PO_4, for 1liter) or use commercial tablets.
2. Bovine serum albumin (BSA) fraction V, pH-adjusted to 7 (cat. no. A2153).
3. Sodium azide (NaN_3): 10% (w/v) stock solution in H_2O. **Caution**: under aqueous acidic conditions sodium azide yields hydrazoic acid, an extremely toxic compound, and should be flushed with large volumes of water during disposal.
4. Staining buffer: PBS with 0.5% (w/v) BSA and 0.1% (w/v) NaN_3 (PAB); 100 mL 10X PBS + 10 mL 10% (w/v) NaN_3 + 890 mL H_2O + 0.5g BSA, filtered (e.g., using a 0.45 µM bottle-top filter) and stored at 4°C.
5. Final wash buffer: PBS with 0.1% (w/v) NaN_3; 100 mL 10X PBS + 10 mL 10% (w/v) NaN_3 + 890 mL H_2O, filtered and stored at 4°C.
6. Paraformaldehyde (PFA) (optional): 1% (w/v) in PBS; heat 80 mL H_2O to 60°C in a fume hood, then add 1g PFA. When completely dissolved, cool and add 10 mL 10X PBS, adjust volume to 100 mL with H_2O, check pH and filter. Best used freshly prepared, but can be stored in aliquots at –20°C. Alternatively, use a commercial fixative, e.g., CellFIX (Becton Dickinson, San Jose, CA). **Caution**: PFA is toxic and inhalation, ingestion, and contact with skin, eyes, and clothing should be avoided.
7. Propidium iodide (optional): 100 µg/mL stock solution in PBS. Store at 4°C in the dark. **Caution**: propidium iodide is a potential carcinogen and should be handled with care.
8. Fluorochrome-conjugated primary monoclonal antibodies (mAbs) and isotype-matched control antibodies, preferably from the same supplier.
9. 5 mL (12×75 mm) Falcon polystyrene tubes (Becton Dickinson, cat. no. 352052)
10. Refrigerated centrifuge with carriers for 12×75 mm tubes.

2.1.2. Indirect Immunofluorescence

All reagents as for direct immunofluorescence, except for the antibodies.

1. Unconjugated or biotinylated primary antibody (mAb or polyclonal antibody).
2. Isotype-matched control antibody (e.g., mouse myeloma proteins, MOPC 21/ IgG1 or UPC 10/IgG2a, from Sigma-Aldrich).
3. Fluorochrome-conjugated secondary antibody (e.g., FITC-conjugated F(ab')$_2$ goat anti-mouse Ig, Dako, Cambridge, UK) or streptavidin.
4. Mouse IgG.

2.2. Reagents for Respiratory Burst Assay

1. Assay buffer: PBS containing Ca^{2+} and Mg^{2+} with 10 mM HEPES, 10 mM glucose and 0.1% (w/v) BSA, pH 7.2–7.4.
2. Dihydrorhodamine 123 (DHR 123) (Molecular Probes, Eugene, OR or Sigma-Aldrich) dissolved in dimethyl sulfoxide (DMSO) at 1 mM, aliquoted and stored at –20°C. Aliquots can be thawed and refrozen several times.
3. 1.2 mL polypropylene cluster tubes (Costar, Cambridge, MA)
4. Water bath at 37°C

3. Methods

3.1. Immunofluorescence Staining of Cell Surface Receptors

3.1.1. Direct Immunofluorescence

Immunostaining of cells is very quick and simple when directly-conjugated mAbs are used. Two or more mAbs, conjugated to different fluorochromes, can be added to the cells simultaneously to detect multiple surface antigens.

1. Place the required number of 5-mL Falcon tubes on ice (*see* **Note 1**) and dilute primary, conjugated mAbs or control antibodies in PAB to give a total volume of 50 μL per tube (*see* **Note 2**).
2. Resuspend cells at 4×10^6/mL to 2×10^7/mL in ice-cold PAB (*see* **Note 3**).
3. Add 50 μL cell suspension to each tube (2×10^5 to 10^6 cells), mix gently but thoroughly and incubate on ice for 20–30 min, preferably in the dark.
4. Add 3 mL cold PBS/0.1% (w/v) NaN$_3$ to each tube and centrifuge at 300g for 5 min at 4°C (*see* **Note 4**).
5. Tip off the wash buffer and blot any remaining at the top of the inverted tube on absorbent paper (*see* **Note 5**).
6. Loosen the cell pellet by flicking the tube and wash once more (i.e., repeat **steps 4** and **5**).
7. Loosen the cells thoroughly, add 200 μL–1 mL ice-cold fixative (to give 10^6 cells/mL) and mix immediately to ensure the cells are dispersed in the fixative and not clumped together. Maintain at 4°C in the dark until the cells can be analyzed on a flow cytometer (*see* **Note 6**).
8. If a significant number of cells are likely to be dead or apoptotic (*see* **Note 7**), instead of fixing the cells after the final wash, resuspend in 200 μL–1 mL PBS/

0.1% (w/v) NaN$_3$, add propidium iodide (*see* **Note 8**) at 5 μg/mL final concentration (5 μL of 100 μg/mL stock solution per tube) and analyze, without washing, after incubating for 5 min (see **Note 9**).

3.1.2. Indirect Immunofluorescence

3.1.2.1. STAINING WITH A SINGLE ANTIBODY/FLUOROCHROME

When directly conjugated antibodies are not available a fluorochrome-conjugated secondary antibody is required to detect binding of the primary antibody. This two-layer method can also be used to amplify the signal if staining with a directly conjugated antibody is weak. If a biotinylated primary antibody is available, fluorochrome-conjugated streptavidin can be used as the secondary reagent and may give lower nonspecific staining than a secondary antibody.

1. Place the required number of 5-mL Falcon tubes on ice (*see* **Note 1**) and dilute the primary antibodies or control antibodies in PAB to give a total volume of 50 μL (*see* **Note 10**).
2. Resuspend cells at 4×10^6/mL to 2×10^7/mL in ice-cold PAB (*see* **Note 3**).
3. Add 50 μL cell suspension to each tube (2×10^5 to 10^6 cells), mix gently but thoroughly and incubate on ice for 20–30 min.
4. Add 3 mL cold PAB to each tube and centrifuge at 300g for 5 min at 4°C (*see* **Note 4**).
5. Tip off the wash buffer and blot any remaining at the top of the inverted tube on absorbent paper (*see* **Note 5**).
6. Add an appropriate, conjugated secondary antibody (e.g., goat antimouse Ig for mouse mAbs or swine antirabbit Ig for rabbit polyclonals) or conjugated streptavidin, to each tube at the predetermined optimal concentration (*see* **Note 11**).
7. Mix gently but thoroughly and incubate on ice for 20–30 min, preferably in the dark.
8. Add 3 mL cold PBS/0.1% (w/v) NaN$_3$ to each tube and centrifuge at 300g for 5 min at 4°C.
9. Tip off the wash buffer as before and loosen the cell pellet.
10. Resuspend the cells thoroughly in 200 μL–1 mL ice-cold fixative (to give 10^6 cells/mL) and maintain at 4°C in the dark until the cells can be analyzed on a flow cytometer (*see* **Note 6**), or in 200 mL–1 mL PBS/0.1% (w/v) NaN$_3$ + 5μL propidium iodide (100 μg/mL stock solution) and analyze after incubating for 5 min (*see* **Notes 7, 8** and **9**).

3.1.2.2. STAINING WITH TWO OR MORE ANTIBODIES/FLUOROCHROMES

Cells can be stained with two unconjugated antibodies simultaneously without modifying the above procedure, if:

1. The primary antibodies are of different isotypes and isotype-specific secondary antibodies can be employed. However, some crossreactivity may occur and the specificity of the secondary antibodies should be verified with appropriate controls.

2. The primary antibodies were raised in different species and species-specific secondary antibodies can be used, although possible crossreactivity between species may be problematic and should also be tested.

Staining with two antibodies of the same species and isotype is possible if one is directly conjugated or biotinylated, and staining with three antibodies is possible if two are conjugated or one is conjugated and one biotinylated, as follows:

1. Perform indirect staining as above with secondary antibody but use PAB for the second wash (*see* **Subheading 3.1.2.1., step 8**).
2. Next, add mouse IgG (if the mAbs are murine) at 50 μg/mL, to saturate free-binding sites on the goat antimouse Ig.
3. After 10 min on ice, incubate with the directly conjugated mAb(s), or conjugated mAb plus biotinylated mAb for 20–30 min and then conjugated-streptavidin after washing once.
4. Wash with PBS/0.1% NaN₃ and resuspend in fixative or PBS/0.1% (w/v) NaN₃ plus propidium iodide and analyze.

3.2. Respiratory Burst Assay

A convenient assay for measuring respiratory burst activity of cells can be performed by flow cytometry using dihydrorhodamine 123(DHR 123), a nonfluorescent molecule that is converted to fluorescent rhodamine 123 when oxidized by hydrogen peroxide (H_2O_2). This assay uses few cells, which do not have to be pure because the relevant population can be selected on the basis of FSC vs SSC or by staining for a phenotypic marker using an antibody conjugated to phycoerythrin (PE), such as anti-CD16-PE to distinguish neutrophils from eosinophils. Only cell-associated, rather than released, H_2O_2 is measured, so the results obtained may not be directly comparable to more conventional methods used to quantify respiratory burst. However, this assay is simple and allows respiratory burst activity to be measured in mixed cell populations.

1. Dilute DHR 123 to 2 nM in assay buffer (*see* **Note 12**).
2. Prepare agonists at 2X concentration and add 50 μL to 1.2 mL polypropylene tubes (*see* **Note 13**).
3. Resuspend cells in assay buffer at 2×10^7/mL, mix an equal volume of cells and DHR 123 (e.g., 1 mL each for 40 tubes) and incubate at 37°C for 5 min.
4. Add 50 μL labeled cell suspension to each tube containing agonist and incubate at 37°C for 15–30 min (*see* **Note 14**).
5. To stop the reaction, put the tubes in an ice-water bath and add 100 μL cold PBS (*see* **Note 15**).
6. Insert the 1.2 mL tubes into 5 mL Falcon tubes to read the samples on the flow cytometer and measure the DHR 123 fluorescence intensity on FL1 (530 nm) (*see* **Fig. 2**).

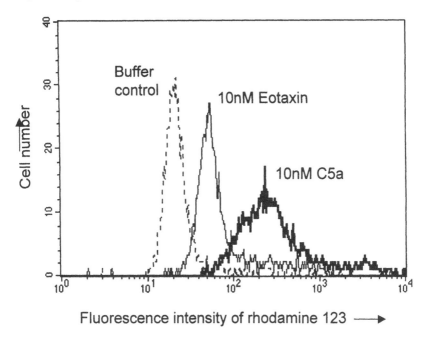

Fig. 2. Relative fluorescence intensity of DHR 123, as an indication of respiratory burst activity, of purified eosinophils. Cells were labeled with DHR 123 and stimulated for 30 min at 37°C with buffer, 10 nM eotaxin or 10 nM C5a. The increase in fluorescence intensity following stimulation with eotaxin or C5a is proportional to the production of H_2O_2 by the cells.

4. Notes

1. Immunonstaining of cells should be performed at 4°C throughout, including centrifugation, in the presence of sodium azide, to minimize the possibility of receptor internalization or shedding.
2. Up to four mAbs conjugated to different fluorochromes may be added simultaneously, depending on the number of fluorescence detectors available on the flow cytometer. Many mAbs can be used at a lower concentration than that recommended by the supplier. Each mAb should be titrated to establish the lowest saturating concentration. For each mAb, the same concentration of an isotype-matched control antibody of irrelevant specificity, conjugated to the same fluorochrome as the test antibody, should be added to a separate aliquot of cells to determine the nonspecific staining.
3. Cultured cell lines, isolated leukocytes or BAL cells are generally washed once before staining. If cells are stimulated in vitro prior to staining, this can be performed with the cells at 4×10^6/mL to 2×10^7/mL in an appropriate buffer (e.g., PBS or RPMI containing up to 0.5% (w/v) BSA or 5–10% (w/v) FCS) and the cells then cooled rapidly and used directly, without washing.

4. A cell pellet may be barely visible on the bottom of the tube after centrifugation.
5. Approximately 100 μL buffer will remain when the tubes are placed upright, but this volume will be consistent between tubes.
6. Cells fixed in PFA should be stable for 24 h or longer, but some cell types may exhibit altered characteristics more rapidly than others. For example, the autofluorescence of eosinophils can increase significantly within 24 h. Therefore, only fix cells if it is not possible to perform flow cytometric analysis within a few hours of staining.
7. Certain samples, for example BAL cells, may contain a number of dead or apoptotic cells and some cell death may occur during the staining procedure. Dead cells bind antibodies and fluorochromes nonspecifically and produce false positive results or an increase in the apparent background, and so it is essential to exclude them from the analysis.
8. Dead cells sometimes exhibit a decrease in FSC, appearing as a separate population, and can be excluded on this basis. However, this is not always the case and it is preferable to use a fluorescent dye, such as propidium iodide, which enters cells that do not have an intact plasma membrane and binds to nucleic acid, to identify dead cells. Propidium iodide can be used together with FITC, or FITC and PE if the flow cytometer has a third detector for red fluorescence. If the flow cytometer being used has a second laser and a fourth detector for red fluorescence, dead cells can be identified using dyes such as TO-PRO-3 (Molecular Probes), which is used in a similar way to propidium iodide and has the advantage of being nontoxic.
9. Data are usually collected for up to 10,000 cells of interest, depending on their frequency in the sample. Cell populations are defined by gating on FSC and SSC parameters and dead cells excluded by gating out propidium iodide positive cell (measured on FL2 or FL3). In T-cell analysis, it is common for antibodies to surface markers to define subsets of cells and therefore a bimodal fluorescence distribution is seen. In this case the results are expressed as percent positive cells, at the 99% or 95% confidence level, that is relative to a marker positioned to include 1% or 5% of the brightest cells stained with control antibody. If the separation between positive and negative populations is not good or if they overlap, the percent positive cells may not be an absolute number but will depend on the staining reagents, procedure, and flow cytometer used. For other leukocytes types, it is more common for surface receptors to be expressed in an all-or-nothing fashion, with a range of receptor expression seen for a positive cell population. Thus, where the fluorescence distribution is unimodal, even if it overlaps with the control sample, it is more appropriate to express the results as mean fluorescence intensity (with control antibody fluorescence subtracted), rather than percent positive cells. Again the fluorescence intensity will be dependent on the reagents used and the flow cytometer and comparisons between samples analyzed at different times requires the staining protocol to be standardized and the flow cytometer to be set up similarly each time *(5)*.

10. Monoclonal antibodies are generally used at concentrations in the region of 10 μg/mL and polyclonal antibodies at 1 μg/mL, but each antibody should be titrated to determine a saturating concentration that gives negligible nonspecific staining. Nonspecific binding of mAbs to the low affinity Fc receptors, FcγRII (CD32), and FcγRIII (CD16) is usually minimal, but is greater to the high affinity receptor, FcγRI (CD64), expressed by monocytes and macrophages, particularly for mouse mAbs of the IgG2a isotype. To prevent nonspecific binding of mAbs to Fc receptors incubate cells with human IgG at 10 μg/mL for 10 min prior to incubation with mAbs.

11. Nonspecific binding of secondary, fluorochrome-conjugated, polyclonal antibodies can be minimized by using $F(ab')_2$ fragments. Each antibody should be titrated to establish the amount that will give the maximum signal with the minimum background. To titrate a secondary antibody, incubate a number of cell samples with a fixed concentration of primary mAb or control antibody, followed by a range of dilutions of the secondary, and choose the concentration that gives a maximal signal with the positive antibody but negligible background with the control antibody. It is important to titrate secondary antibodies, as suppliers normally suggest a range of dilutions, and the same dilution may not be optimal for every application. Minimizing background fluorescence is very important for obtaining the best results.

12. The optimal final concentration of DHR 123 for measuring eosinophil respiratory burst was found to be 1 n*M*, which is a modification of the published method for neutrophils in which 1 μ*M* DHR 123 was used *(6)*. The use of 1 n*M* DHR 123 appears to give similar results, but with lower background fluorescence.

13. The 1.2 mL polypropylene tubes enable smaller volumes to be used and do not adsorb agonists that bind well to polystyrene tubes.

14. Unlike other assays for respiratory burst, the reaction product is cumulative rather than transient, so a single end-point measurement can be made to indicate the magnitude of the response, but no kinetic data are obtained.

15. To distinguish neutrophils from eosinophils in mixed granulocytes, 1–2 μL anti-CD16-PE (Dako) can be added to each tube before the cold PBS (300 μL rather than 100 μL), which is then added after incubating on ice for 10 min, and the samples analyzed without washing.

References

1. Hartnell, A., Moqbel, R., Walsh, G.M., Bradley B., and Kay, A.B. (1990) Fcγ and CD11/CD18 receptor expression on normal density and low density human eosinophils. *Immunology* **69,** 264–270.
2. Corrigan, C.J., Hartnell A., and Kay, A.B. (1988) T lymphocyte activation in acute severe asthma. *Lancet* **i,** 1129–1132
3. Robinson, D.S., Bentley, A.M., Hartnell, A., Kay, A.B., and Durham, S.R. (1993) Activated memory T helper cells in bronchoalveoler lavage fluid from patients with atopic asthma—relation to asthma symptoms, lung function and bronchial responsiveness. *Thorax* **48,** 26–32

4. Hartnell, A., Robinson, D.S., Kay, A.B., and Wardlaw, A.J. (1993) CD69 is expressed by human eosinophils activated in vivo in asthma and in vitro by cytokines. *Immunology* **80,** 281–286

5. Parks, D.R., Lanier, L.L., and Herzenberg, L.A. (1986) Flow cytometry and fluorescence activated cell sorting (FACS). In *Handbook of Experimental Immunology, 4th ed.* vol 1,Weir, D.M., ed. Blackwell Scientific Publications, Oxford, UK, p 29.1–29.21.

6. Emmendorffer, A., Hecht, M., Lohman-Matthes, M.-L., and Roesler, J. (1990) A fast and easy method to determine the production of reactive oxygen intermediates by human and murine phagocytes using dihydrorhodamine 123. *J. Immunol. Methods* **131,** 269–75. [Addendum: *J. Immunol. Methods* **138**:133–135]

7. Sabroe, I., Hartnell, A., Jopling, L.A., Bel, S. Ponath,, P.D., Pease, J.E., Collins P.D., and Williams T.J. (1999) Differential regulation of eosinophil chemokine signalling via CCR3 and non-CCR3 pathways. *J. Immunol.* **162,** 2946–2955.

26

Measurement of Granulocyte Pharmacodynamics in Whole Blood by Flow Cytometry

Shannon A. Bryan, Margaret J. Leckie, Gavin Jenkins, Peter J. Barnes, Timothy J. Williams, Ian Sabroe, and Trevor T. Hansel

1. Introduction

During the Phase I/II assessment of new therapies with the potential to suppress eosinophil and neutrophil inflammation, there is a need to assess the peripheral blood pharmacokinetic (PK) and pharmacodynamic (PD) profiles of the drug. This has relevance in respiratory disease since drugs that target eosinophillic inflammation are in development for asthma; whereas neutrophil-directed therapies are being introduced for treatment of chronic obstructive airways disease (COPD). Pharmacokinetic evaluation is required to determine the concentration of drug substance (and possibly metabolites) in peripheral blood at intervals following single or repeated dosing. Pharmacodynamic assessment is also required since many drug substances have a duration of action which is prolonged beyond the time when drug substance is detectable in the blood (*see* **Fig. 1**).

1.1. Whole Blood Gated Autofluorescence Forward Scatter (GAFS) Assay

Granulocytes are recruited into the tissue from the circulation in response to mediators, including chemoattractant cytokines ("chemokines"). Rearrangement of the cell cytoskeleton is a fundamental component of the mechanisms involved in the migration of leukocytes along concentration gradients of chemokines, and is dependent upon polymerization of cytoplasmic monomeric actin (G-actin) to microfilamentous actin (F-actin) *(1)*. Along with other

From: *Methods in Molecular Medicine, vol. 56:*
Human Airway Inflammation: Sampling Techniques and Analytical Protocols
Edited by: D. F. Rogers and L. E. Donnelly © Humana Press Inc., Totowa, NJ

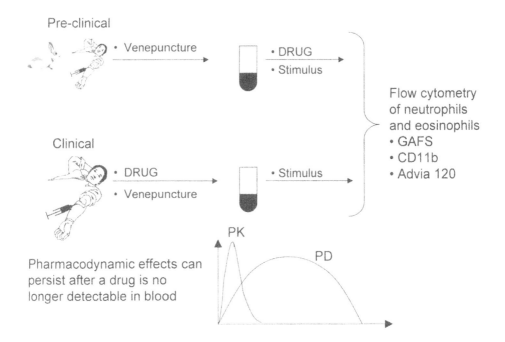

Fig. 1. Whole blood pharmacodynamics. In preclinical studies, animal or human blood is treated with test agents. In clinical studies, human subjects are treated with drug and blood removed for analysis. GAFS, gated autofluorescence forward scatter; PK, pharmacokinetics; PD, pharmacoldynamics.

changes in the cell, this reorganization allows cells to adhere to and migrate through blood vessel walls as well as to infiltrate the tissues where inflammation occurs (2). Shape change can be induced by chemokines such as eotaxin in eosinophils, as well as by nonchemokine mediators such as C5a in neutrophils and eosinophils (3). Chemokines bind to 7-transmembrane, G-protein coupled receptors on the cell membrane which can stimulate multiple signaling pathways including activation of phospholipase C (PLC), intracellular calcium (Ca^{2+}) flux, mitogen activated protein kinase (MAPK) and phosphatidyl inositol-3 kinase (PI_3K). Using a flow cytometer, the shape of cells can be evaluated before and after stimulation, by measuring the forward scatter of light generated when the cell is passed through a laser beam. This principle has been established in the GAFS assay using mixed granulocytes (3) and the method has been adapted for use in whole blood.

1.2. CD11b Measurement in Whole Blood

CD11b forms the α-chain of dimeric complement receptor 3 (CR3) and is commonly associated with CD18 (CD11b/CD18 or Mac-1). CR3 mediates the phagocytosis of opsonized particles, but also has an important role in leukocyte recruitment to sites of infection and inflammation. After an initial rolling adhesion phase through the interaction of selectin molecules with their counter-ligands, chemokines induce leukocytes to upregulate adhesion molecule avidity and expression, mediating firm arrest of the leukocyte on the endothelium prior to diapedesis into the tissues. CD11b is stored in cytoplasmic granules and can be rapidly upregulated upon activation by inflammatory mediators *(4)*. McCarthy and Macey *(5)* have developed a method of measuring CD11b by flow cytometry using whole blood. This is preferable to performing markers on isolated cells since CD11b surface expression can be upregulated ex vivo by merely cooling and warming *(6)*, centrifugation and fixation. The binding of certain anti-CD11b monoclonal antibodies to CD11b antigen is calcium-dependent *(7)*, and binding may be reduced in the presence of the anticoagulant ethylenediaminetetraacetic acid (EDTA) that chelates calcium and divalent cations. Efforts have been made to use an anticoagulant that does not effect monoclonal antibody binding to cell-surface epitopes, and leupeptin is an enzyme inhibitor that inhibits early steps in the coagulation cascade *(8,9)*. Ex vivo upregulation of CD11b by chemokines may be affected by the anticoagulant through mechanisms such as antibody binding as described above. However, upregulation of CD11b on leukocytes in response to chemokines has been described in blood anticoagulated with EDTA *(10)*. The dye LDS-751 can be used to discriminate nucleated leukocytes from red blood cells and platelets by their DNA content *(11)*. LDS-751 stains DNA and is excited at 488 nm and emits at >640 nm; this is detected in the far-red fluorescence channel leaving the first two channels of a Becton Dickinson FACScan flow cytometer available for detection of fluorescein isothiocyanate (FITC) and phycoerythrin (PE) labeled antibodies. This technique enables direct ex vivo measurement of leukocyte surface antigens with minimal modulation of the expression and antigenicity of the marker of interest. We recommend that preliminary experiments should be performed with particular anti-CD11b monoclonal antibodies binding to particular cell types, using different anticoagulants, in relation to defined ex vivo stimulation conditions. In this chapter we describe anticoagulation of blood with the enzyme inhibitor leupetin hemisulfate, stimulation of whole blood with n-formyl-methionyl-leucyl-phenyialanine (fMLP), and use of monoclonal antibodies (MoAbs) against CD11b (FITC) and CD16 (PE) in conjunction with LDS-751 to differentiate eosinophils and neutrophils.

1.3. Advia 120 for Granulocyte Pharmacodynamic Assays

The Advia 120 (Bayer) hematology analyzer counts leukocytes on the basis of peroxidase staining and a flow cytometric procedure to measure absorption and scatter of light by individual cells. A leukocyte peroxidase dot-plot is produced with light absorption and scatter plotted on the *x*- and *y*-axes, respectively. This

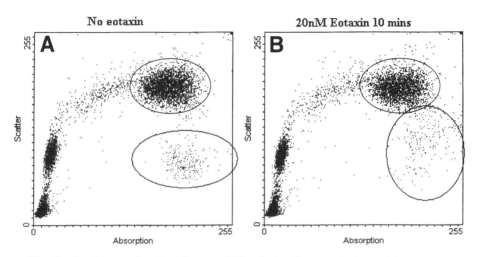

Fig. 2. Leukocyte dotplot of normal blood. **A**. Characteristic position of neutrophils (upper "cloud") and eosinophils (lower cloud) prior to stimulation using Advia 120. **B**. Effect of stimulation with eotaxin 20 n*M* for 10 min using Advia 120.

is routinely used to determine the total and differential leukocyte count in anticoagulated blood. The position of the neutrophil cluster is determined automatically by gating using the Advia software. We have adapted this analyzer by using the WinMDI flow cytometry computer software package to gate the eosinophil population. This enables analysis of both absorption (*x*-axis) and scatter (*y*-axis) coordinates of eosinophils on the peroxidase dot plot. (*see* **Fig. 2**). Neutrophil and eosinophil activation is measured in terms of light absorption and scatter, which reflect granularity and morphology, respectively. This automated whole blood method requires minimal sample processing, and results are available within minutes of sample acquisition. This method can be applied to preclinical samples since software packages are available for most mammalian species including rats, rabbits, and monkeys. The analyzer is calibrated daily for neutrophil light absorption and scatter using Testpoint calibrant (Bayer). The neutrophil and eosinophil-specific chemokines interleukin-8 (IL-8) and eotaxin, respectively, have been added in an in vitro assay to determine the effects of these stimulants on neutrophil and eosinophil size, shape, and granularity. Shape changes in neutrophils can be produced following stimulation with IL-8 (*see* **Fig. 3B**), and in eosinophils (*see* **Figs. 2B** and **3A**) following stimulation with eotaxin.

2. Materials
2.1. Whole Blood GAFS Assay

1. Assay buffer: 10 m*M* HEPES (Life Technologies, Paisley, UK), 10 m*M* glucose (Sigma, Poole, UK), 0.1% BSA (Sigma) in 10 m*M* phosphate buffered saline containing calcium and magnesium pH 7.2 – 7.4 (Life Technologies,).

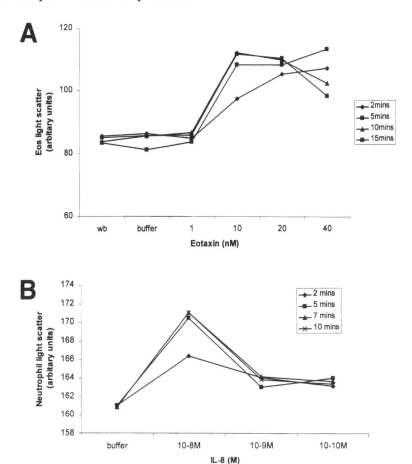

Fig. 3. Effect of chemokines on leukocytes. **A**. Concentration-response to eotaxin on eosinophil light scatter at different time points, using Advia 120. **B**. Concentration-response to IL-8 on neutrophil light scatter at different time points, using Advia 120.

2. Ammonium chloride lysis solution: Make up 10x stock solution prior to the day of the experiment and keep at 4°C: 8.29 g NH_4Cl, 1.001 g $KHCO_3$ in 100 mL sterile water (Sigma,). On the day of the assay, make up a 1X solution (1 part stock solution + 9 parts sterile water). Keep on ice.

3. Optimized fixative: 1X Cellfix in water (Becton Dickinson, Mountain View, CA), made up to a 1 in 4 dilution with ice-cold Facsflow (Becton Dickinson). Keep on ice.

4. Agonists: The freeze-dried chemokine (PeproTech, London, UK) should be reconstituted in PBS and stored in aliquots at –20°C at high concentrations (e.g., 10^{-5} M) before being made up to appropriate concentrations on the day of the assay. Chemokine dilutions are reconstituted in assay buffer (final concentration 0 – 40 n*M*) and kept on ice. The dilutions should not be prepared more than 4 hours prior to the assay.

5. Polypropylene 1.2 mL cluster tubes (Costar, Cambridge, MA).
6. Polystyrene round bottom flow cytometry tubes (Becton Dickinson Labware, Franklin Lakes, NJ).
7. Water bath at 37°C.
8. Flow cytometer (Becton Dickinson), acquisition and analysis software—Cell Quest or WinMDI.

2.2. CD11b Measurement in Whole Blood

1. Antibodies: CD11b (FITC) conjugate (Serotec), CD16 phycoerythrin (PE) conjugate, mouse-antihuman (DAKO, Denmark). Store at 4°C in the dark.
2. LDS-751: far-red fluorescent DNA dye, (2-[4-[4-(dimethylamino)phenyl]-1,3-butadienyl]-3-ethylbenzothiazolium perchlorate) (Molecular Probes, Eugene, Oregon, USA). Dissolve 0.001 g of LDS-751 into 5 mL of methanol for a 0.02% stock solution. Store at 4°C, in the dark.
3. Anticoagulants: Lithium heparin 2 mL Pediatric tube or Leupeptin hemisulfate (Sigma, Poole). Prepare 2mg/mL stock. Store at -20°C. Prepare Eppendorf tubes with 10 μL of Leupeptin stock to which 1μL of whole blood is added (final concentration of 20 μg/mL).
4. Dulbeccos' PBS (Sigma, Poole). Store at 4°C.
5. Polystyrene round bottom flow cytometry tubes (Becton Dickinson Labware)
6. Flow cytometer — Becton Dickinson FACScan. Acquisition and analysis software — Cell Quest or Win MDI.

2.3. Advia 120 for Granulocyte Pharmacodynamic Assays

1. Whole blood in EDTA tube (Vacutainer, UK).
2. Advia 120 (Bayer Diagnostics, Tarrytown, NY) hematology analyzer.
3. Advia 120 software package (Bayer Diagnostics).
4. WinMDI software package (http://facs.scripps.edu/software.html).
5. IL-8 (Sigma) diluted to 10^{-8}M using PBS (Sigma-Aldrich, Irvine, UK).
6. Eotaxin (Peprotech, London, UK) diluted to 0-40 nM using buffer (10 mM HEPES (Life Technologies, Paisley, UK), 10 mM glucose (Sigma), 0.1% BSA (Sigma) in 10 mM phosphate buffered saline containing calcium and magnesium pH 7.2 – 7.4 (Life Technologies).
7. Water bath at 37°C.

3. Methods
3.1. Whole Blood GAFS Assay

1. The following are prepared freshly in advance of blood sampling as above:
   a. ammonium chloride lysis solution (NH_4Cl).
   b. Assay buffer.
   c. Optimized fixative solution.
   d. Agonist concentrations.
2. NH_4Cl is aliquoted into each round bottom polystyrene tube and kept on ice (volume = 5 × volume of blood + fixative).

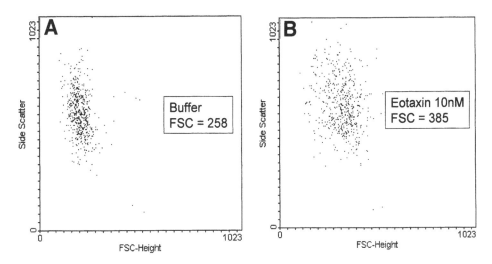

Fig. 4. Flow cytometer dotplot showing FSC in an eosinophil population before (**A**) and after (**B**) stimulation with eotaxin (10 n*M*), using the whole blood GAFS assay.

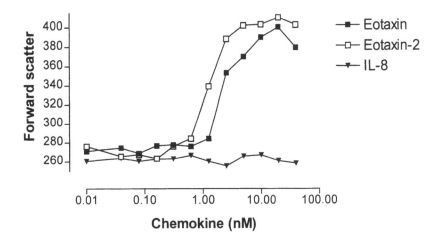

Fig. 5. Typical concentration-response curves showing eosinophil shape change in response to different chemokines using the whole blood GAFS assay.

3. Aliquots of respective doses of agonist or buffer for a dose response curve are placed in each 1.2 mL polypropylene cluster tube.
4. Blood is collected by syringe and anticoagulated using 3.8% trisodium citrate (1 part anticoagulant, 9 parts blood) (*see* **Note 1**).
5. Aliquots of blood (typically 90 µL) are added to agonist or buffer to a final volume of 100 µL. Where the properties of antagonists of cell function are investigated ex-vivo, typically the whole blood is incubated with the antagonist 10 min at room temperature before being added to the agonist and the method continued as below.

6. Mix gently and incubate at 37°C for 4 min in a shaking water bath.
7. On completion of incubation, the tubes are placed directly on ice.
8. 250 µL optimized cold fixative is added quickly to each tube mixed gently and left on ice for 1 min.
9. The samples are then gently individually transferred into the cold NH$_4$Cl in flow cytometer tubes and left on ice in the lysis solution for 20 min to achieve uniform red cell lysis (*see* **Note 2**).
10. Forward scatter data is acquired on a flow cytometer (*see* **Fig. 4**). The eosinophils are identified and differentiated from neutrophils by their higher autofluorescence signal, which is acquired on the FL-2 fluorescent channel. Typically, 500 eosinophils per sample were measured. Depending on the percentage of eosinophils in the sample, acquiring the data took between 20 s and 2 min per sample (*see* **Note 3**).
11. Data analysis is performed using Cell Quest software to calculate mean forward scatter (FSC) values for the neutrophil and eosinophil populations and a dose response curve is generated for each chemokine (*see* **Fig. 5**).

3.2. CD11b Measurement in Whole Blood

1. Blood collection: Collect blood into tubes containing anticoagulant and mix gently. Use precooled (4°C) tubes if a stimulation step is not being performed.
2. If an agonist is being used to induce CD11b upregulation, such as fMLP, it is added to the blood at this stage. Add fMLP to a final concentration of 10^{-8}M and incubate for 10 min at 37°C.
3. After stimulation, add 5µL of each monoclonal antibody to 20µL anticoagulated blood within 20 min of collection. Vortex for no more than 1 s and allow to incubate at 4°C in the dark for 20 min.
4. Dilute the sample by adding 3 mL cold PBS.
5. To the stained blood add 3 µL LDS-751 methanol stock to give a final concentration of 0.0002% LDS-751. Vortex (<1 s) and allow the sample to stand for 2 min.
6. Vortex the sample (<1 s) and acquire data on Becton Dickinson FACScan. Use low flow rate to prevent flow cell clogging. Set-up an "acquisition gate" with side scatter (SSC) against FL3 fluorescence (far-red) to count only LDS-751 positive events (*see* **Notes 4, 5** and **6**).

3.3. Advia 120 for Granulocyte Pharmacodynamic Assays

1. Whole blood (200 µL) is introduced into the analyzer within 30 min of sampling (*see* **Notes 7** and **8**). Following continuous flow analysis of 500–2000 cells per second, the analyzer automatically creates a peroxidase leukogram consisting of a dot plot of individual cells (*12*). Neutrophil cluster position in terms of light absorption and scatter (*x* and *y* axes, respectively) is calculated automatically (*13*).
2. Data from each sample is saved and later played-back using the Advia software package on WinNT.

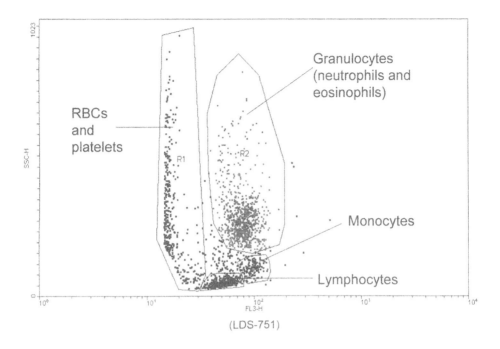

Fig. 6. Identification of leukocyte populations with LDS-751 staining. RBCs, red blood cells.

3. Following playback, WinMDI software is applied to the leukocyte dotplots. Eosinophil populations are gated on the basis of their position, gates being applied around clusters, aiming to include at least 95% of cells in a given gate.
4. In vitro activation of whole blood: 10^{-8}M IL-8 (100 µL), or $10^{-9}M$ eotaxin (100 µL) is added to whole venous blood (900 µL) and incubated at 37°C for 2–10 min. Samples are run through the analyzer after different time intervals. Neutrophil populations are gated automatically by the Advia 120 while eosinophil populations are gated using WinMDI.

4. Notes

1. Always use freshly sampled blood. If the blood is "older" than 30 min, the baseline FSC of the neutrophils and eosinophils is increased. Therefore, ensure that all the buffers and reagents are prepared in advance of blood sampling so that once the sample has been collected, it can be used immediately.
2. While acquiring data on individual samples, keep the remaining samples on ice. This will help to maintain the shape of the cells in the samples not yet analyzed.
3. Since the sample is a whole blood sample, it is impossible to standardize the number of cells per sample. If eosinophils are to be analyzed, acquiring 500 eosinophils may take longer in some samples than others. If the sample takes longer than 2 min to acquire, it is advisable to count fewer eosinophils per sample (for example 250 cells). It is also therefore advised that a smaller sample number

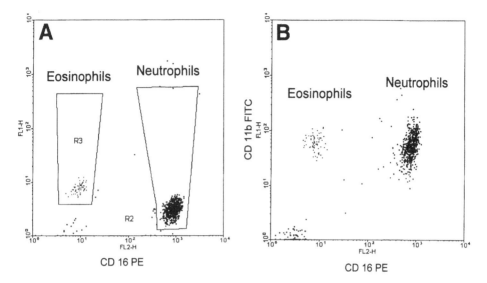

Fig. 7. **A**. LDS +ve granulocytes stained with CD16. Eosinophils (CD16 –ve) and neutrophils (CD16 +ve) in the FL-2 channel. **B**. Granulocytes stained with CD11b and CD16. All R1 events are removed ("NOT" gate logic). Eosinophils (CD16 –ve) and neutrophils (CD16 +ve) both show CD11b staining in FL-1.

    be assayed. These precautions are taken because the cell shape may alter if left for longer than 1 h after the lysis step.

4. Do not acquire data for more than 10 min. After this time the LDS-751 nuclear stain is absorbed by red blood cells and staining is increased in the leukocytes. This pollutes the acquisition gate.

5. Identifying leukocyte populations: **Fig. 6** shows a dotplot gated on LDS-751 positive events only. Along the x-axis is the FL-3 channel, in which LDS-751 staining is visualized most strongly. The y-axis is SSC. This dotplot excludes most of the red blood cells reducing data files to a more manageable size. The red blood cells shown in the R1 region represent the right leading edge of the whole red blood cell population. The main leukocyte populations are clearly positive in the FL-3 channel.

6. Neutrophils and eosinophils can be differentiated by CD16 staining in the FL-2 channel. Neutrophils stain positively for CD16 and eosinophils can be visualized as a small CD16 negative population in a FL-1 against FL-2 dotplot (*see* **Fig. 7A**). Double staining with CD11b and CD16 is shown in **Fig. 7B**. Red blood cells and lymphocytes do not stain with CD11b or CD16. Monocytes do stain with CD11b, but are gated out of the granulocytes. On stimulation with fMLP the increase in CD11b-FITC fluorescence can be measured and quantified.

7. Blood should be analyzed within a few minutes of sampling and kept at 37°C during activation.

8. Analyzer should be calibrated on a daily basis using Testpoint calibrant (Bayer) to ensure stability of cluster positions.

References

1. Howard, T.H. and Watts, R.G. (1994) Actin polymerisation and leukocyte function. *Curr. Opin. Haematol.* **1,** 61–68.
2. Springer, T.A. (1994) Traffic signals for lymphocyte recirculation and leukocyte emigration: the multistep paradigm. *Cell* **76,** 301–314.
3. Sabroe, I., Hartnell, A., Jopling, L.A., Bel, S., Ponath, P.D., Pease, J. E., et al. (1999) Differential regulation of eosinophil chemokine signalling via CCR3 and non-CCR3 pathways. *J. Immmunol.* **162,** 2946–2955.
4. O'Shea, J.J., Brown, E.J., Seligmann, B.E., Metcalf, J.A., Frank, M.M., Gallin, J.I. (1985) Evidence for distinct intracellular pools of receptors for C3b and C3bi in human neutrophils. *J. Immunol.* **134,** 2580–2587.
5. McCarthy, D.A. and Macey, M.G. (1993) A simple flow cytometric procedure for the determination of surface antigens on unfixed leucocytes in whole blood. *J. Immunol. Methods* **163,** 155–160.
6. Forsyth, K.D. and Levinsky, R.J. (1990) Preparative procedures of cooling and re-warming increase leukocyte integrin expression and function on neutrophils. *J. Immunol. Methods* **128,** 159–163
7. Leino,L. and Sorvajarvi, K. (1992) CD11b is a calcium-dependent epitope in human neutrophils. *Biochem. Biophys. Res. Commun.* **187,** 195–200.
8. Repo, H., Jansson, S.E., and Leirisalo-Repo, M. (1995) Anticoagulant selection influences flow cytometric determination of CD11b upregulation in vivo and ex vivo. *J. Immunol. Methods* **185,** 65–79.
9. McCarthy, D.A. and Macey, M.G. (1996) Novel anticoagulants for flow cytometric analysis of live leucocytes in whole blood. *Cytometry* **23,** 196–204.
10. Conklyn, M.J., Neote, K., and Showell, H.J. (1996) Chemokine-dependent upregulation of CD11b on specific leukocyte subpopulations in human whole blood: effect of anticoagulant on RANTES and MIP-1β stimulation. *Cytokine* **8,** 762.
11. Terstappen, L.W. and Loken, M.R. (1988) Five-dimensional flow cytometry as a new approach for blood and bone marrow differentials. *Cytometry* **9,** 548–556.
12. Saunders, A.M. (1972) Development of automation of differential leukocyte counts by use of cytochemistry. *Clin. Chem.* **18,** 783–788.
13. Simson, E. and Groner, W. (1994) The state-of-the-art for the automated WBC differential Part 1: Analytical performance. *Lab. Hematol.* **1,** 13–22.

27

Current In Vitro Models of Leukocyte Migration

Methods and Interpretation

Jennifer R. Allport, Guillermo García-Cardeña, Yaw-Chyn Lim, and Francis W. Luscinskas

1. Introduction

A large component of airway inflammatory disease is the recruitment of activated leukocytes (primarily eosinophils and T lymphocytes) from the lung vasculature into the bronchial walls resulting in lung edema. Ultimately, many of the infiltrating leukocytes progress across the airway epithelium into respiratory bronchioles, compromising lung capacity *(1,2)*. In the case of an infection, such as pneumonia, leukocytes (primarily neutrophils and monocyte/macrophages) are recruited to alveolar air spaces reducing the capacity for gaseous exchange. In both cases, resident leukocytes then release further factors that promote additional leukocyte recruitment. During an inflammatory response in the peripheral microvasculature leukocyte recruitment takes place predominantly in the postcapillary venules via the multistep adhesion cascade (reviewed in *3,4,5*). In the lung, however, leukocyte extravasation takes place via capillaries. This may be due to the specialized architecture of the lung vasculature (e.g., large numbers of branch points), or because of the differing expression of surface adhesion molecules that are required for leukocyte recruitment *(1,6)*. In addition, local concentrations of cytokines, chemokines or other chemoattractant factors will play a role in the site and degree of leukocyte infiltration *(7,8)* through acute local activation of endothelial cells.

Continuous tissue damage, particularly in chronic disorders, results in activation of the endothelial cells *(9)* and surrounding smooth muscle cells.

From: *Methods in Molecular Medicine, vol. 56:*
Human Airway Inflammation: Sampling Techniques and Analytical Protocols
Edited by: D. F. Rogers and L. E. Donnelly © Humana Press Inc., Totowa, NJ

Although leukocytes are specialized for locomotion, in most tissue cells (endothelium, smooth muscle), the capacity for locomotion normally is repressed. A variety of external stimuli, however, (e.g., wounding) can induce activation of smooth muscle cells or endothelial cells which are then capable of migration resulting in tissue remodeling (e.g., granulation tissue; *[6]*).

Cell migration is undoubtedly complex, requiring coordinated activity of cytoskeletal, membrane, and adhesion systems. Thus, dynamic interactions between cell surface adhesive receptors, organization of the actin cytoskeleton and the turnover of focal adhesions are all key processes in cell locomotion and migration *(10)*. In addition, cytokines and growth factors influence cell motility in several ways:

1. Either enhance or retard the rate of migration (chemokinesis).
2. Change the average amount of cell migration observed before the cell turns.
3. Increase the direction of movement by limiting the number of turns made by the cells *(11)*.

Many chemotactic factors have been identified, but the signaling mechanisms that mediate their induced cell movement have only recently begun to be studied. The mechanisms that mediate cell migration have been investigated using several types of in vitro migration assays. In this chapter, we will describe modified Boyden chamber techniques that we and others have used extensively as a quantitative approach to the study of net cell migration *(12–17)*, and are suitable for migration studies with both leukocytes or vascular cells. The role of cytokines or chemokines in migration of leukocytes can be addressed also using these methods. Importantly, the quantification and interpretation of the data will be discussed.

2. Materials

2.1. Reagents

1. Membrane filters. For leukocyte studies these can either be a thin (<20 μM thickness) isopore polycarbonate filter, or a thicker (>100 μM thickness) cellulose nitrate filter (Millipore, Corp., Bedford, MA). For endothelial or smooth muscle cell studies use polyvinylpyrrolidine (PVP)-free filters (25 × 80 mm, Corning Separations, Corning, NY). The investigator must select the pore size of the filter depending on the size of the cells being studied (*see* **Note 1**). Filters must be kept sterile to prevent the influence of bacterial factors on the chemotaxis assay.
2. Collagen Type I (Collaborative Research, Bedford, MA) 100 mg/mL in 0.2 M acetic acid, sterile, stored at 4°C.
3. Suitable buffer (e.g., Hanks balanced salt solution (HBSS) containing 0.1% (w/v) bovine serum albumin (BSA) (fraction V fatty-acid free), 25 mM HEPES, pH 7.2). For longer term experiments with endothelial cells or smooth muscle cells, a more complete serum-free media such as M199 should be used.

4. Trypsin/EDTA or Cell Dissociation Buffer (Gibco-BRL, Rockville, MD) to remove adherent cells from culture (*see* **Note 2**).
5. Chemoattractant of interest, (e.g., fMLP or platelet activating factor for leukocytes; vascular endothelial growth factor (VEGF) or platelet derived growth factor (PDGF) for endothelium) at suitable concentrations in an assay buffer containing 0.1% BSA.
6. Staining kit such as Diff-Quik (Fisher Scientific, Springfield, NJ) or Wright-Giemsa (Sigma Chemical Co., St. Louis, MO) prepared according to the manufacturer's instructions.
7. Mounting media, such as DePex (Sigma) or Permount (Fisher).
8. Ethanol, butanol, and xylene for fixation of cellulose nitrate filters.

2.2. Equipment

1. 48-well chemotaxis chamber (Neuroprobe Inc., Gaithersburg, MD).
2. Glass slides (25 × 80 mm), sterile scalpel blades and a clean glass plate.
3. Plastic box with lid. Dimensions should be greater than those of the chamber.

3. Methods

Boyden chambers are used to study the directed movement (chemotaxis) of a specific cell type in response to a chemoattractant gradient. The 48-well chamber comprises two halves that are clamped together on either side of a microporous filter barrier. The method relies on the migration of cells placed in an upper chamber through the filter into a lower chamber filled with a chemoattractant. Thus, the specific effect of doses of a chemoattractant can be assessed in the absence of contributing factors from other cell types. The main disadvantage of this method is that it can be time consuming and may not closely mimic the relevant physiological setting of the cell under investigation. Hence, a particular factor might be chemotactic for specific leukocytes or endothelial cells in vitro, but may not play a significant role in the in vivo setting where other factors are contributing.

3.1 Protocols

3.1.1. Protocol for Leukocyte Chemotaxis

1. Prepare dilutions of the chemoattractant of interest in the assay buffer. The suggested range is from 0.1 n*M* to 10 μ*M*. Always use a positive control (known chemoattractant) and negative control (buffer alone) if possible.
2. Using a sterile scalpel blade and a clean glass plate as support cut a filter to fit the chamber (use a 25 × 80 mm glass slide as a template). Mark the orientation of the filter by cutting across one corner. If using polycarbonate filters, there is no need to presoak the filter in the assay buffer. If using cellulose nitrate filters, place the filter on the surface of 10-mL assay buffer in a Petri dish and allow it to absorb the buffer (*see* **Note 3**).
3. Pipet chemoattractant into the lower wells (25 μL), taking care to avoid bubbles (*see* **Note 4**). Fill the wells quickly so that they do not dry out. Fill all the wells,

Table 1
Suggested Migration Times for Boyden Chambers

Leukocyte	Filter Type (thickness)	
	Polycarbonate (20 µM)	Cellulose Nitrate (140 µM)
neutrophil	30–60 min	60–120 min
monocyte	60 + min	90 + min

whether you are using them or not, or you will get leaching into the dry wells. Intersperse chemoattractant filled wells with buffer filled wells to check for leaching of the chemoattractant.

4. Immediately after the wells are filled, pick up the membrane at both ends with forceps and place it on to the chamber. If using polycarbonate filters, make sure the PVP side (nonshiny side) is facing the lower chamber, i.e., the shiny side must face upwards. For cellulose nitrate filters there is no orientation requirement. Place the center down first, and then the edges. Take care not to shift the filter around which could spread the chemoattractant.

5. Immediately place the gasket firmly on the filter and clamp the upper chamber tightly on the top.

6. Place a glass slide over the upper wells to prevent evaporation and place the whole chamber in a plastic box with a lid, and place in the cell culture incubator (37°C) for 15 min to warm.

7. Suspend the leukocytes of interest at 2×10^6/mL in the assay buffer. Once the chamber is warm, pipet 50 µL of cell suspension into each well, taking care to avoid bubbles between the cell suspension and the filter (*see* **Note 5**).

8. Replace the glass slide and replace the chamber in the cell culture incubator.

9. Allow the cells to migrate for the required time. Migration time depends on the thickness of the filter and the leukocyte type. Suggested times are shown in **Table 1**, but individuals should optimize the assay for their cells and chemoattractant (*see* **Note 6**).

10. At the end of the migration time, remove the chamber from the incubator, remove the upper chamber and the gasket. Take the membrane filter and using the clamps and scraper provided, scrape the cells from the upper surface. These cells have merely sedimented on to the surface of the membrane and should be removed to prevent misinterpretation of the data. It is essential to keep the filter wet at all times.

11. If using a polycarbonate filter the migrated cells will have stuck to the underside of the filter and these can be counted on a microscope. Fix and stain the filter using the Diff-Quik or Wright-Giemsa staining kit, and mount on to glass slides using a suitable mounting medium. Count four to five random high power fields for each well (40× objective).

12. If using a cellulose nitrate filter, the migrated cells will be part way through the filter because of its greater thickness. To fix and stain these filters use the following protocol in sequence:

1. 70% (v/v) ethanol	5 min	fixative
2. Distilled H_2O	1 min	wash
3. Hematoxylin	45 s	stains nuclei
4. Distilled H_2O	1 min	wash
5. Running tap water	2-3 min	wash
6. 70% (v/v) ethanol	2 min	dehydration
7. 95% (v/v) ethanol	2 min	dehydration
8. 8:2 ethanol:butanol	5 min	dehydration
9. 100% (v/v) xylene	indefinitely	clearing

The hematoxylin step can be replaced by Wright-Giemsa staining if cytosolic staining is desired. The cellulose nitrate filters are opaque and must be cleared in xylene before the cells can be counted. Filters are then mounted on to glass slides in DePex mounting medium and counted. The stained filters can be left indefinitely in xylene until counting as exposure to air will render them once more opaque. Hence, do not mount filters until you are ready to count them.

3.1.2. Tissue Cell Chemotaxis

1. Prepare the PVP-free filters by presoaking in 0.2 *M* acetic acid for 30 min. Transfer the filters to a 100 mm culture dish and cover them with collagen I solution. Place up to 5 filters in each dish. Soak for 24 h (*see* **Note 7**). Remove the excess collagen solution and place the filters on sterile KimWipes under a laminar hood until completely dry. Individual filters should be stored at 4°C in sterile tissue culture dishes.
2. Dilute the chemoattractants (e.g., vascular endothelial growth factor, platelet derived growth factor, leptin) in medium (e.g., M199) containing 0.1% (w/v) BSA and add to the lower wells of the Boyden chamber, ensuring a continuous contact between the lower surface of the filter and the solution (*see* **Note 4**).
3. Screw the gasket and the upper chamber into place. There is no need to prewarm the chamber, owing to the long incubation time for the experiment (>4 h).
4. Trypsinize the adherent cells briefly (or use cell dissociation media) and resuspend in medium (M199) containing 0.1 % (w/v) BSA at 3×10^5/mL (*see* **Notes 2** and **8**). Add 50 µL of the cell suspension to each upper chamber taking care to avoid filter perforation (*see* **Note 5**).
5. Incubate the chamber in a cell culture incubator at 37°C in 5% (v/v) CO_2 for 4 h.
6. Unlock the chamber and remove the filter, scrape the upper side of the filter with a rubber wiper to remove all of the nonmigrated cells. Repeat this process two more times.
7. Fix the migrated cells by placing the filter in 100% methanol overnight.
8. Stain the filter with Wright-Giemsa solution for 1–2 h, wash three times with PBS and once in water to remove salt. Leave to dry. Mount the filters on glass slides using suitable mounting medium.
9. Count the number of cells/microscopic field (40× objective) in 10 random fields/well.

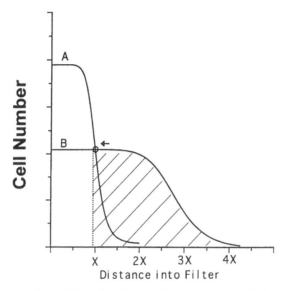

Fig. 1. Examples of possible migration patterns across a cellulose nitrate filter. At distance X into the filter, the same number of cells are present in both **A** and **B**. At distance 2X, there are no cells present in **A**, but many cells present in **B**. If cells at distance X only are counted, there will be no apparent difference between **A** and **B**. For counting by the leading front method, count all cells present in the filter after a set distance (shaded area). By the leading front method, many more cells are present in **B** than in **A**.

3.2. Quantification and Interpretation

1. Always intersperse chemoattractant filled wells with buffer wells to account for leaching of the chemoattractant.
2. Distinguish between chemotaxis (the unidirectional migration of a cell toward an increasing concentration of the factor) and chemokinesis (nondirectional migration of cells because of activation by the factor) using checkerboard assays. In checkerboard assays chemoattractant is placed on either side of the filter (on either the opposite side from the leukocytes [lower chamber] or the same side as the leukocytes [upper chamber]) or on both sides of the filter (both lower and upper chambers). Chemokinesis (nondirected migration, equal in all directions) will occur under any circumstance, providing the chemoattractant is at the optimal concentration for cell activation. True chemotaxis (directed movement), however, will only occur when the concentration of the chemoattractant in the lower chamber is optimal, and there is no chemoattractant in the upper chamber. By trying a range of conditions, the investigator can determine if the factor is chemokinetic or chemoattractant.
3. When counting the migrated cells in cellulose nitrate filters, use a leading front method. Select a distance into the filter where there are reasonable numbers of leukocytes/field (e.g., 200 cells/X40 field), and count all cells that have migrated from that point onwards (*see* **Fig. 1**, shaded area). Counting only the cells at the

selected distance may misrepresent the numbers. In both A and B, there are equal numbers of cells at distance X, but at 2 X there are no cells in A and many cells in B. Counting cells only at distance X would produce the same data for A and B, when in fact more cells migrated further in B than in A.

4. When counting migrated cells using polycarbonate or PVP-free filters, it is important to stop the experiment early enough, do not allow the migration to continue once the underside of the filter is covered with leukocytes. At this time, newly migrating cells will knock the existing cells into the chamber below, hence you may observe the same number of leukocytes for migration times of 30 min or 60 min when only the filter is examined.

4. Notes

1. Suggested pore sizes are shown below.
   3 μM pore size, neutrophils, eosinophils; 5 μM pore size, lymphocytes, monocytes; 8 μM pore size, macrophages, mast cells, tumor cells, endothelial cells or smooth muscle cells.

2. Trypsinization of adherent cells may strip the plasma membrane of receptors or other signaling molecules required by the cell to sense or respond to a chemotactic gradient. If you are unsure if your receptor or pathway of interest is trypsin sensitive, cell dissociation media should be used to suspend adherent cells. The cell dissociation media does not contain any proteases or EDTA that could disrupt receptor structural integrity. Before resuspending cells in the assay buffer/media they should be washed to remove traces of trypsin or the cell dissociation buffer.

3. Clean the glass plate and slide with 70% (v/v) ethanol to sterilize. Multiple filters can be cut at the same time provided they are cut under sterile conditions and stored in a sterile Petri dish to prevent bacterial contamination.

4. While pipeting the medium containing the chemoattractants check that the volume of medium is enough to create a slight positive meniscus when the well is filled; this prevents air bubbles from being trapped when the filter is applied. You may find that fine tipped pipet tips work best (e.g., Sigma 200 μL microcapillary round tips). The wells hold 25 μL, so we suggest setting the pipet to 27 μL to allow "doming" of the buffer, and avoid a meniscus. Complete the filling in no more than 5 min to prevent excessive evaporation. If necessary, once the chamber is filled, top off wells where evaporation has occurred.

5. Check for trapped bubbles in the upper wells. Again, fine tips work best. If 50 μL of cell suspension appears not to fit in the well, this is a good indication of a bubble. Use a vacuum line to aspirate out the cells and then refill the well. Take care not to puncture the filter with the pipet tip.

6. Migration times for leukocytes across polycarbonate filters tend to be very short owing to the minimal thickness of the filter and the high degree of leukocyte motility. It is very important, therefore, not to allow the cells to migrate for too long or leukocytes will pile up on the underside of the filter and newly migrating cells will knock them into the well below.

7. When preparing the collagen-coated filters for endothelial cell or smooth muscle cell migration, keep all reagents and filters sterile throughout to prevent bacterial contributions to the migration assay.

8. A critical point of this procedure is the resuspension of cells after trypsinization. Failure to obtain a homogenous single cell suspension will result in cell clusters that will produce artifacts such as cell-to-cell adhesion, giving the impression of reduced migration. In addition, the attachment of these cell clusters to the filters may interfere with quantification of cell numbers.

References

1. Martin, T.R. (1997) Leukocyte migration and activation in the lungs. *Eur.Respir.J.* **10,** 770–771.

2. Liu, L., Mul, F.P., Kuijpers, T.W., Lutter, R., Roos, D., and Knol, E.F. (1996) Neutrophil transmigration across monolayers of endothelial cells and airway epithelial cells is regulated by different mechanisms. *Ann. N.Y. Acad. Sci.* **796,** 21–29.

3. Butcher, E.C. (1991) Leukocyte-endothelial cell recognition; three (or more) steps to specificity and diversity. *Cell* **67,** 1033–1036.

4. Luscinskas, F.W. and Lawler, J. (1994) Integrins as dynamic regulators of vascular function. *FASEB J.* **8,** 929–938.

5. Symon, F.A. and Wardlaw, A.J. (1996) Selectins and their counter receptors; a bitter sweet attraction. *Thorax* **51,** 1155–1157.

6. Cotran, R.S. and Mayadas-Norton, T. (1998) Endothelial adhesion molecules in health and disease. *Pathol. Biol. (Paris)* **46,** 164–170.

7. Rothenburg, M.E., Zimmermann, N., Mishra, A., Brandt, E., Birkenberger, L.A., Hogan, S.P. and Foster, P.S. (1999) Chemokines and chemokine receptors: their role in allergic airway disease. *J. Clin. Immunol.* **19,** 250–265.

8. Strieter, R.M., Kunkel, S.L., Keane, M.P., and Standiford, T.J. (1999) Chemokines in lung injury: Thomas A. Neff lecture. *Chest* **116,** 103S–110S.

9. Zimmerman, G.A., Albertine, K.H., Carveth, H.J., Gill, E.A., Grissom, C.K., Hoidal, J.R., et al. (1999) Endothelial Activation in ARDS. *Chest* **116,** 18S–24S.

10. Sheetz, M.P., Felsenfeld, D.P., Galbraith, C.G. (1998) Cell migration: regulation of force on extracellular matrix-integrin complexes. *Trends Cell Biol.* **8,** 51–54.

11. Parent, C.A. & Devreotes, P.N. (1999) A cell's sense of direction. *Science* **284,** 765–770.

12. Wilkinson, P.C. (1988) Micropore methods for leukocyte chemotaxis. *Methods Enzymol.* **162,** 38–50.

13. Muir, D., Sukhu, L., Johnson, J., Lahorra, M. A., and Maria, B. L. (1993) Quantitative methods for scoring cell migration and invasion in filter-based assays. *Anal. Biochem.* **215,** 104–109.

14. Kundra, V., Escobedo, J.A., Kazlauskas, A, Kim, H.K., Rhee, S.G., Williams, L.T., and Zetter, B.R. (1994) Regulation of chemotaxis by the platelet-derived growth factor receptor-beta. *Nature* **367,** 474–476

15. Allport, J.R., Donnelly, L.E., Hayes, B.P., Murray, S., Rendell, N.B., Ray, K.P., and MacDermot, J. (1996) Reduction by inhibitors of mono(ADP-ribosyl)trans-

ferase of chemotaxis in human neutrophil leucocytes by inhibition of the assembly of filamentous actin. *Br. J. Pharmacol.* **118,** 1111–1118.

16. Sierra-Honigmann, M.R., Nath, A.K., Murakami, C., Garcia-Cardena, G., Papapetropoulos, A., Sessa, W.C., et al. (1998) Biological action of leptin as an angiogenic factor. *Science* **281,** 1683–1686.
17. Papapetropoulos, A., Garcia-Cardena, G., Dengler, T.J., Maisonpierre, P.C., Yancopoulos, G.D., and Sessa, W.C. (1999) Direct actions of angiopoietin-1 on human endothelium: evidence for network stabilization, cell survival, and interaction with other angiogenic growth factors. *Lab. Invest.* **9,** 213–223.

28

Tracing Intracellular Mediator Storage and Mobilization in Eosinophils

Salahaddin Mahmudi-Azer, Paige Lacy, and Redwan Moqbel

1. Introduction

In this chapter, we will describe two different techniques used to trace storage and mobilization of intracellular granule-derived mediator proteins in eosinophils. The first is confocal laser scanning microscopy (CLSM) used to investigate immunofluorescence labeling in cytospins, and the second is subcellular fractionation, leading to the generation of fractions that may be analyzed for their organelle elution profiles using appropriate protein, enzyme, and organelle marker assays.

1.1. Confocal Laser Scanning Microscopy

CLSM systems are based on the principle that both the illumination and detection (imaging) systems are focused on a single point within a focal plane (volume element) of a specimen *(1–3)*. CLSM image collection occurs by directing a laser-generated excitation light, at or near the appropriate excitation wavelength for the fluorochrome in use, toward the specimen. The excitation light passes through a scanning system and a dichroic mirror to reach the microscope objective, which focuses the scanning beam onto a single spot on the specimen. Fluorescent emission deriving from the fluorochrome present within the focal plane of the specimen then returns via the objective and is reflected off the dichroic mirror onto a detector. A spatial filter containing an aperture (the detection pinhole) defines the area within the volume element of the specimen by removing all out-of-focus information. Thus, the illumination, specimen, and detector all have a single focus, i.e., they are confocal (*see* **Fig. 1**). To form a two-dimensional image, the laser beam is scanned repeatedly across

From: *Methods in Molecular Medicine, vol. 56:*
Human Airway Inflammation: Sampling Techniques and Analytical Protocols
Edited by: D. F. Rogers and L. E. Donnelly © Humana Press Inc., Totowa, NJ

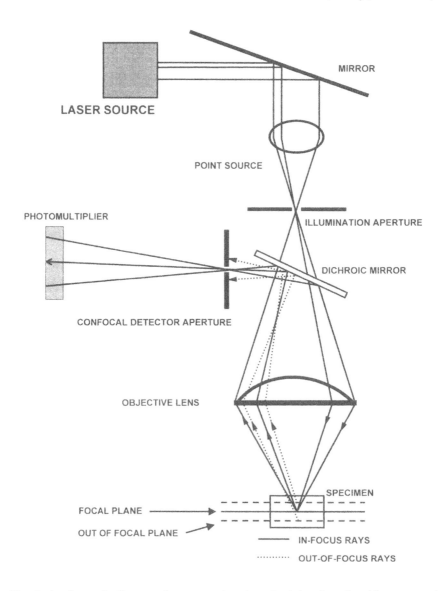

Fig. 1. A schematic diagram demonstrating the principle of confocal laser scanning microscopy. Excitation of the fluorochrome-labeled specimen is achieved by the passage of light emitted at the excitation maximum appropriate for the fluorochrome through an illumination aperture. This light passes through a dichroic mirror and is focused on the specimen through the objective lens. Fluorochrome excitation leads to the emission of a longer wavelength light (fluorescence), which returns via the objective and reflects off the dichroic mirror through the imaging aperture (the detection pinhole), and is detected by a photomultiplier tube. Light from above and below the plane of focus is blocked by the pinhole. Thus, out-of-focus light is virtually eliminated from the final confocal image.

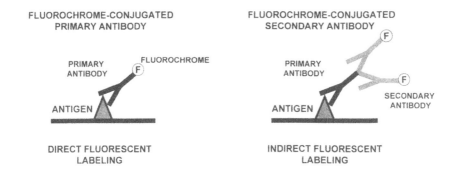

Fig. 2. Direct and indirect immunofluorescent labeling. In the direct method, a fluorochrome-conjugated primary antibody is used to detect and visualize the antigen of interest. In the indirect method, a fluorochrome-conjugated secondary antibody is used which binds to and detects a primary antibody, which is specific for the antigen of interest.

the specimen, enabling a computer to rasterize the emitted fluorescence onto a computer monitor.

1.2. Immunofluorescent Labeling and CLSM

Immunofluorescent labeling can be considered as the detection and visualization of proteins of interest in cell preparations (tissue sections, cytospins, or smears) by the use of specific antigen-antibody interactions. A fluorochrome-conjugated antibody is used to detect sites of immunoreactivity. The aim of the procedure is to consistently and reproducibly visualize a particular antigen, with minimum background staining, while preserving the integrity of cell architecture.

Two different immunofluorescent labeling approaches, direct and indirect labeling, may be used to localize antigens (*see* **Fig. 2**). The choice of either depends on the availability of reagents, degree of sensitivity required, and achievement of the desired signal-to-noise ratio, among others. In the direct technique, the primary antibody, which may be monoclonal (rat, mouse) or polyclonal (goat, rabbit), is directly conjugated to a fluorochrome, allowing immediate visualization of the protein of interest. In the indirect labeling method, the primary antibody is visualized after binding of a secondary antibody conjugated to a fluorochrome. The secondary antibody is normally polyclonal and recognizes the immunoglobulin class of the primary antibody in a species-specific manner. For example, fluorochrome-conjugated rabbit antimouse IgG may be used if the primary antibody is a mouse monoclonal IgG. Although indirect labeling is generally more sensitive than direct labeling because of amplification of the signal using a polyclonal secondary antibody,

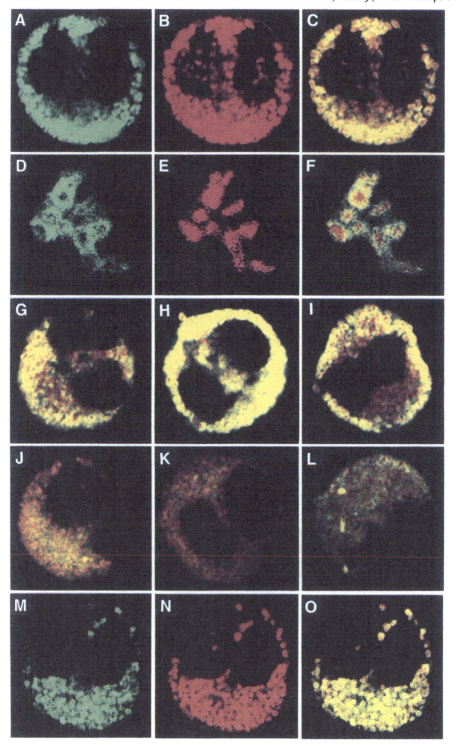

it is also susceptible to a poor signal-to-noise ratio because of increased nonspecific binding by antibodies. Up to three proteins may be labeled in the specimen, depending on the capacity of the confocal imaging system, so that the combined images may reflect the overlapping distribution of components of interest.

Recently, CLSM was used by our group for the localization and tracing of intracellular mediators, specifically interleukin-6 (IL-6) and regulation on activation normal T-cell expressed and secreted chemokine (RANTES), stored within small secretory vesicles and crystalloid granules in eosinophils *(4–6)*. The distribution of these proteins was examined in resting and stimulated human peripheral blood eosinophils using interferon-γ (IFNγ) as the agonist (*see* **Fig. 3**).

1.3. Subcellular Fractionation

Another method used for intracellular localization and tracing of mediators is the technique of subcellular fractionation. This procedure involves the disruption of cellular structures and separation of resulting intracellular organelles across a density gradient following ultracentrifugation. Subcellular fractionation is a well-established procedure in many cell types *(7)*, and was recently modified for use with guinea pig eosinophils *(8)*. This method was further optimized for human eosinophils *(9)*. One of the modifications involved the use of a specialized ball-bearing stainless steel cell homogenizer known as a cell cracker, which is essential for maintaining the integrity of delicate intracellular organelles. Secondly, Nycodenz density gradient media, a nonionic tri-iodinated media resembling metrizamide *(10)*, was employed for organelle separation. Nycodenz is superior to other types of density gradient media (sucrose, glycerol) because of its relative isotonicity and low viscosity.

Fig. 3. CLSM images of single-and double-immunofluorescent staining of peripheral blood eosinophils with antibodies for MBP combined with RANTES, (**A–L**) and MBP combined with IL-6 (M-O). (**A–C**) Unstimulated eosinophils labeled with BODIPY FL indicating RANTES immunoreactivity (**A**), Rhodamine Red corresponding to MBP (**B**), and combined images (**C**). (**D–F**) Higher magnification of eosinophil crystalloid granules showing matrix-associated doughnut-shaped RANTES immunoreactivity (**D**), surrounding red-labeled cores of MBP immunoreactivity (**E**), and combined images of the same structure (**F**). (**G–L**) Combined images of RANTES and MBP, depicting time course of IFNγ (500 U/mL) stimulation, comparing (**G**) unstimulated cells with those stimulated for 5 min (**H**), 10 min (**I**), 30 min (**J**), 60 min (**K**), and 16 h (**L**).
(**M–O**) Unstimulated eosinophils labeled with BODIPY FL indicating IL-6 immunoreactivity (**M**), Rhodamine Red corresponding to MBP (**N**), and combined images (**O**).

The procedure outlined in **Subheading 3.2.** contains the most recent version of the subcellular fractionation technique used for human peripheral blood eosinophils.

2. Materials

2.1. Reagents

2.1.1. Double-Labeling and CLSM

The following buffers may be prepared as 10× stocks and stored at 4°C for many months. All general chemicals are of the highest quality available from commercial sources (Sigma-Aldrich Canada, Mississauga, ON; BDH Inc, Toronto, ON; Fisher Scientific, Fair Lawn, NJ; and ICN Biomedicals Inc, Aurora, OH).

1. Phosphate-buffered saline (PBS) 10X stock solution: 80 g/L NaCl, 2 g/L KCl, 21.71 g/L Na$_2$HPO$_4$.7H$_2$O, 2 g/L KH$_2$PO$_4$, pH 7.2–7.4. Filter through 0.22 m before storage. Final concentration of 1X solution: 137 mM NaCl, 2.7 mM KCl, 8.1 mM Na$_2$HPO$_4$, 1.4 mM KH$_2$PO$_4$. Adjust pH of 1X solution to 7.2–7.4 if necessary.
2. Tris-buffered saline (TBS) 10X stock solution: 60.7 g/L Tris-HCl, 87.66 g/L NaCl, pH 7.6. Pass through 0.22 μm filter before storage. Final concentration of 1X solution: 100 mM Tris,150 mM NaCl. Adjust pH of 1X solution to 7.6 if necessary.
3. RPMI-1640 (BioWhittaker, Walkersville, MD).
4. 2% Paraformaldehyde (Fisher Scientific) in PBS. Prepare this solution just before use. Weigh out 5 g paraformaldehyde, add 250 mL 1X PBS, and heat to 55–60°C while stirring on a heating platform until fully dissolved. Filter through 0.22 μm after cooling the solution to room temperature. **Caution:** Paraformaldehyde solutions should be prepared in a fume hood as these release toxic formaldehyde gas upon overheating. In addition, take care not to overheat as formaldehyde solutions are flammable.
5. Bovine serum albumin (ICN Biomedicals, Inc., Aurora, OH).
6. Fetal calf serum (FCS) (Gibco-BRL Life Technologies, Grand Island, NY).
7. Antibleaching solution. Add 250 μL 10X TBS, 1.87 g glycerol, and 10 mg *n*-propyl gallate (Sigma-Aldrich) to a graduated test tube, and make up to 2.5 mL with double-distilled water. Dissolve by vortexing.
8. Dextran (~110,000 Da, Fluka BioChemika, Buchs, Switzerland).
9. Ficoll-Paque Plus (Amersham Pharmacia Biotech AB, Uppsala, Sweden)
10. Anti-CD3, CD14, and CD16-coated immunomagnetic beads (MACS beads; Miltenyi Biotec, Bergisch-Gladbach, Germany).
11. Mouse monoclonal (IgG1) antihuman MBP antibody (BMK-13, generated in-house).
12. Mouse monoclonal (IgG2) antihuman IL-6 antibody (Immunotech, Westbrook, ME).
13. Mouse monoclonal (IgG2) antihuman RANTES antibody (Molecular Probes, Eugene, OR).
14. Goat antimouse IgG2 antibody (Molecular Probes).
15. Rhodamine Red-labeled goat polyclonal antimouse IgG antibody (Jackson ImmunoResearch Laboratories Inc, West Grove, PA).

16. BODIPY FL-conjugated goat polyclonal antimouse IgG antibody (Molecular Probes).

2.1.2. Subcellular Fractionation

All reagents are from Sigma-Aldrich Canada (Mississauga, ON) unless otherwise specified.

1. Sucrose buffer (Buffer A): 0.25 M sucrose, 10 mM HEPES (pH 7.4), 1 mM ethyleneglycol-*bis*(β-aminoethylether)-N,N,N^1,N^1-tetraacetic acid(EGTA) (prepared as a stock of 100 mM, pH adjusted to 7.0 by addition of NaOH; add 10 mL to each liter of buffer), adjust pH to 7.4 and filter through 0.45 μm disposable filter prior to storage of 50 mL aliquots at –20°C. Usually only need to prepare 100–200 mL at a time.
2. Protease inhibitors: 10 mg/mL phenylmethylsulfonylfluoride (PMSF) in isopropanol, stored at room temperature for up to 6 mo. **Caution:** Take care in handling PMSF as it is extremely toxic (cholinesterase inhibitor); use gloves when weighing out samples.
3. Protease inhibitor cocktail: 5 mg/mL each of leupeptin, aprotinin, and *N*-α-*p*-tosyl arginine methyl ester (TAME) in dimethyl sulfoxide (DMSO) and stored at –20°C in 20 μL aliquots.
4. Sucrose buffer (Buffer B): Buffer A with 2 mM MgCl$_2$, 1 mM adenine triphosphate (ATP) (prepared as stock at 100 mM in 0.2 M Tris, stored at –20°C), 100 μg/mL PMSF, 5 μg/mL protease inhibitor cocktail.
5. 45% w/v Nycodenz density gradient solution: add 45 g Nycodenz (Nycomed Pharma AS, Oslo, Norway) to 50 mL Buffer A, stir for approx. 1–2 h, then make up to 100 mL, and filter through 0.45 μm before storing 10 mL aliquots at –20°C.

2.2. Apparatus

2.2.1. Double-Labeling and CLSM

1. Cytospin two centrifuge (Shandon Ltd, Astmoor, Runcorn, UK) for slide preparation.
2. Leica confocal laser scanning microscope system (Leica Lasertechnik GmbH, Heidelberg, Germany), equipped with a krypton/argon laser to allow simultaneous scanning of up to three excitation wavelengths (488, 568, and 647 nm), in order to acquire multiple images from a single pass and reduce bleaching of photosensitive fluorochromes.

2.2.2. Subcellular Fractionation

1. Stainless steel ball-bearing cell cracker containing an 8.020 mm bore, plus ball bearings with sizes between 8.002–8.010 mm (increments of 0.002 mm) (Precision Engineering, European Molecular Biology Laboratory, Heidelberg, Germany).
2. Beckman SW40.1 Ti swing-out rotor and buckets for ultracentrifugation (Beckman Instruments, Palo Alto, CA).
3. Beckman Optima XL-90 ultracentrifuge (Beckman Instruments).

3. Methods

3.1. Double-Labeling and CLSM

3.1.1. Eosinophil Purification

1. Collect samples of peripheral blood (50–100 mL), from atopic subjects exhibiting a mild eosinophilia (>5%) not receiving oral corticosteroids, in heparinized tubes.
2. Add 10 mL 5% dextran to whole blood and thoroughly mix in 50-mL syringes before allowing settling of erythrocytes by gravitation. Sediment erythrocytes for no more than 45 min at room temperature. Dextran acts by promoting rouleaux formation of erythrocytes.
3. Remove the upper phase of the leukocyte-rich plasma and layer the plasma onto a 15-mL Ficoll-Paque Plus cushion in a sterile 50-mL Falcon conical centrifuge tube. Centrifuge the gradient for 25 min at 1000*g* at room temperature.
4. Remove excess clarified plasma, mononuclear layer, and excess Ficoll until <1 mL remains above the granulocyte pellet.
5. Contaminating erythrocytes may be optionally removed by hypotonic lysis on ice by adding 2–3 mL sterile H_2O to the granulocyte pellet for a few seconds, followed by a rapid addition of 10–15 mL ice-cold RPMI-1640 and centrifugation.
6. Resuspend the cell pellet in 300 µL RPMI immediately after washing, and add 12 µL anti-CD16-coated immunomagnetic beads for every 50×10^7 cells, plus 10 µL anti-CD3 and 10 mL anti-CD14-coated immunomagnetic beads to the total cell suspension.
7. Incubate the mixture for 45 min at 4°C. It is important not to incubate the beads with cells on ice, as this will reduce the binding ability of the antibody-conjugated beads. This procedure will remove contaminating neutrophils, lymphocytes, and monocytes, respectively, by negative selection.
8. Add the mixture to a freshly prepared magnetic column according to the manufacturer's instructions (Miltenyi Biotec) and elute purified eosinophils in a sterile 50-mL Falcon conical tube. Provided that the flow through the column is carefully monitored, the resulting eosinophil purity should be greater than 97% *(9)*.

3.1.2. Slide Preparation and Immunofluorescent Labeling

The method below will describe double labeling of eosinophil cytospins using the indirect labeling approach.

1. Prepare cytospins of eosinophils by spinning $3–5 \times 10^4$ cells (suspended in 100 µL 20% FCS in RPMI-1640) in a Cytospin 2 centrifuge at 800 rpm for 2 min.
2. Air-dry slides for at least 1 h at room temperature in order to permeabilize cells (*see* **Note 1**). Wrap slides individually in foil and store at –20°C until needed.
3. Fix cytospin slides for 10 min in freshly prepared 2% paraformaldehyde in PBS and rinse five times in TBS.
4. Block slides by adding 60 µL 3% FCS in TBS and incubating a humidified container for 30 min at room temperature (*see* **Note 2**).
5. For the first labeling step, wash slides with TBS and incubate for 1 h at room temperature with 60 µL primary antibody, e.g., 1% mouse monoclonal antihu-

man MBP (i.e., BMK-13) prepared in TBS containing 1% BSA (*see* **Note 3**). An isotype control, for example, approx. 5 µg/mL mouse monoclonal IgG1, should be used in place of this antibody on a separate cytospin slide to provide a negative control for the immunofluorescence.

6. Wash slides and incubate with 50 µg/mL Rhodamine Red-labeled goat antimouse IgG antibody in TBS containing 1% BSA (60 µL) for 1 h at room temperature.

7. Following another washing step, block slides again for 2 h at room temperature using 50 µg/mL goat antimouse IgG in TBS containing 1% BSA (60 µL). This blocking step is necessary for preventing crossreaction of the primary antibody used in **step 5** with the secondary antibody used in **step 9** of this method.

8. Double-labeling may be carried out by adding 60 µL primary mouse monoclonal antihuman IL-6 or RANTES (5 µg/mL) in TBS containing 1% BSA and incubating for 1 h at room temperature (*see* **Note 3**). Another isotype control antibody incubation step should be included in place of this antibody (5 µg/mL mouse monoclonal IgG1) on the same slide used in **step 5** as the negative control for double-labeling.

9. Wash slides and add 20 µg/mL BODIPY FL-conjugated goat antimouse IgG in TBS containing 1% BSA (60 µL) and incubate for 1 h at room temperature to detect anti-RANTES antibody binding.

10. Add 10 µL antibleaching agent prior to cover slip application. Seal cover slips using nail polish.

3.1.3. Confocal Laser Scanning Microscopy

Examine the immunofluorescent staining of eosinophils using a Leica CLSM equipped with a krypton/argon laser, which excites at three major wavelengths (488, 568, and 647 nm). We used the highest magnification available with a Plan Apo ×100/1.32 oil immersion objective on this system in order to fully resolve the structure of immunolabeled intracellular organelles. Optimize the image acquisition settings using the required pinhole size, photomultiplier gain, and offset. It is possible to achieve a higher spatial resolution by using the appropriate zoom setting on the computer. Following subtraction of eosinophil autofluorescence and nonspecific binding by the use of the isotype control-labeled cytospin slides, process and save images using the Multi-user Multi-tasking Image Analysis software. This software was developed by Leica Lasertechnik GmbH using the Motorola 68030 CPU workstation and an OS9 operating system. Store images on the computer and transfer these as TIF files to Adobe Photoshop software (Adobe Systems, Inc., Mountain View, CA) for further image processing.

3.2. Subcellular Fractionation

On the day of fractionation, prepare at least 5×10^7 eosinophils for this procedure, purified as described in **Subheading 3.1.** All steps in the present section should be carried out on ice and at 4°C.

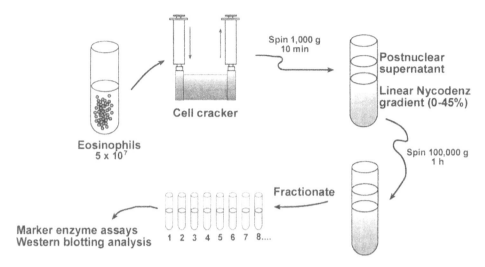

Fig. 4. Subcellular fractionation technique for eosinophils using a cell cracker and a 0–45% Nycodenz linear gradient. Approximately 5×10^7 cells are resuspended at $1–1.5 \times 10^7$ cells/mL before subjecting to homogenization through a cell cracker. The postnuclear supernatant is then layered on the Nycodenz gradient which is spun and fractionated for later analysis.

1. Assemble the cell cracker with 2×3-mL syringes and the required ball bearing (usually 8.010 mm for eosinophils) and place on ice.
2. Prepare a Nycodenz gradient by pipeting 0.5 mL 45% Nycodenz (*see* **Note 4**) into a Beckman UltraClear tube (14×89 mm, Beckman Instruments) before pouring a continuous linear gradient mixed from 4 mL Buffer A (*see* **Note 5**) and 4 mL 45% Nycodenz (containing 5 µg/mL protease inhibitor cocktail) using a stirring platform and peristaltic pump or a gradient mixer. The gradient should be increasing in density from the top to the bottom of the tube. The total volume of the 0–45% Nycodenz gradient will be approx 8 mL.
3. Resuspend eosinophils (5×10^7) in 10 mL ice-cold Buffer A. Centrifuge at $250g$ for 5 min at 4°C.
4. Resuspend eosinophils to a density of $1–1.5 \times 10^7$ cells/mL in Buffer B. Load one of the syringes (with the plunger removed) on the cell cracker with 2.5–3 mL cell suspension using a plastic disposable pipete (*see* **Fig. 4**). Attach the syringe plunger to the top of the cell suspension.
5. Apply pressure to the syringe plunger while pulling up simultaneously on the receiving syringe. Push cells with steady pressure at least 10–15 times through the cell cracker. The viscosity of the homogenate should increase during passaging, resulting in greater force required to depress syringe plungers. This indicates that cell rupture is occurring. Briefly reverse the flow at intervals to prevent clogging of the bore. The number of passages required for full homogenization

depends on the viscosity of the solution. If it becomes very difficult to push the homogenate through the cell cracker, stop the homogenization and check cell density (*see* **Note 6**).

6. Remove one plunger and take a small sample of the cell homogenate to check disruption of cells by light microscopy. A small amount of 1 m*M* ethidium bromide (~1 µL) may also be added to this sample to check for free nuclei and partly broken cells under fluorescence. Cells should be completely broken with organelles moving by Brownian motion. Contaminating red blood cells will be mostly intact.

7. If there are still intact eosinophils in the homogenate, passage the cells two more times through the cell cracker until whole eosinophils are rarely observed by microscopy.

8. Remove plungers and transfer homogenate to a 15-mL conical centrifuge tube.

9. Centrifuge at 400*g*, 10 min at 4°C to remove nuclei, red blood cells, large mitochondria, and unbroken cells. Retain the supernatant, and label this the postnuclear supernatant.

10. Layer the postnuclear supernatant onto the top of the 0–45% Nycodenz gradient by very gentle hand pipeting. The total volume of the gradient plus the supernatant will be between 12–13 mL.

11. Insert the tube into a rotor bucket (SW 40.1 Ti, Beckman Instruments) and balance with the opposite tube (containing water) and bucket by weighing these on a microbalance.

12. Attach caps to each bucket and place these on a precooled rotor head. Note that all buckets, empty or full, must be loaded onto the rotor for safety. Spin the tubes at 100,000*g* for 1 h at 4°C in a Beckman Ultracentrifuge (XL-90 Optima). This allows elution of organelles at their respective equilibrium densities.

13. Remove the centrifuge tube containing the gradient and insert a glass capillary tube (*see* **Note 7**) attached to a peristaltic pump and fraction collector (Gilson Model 205, Middleton, WI). Ideally the fraction collector should be modified to hold a 96-well rack from a Costar cluster tube system (Corning Costar, Cambridge, MA) which can contain up to 96 microtubes (Corning Costar), allowing the use of 8-channel multipipets to aliquot samples and assay for marker activities. The fraction collector should be set to monitor drop numbers rather than collection time to prevent the loss of material between tubes.

14. Collection of fractions will depend on the requirements of the later stages of the technique; generally, between 15 × 0.75 mL to 24 × 0.5 mL fractions may be collected. For collection of 15 × 0.75 mL fractions, set the fraction collector to count 30 drops per tube.

15. Fractions may be frozen as aliquots at –80°C for very long periods with little loss of activity (up to 2 yr) (*see* **Note 8**).

16. Enzyme assays *(11–14)*, ELISA *(5,6,9)*, dot blot analysis for CD9 immunoreactivity *(5,6,9)*, and Western blot analysis *(8,14)* should be carried out on fractions to determine the elution profiles of organelles and proteins of interest, shown in **Figs. 5** and **6**.

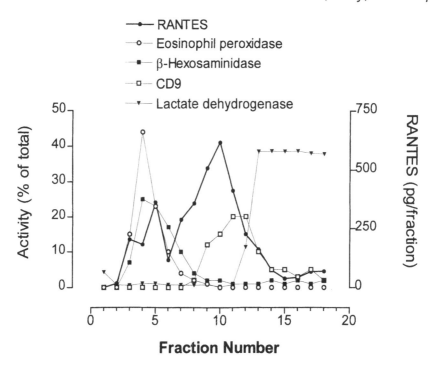

Fig. 5. Fractions were collected from a 0–45% linear Nycodenz gradient and analyzed for marker enzyme activities to obtain profiles of subcellular compartments.
Marker assays used were eosinophil peroxidase (secretory granules), β-hexosaminidase
(secretory granules and lysosomal granules), CD9 (plasma membrane), and lactate
dehydrogenase (cytosol). Quantification of RANTES was carried out by ELISA for
each fraction and is expressed as pg/fraction. Reproduced with permission from the
American Hematological Society (*Blood* [1999] 94:23).

4. Notes

The following notes are critical points to bear in mind when investigating
intracellular mediator detection and localization using immunofluorescent
staining and CLSM and subcellular fractionation. In subcellular fractionation,
the most critical step is the preparation of the homogenate using the cell cracker.
If excessive force is used to prepare the homogenate, then intracellular
organelles may disintegrate into random structures. Although other homogenization procedures, such as sonication, have not been tested with this technique,
it is strongly recommended that the cell cracker be used since this type of
homogenization allows the retention of delicate organelle structures.

1. In our hands, air-drying of eosinophil cytospins has been found to be the optimal
   permeabilization technique for preserving cellular morphology. Addition of
   permeabilization agents, such as saponin, at later stages has been found to induce
   a marked deterioration in cell morphology.

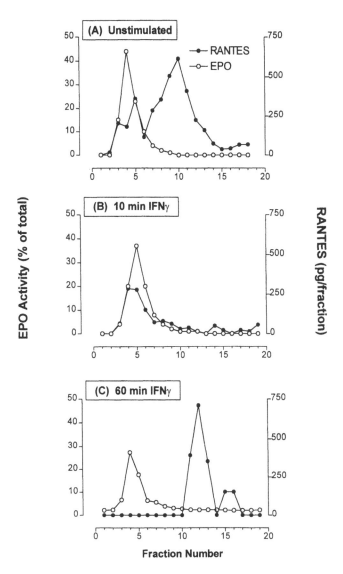

Fig. 6. Subcellular fractionation of resting and IFNγ-stimulated eosinophils (~5 × 10⁷ per fractionation). These experiments were conducted at different times using purified blood eosinophils from the same donor. Immunoreactivity to RANTES was determined in individual fractions by ELISA and expressed as pg/fraction. Profiles of EPO activity are shown here for comparison. (**A**) Unstimulated eosinophils, followed by eosinophils stimulated for (**B**) 10 min and (**C**) 60 min with 500 U/mL recombinant human IFNγ. This study demonstrated a shift in the profile of the RANTES peak of activity (detected by specific ELISA) in human eosinophils at different time points after stimulation with IFNγ. These changes in localization were also observed by CLSM (*see* **Fig. 3 G–L**). Reproduced with permission from the American Hematological Society (*Blood* [1999] 94:23).

2. Care should be taken to reduce autofluorescence and block nonspecific antibody binding through the use of appropriate blocking conditions. In addition, eosinophil granule proteins are highly positively charged, and therefore are readily stained by anionic fluorochromes, such as fluorescein and FITC unless blocked by expensive and stringent blocking proteins (e.g., human IgG). Thus, the use of anionic fluorochromes in staining eosinophils should be avoided. Instead, antibodies conjugated to neutral fluorochromes, such as BODIPY and Rhodamine Red, should be employed for eosinophil immunofluorescence studies. Provided that these neutral fluorochromes are used in these studies, it is possible to use conventional blocking conditions (e.g., FCS, goat serum) with eosinophils.

3. The optimal concentration of primary monoclonal antibody preparations in immunofluorescence must be determined by titration. For most antibodies, a good starting concentration will be in the range of 1–50 µg/mL. Optimization of the antibody label is only possible by comparison with a suitable negative control by the use of an appropriate isotype control antibody at the same concentration.

4. To obtain optimal sedimentation of intracellular organelles, buffers and the Nycodenz gradient media must be filtered through 0.45 µm filters.

5. Do not use Buffer B to construct the gradient since the supplements in this buffer alter the sedimentation properties of organelles. In addition, do not add PMSF to the Nycodenz gradient media, since the solvent (isopropanol) used to prepare this can cause gradient failure (organelles are not fully separated across the gradient).

6. If the cell suspension is difficult to pass through the cell cracker, check the cell density and ensure that it is between $1–1.5 \times 10^7$/mL in the starting material. A cell density higher than this will result in clogging of the cell cracker. Conversely, lower cell density values will not result in sufficient breakage of cells. Inadequate cell density may be determined by the lack of increase in viscosity of the cell suspension during repeated passages.

7. Care should be taken during the insertion of the glass capillary tube into the final centrifuged density gradient. Too much disturbance of the gradient may result in mixing of the different organelle populations.

8. The refractory index of each fraction should be determined during the initial stages of optimization. Refractory index measurements may be converted to density units (g/mL) by the equation $\rho = 3.410h - 3.555$, as specified in the Nycodenz specification sheet, where η represents the refractive index measurement and ρ indicates density.

References

1. Inoue, S. (1989) *The handbook of biological confocal microscopy* (Pawley,J., ed.), IMR Press, Madison, WI, pp. 1–13.
2. White, J. G., Amos, W. B., Durbin, R., and Fordham, M. (1990) *Optical microscopy for biology* (Herman, B. and Jacobson,K., eds.), Alan R. Liss, New York, pp. 1–18.
3. Wilson, T. and Sheppard, C. J. R. (1984) *Theory and practice of scanning optical microscopy.* Academic Press, New York, p 213.

4. Mahmudi-Azer, S., Lacy, P., Bablitz, B., and Moqbel, R. (1998) Inhibition of nonspecific binding of fluorescent-labeled antibodies to human eosinophils. *J. Immunol. Methods* **217,** 113–119.

5. Lacy, P., Levi-Schaffer, F., Mahmudi-Azer, S., Bablitz, B., Hagen, S. C., Velazquez, J., et al. (1998) Intracellular localization of interleukin-6 in eosinophils from atopic asthmatics and effects of interferon γ. *Blood* **91,** 2508–2516.

6. Lacy, P., Mahmudi-Azer, S., Bablitz, B., Hagen, S., Velazquez, J., Man, S. F. P., and Moqbel, R. (1999) Rapid mobilization of intracellularly stored RANTES in response to interferon-γ in human eosinophils. *Blood* **94,** 23–32.

7. Evans, W. H. (1992) Isolation and characterization of membranes and cell organelles. In: *Preparative Centrifugation: A Practical Approach* (Rickwood, D., ed.), IRL Press, Oxford, pp. 233–270.

8. Lacy, P., Thompson, N., Tian, M., Solari, R., Hide, I., Newman, T., and Gomperts, B. (1995) A survey of GTP-binding proteins and other potential key regulators of exocytotic secretion in eosinophils. *J. Cell Sci.* **108,** 3547–3556.

9. Levi-Schaffer, F., Lacy, P., Severs, N. J., Newman, T. M., North, J., Gomperts, B., et al. (1995) Association of granulocyte-macrophage colony-stimulating factor with the crystalloid granules of human eosinophils. *Blood* **85,** 2579–2586.

10. Rickwood, D. (1993) *Iodinated Density Gradient Media: A Practical Approach* (Rickwood, D., ed.), IRL Press, Oxford, pp. 1–21.

11. White, S. R., Kulp, G. V., Spaethe, S. M., Van Alstyne, E., and Leff, A. R. (1991) A kinetic assay for eosinophil peroxidase activity in eosinophils and eosinophil conditioned media. *J. Immunol. Methods* **144,** 257–263.

12. Storrie, B. and Madden, E. A. (1990) Isolation of subcellular organelles. *Methods Enzymol.* **182,** 203–225.

13. Cromwell, O., Bennett, J. P., Hide, I., Kay, A. B., and Gomperts, B. D. (1991) Mechanisms of granule enzyme secretion from permeabilized guinea pig eosinophils. Dependence on Ca^{2+} and guanine nucleotides. *J. Immunol.* **147,** 1905–1911.

14. Lacy, P., Mahmudi-Azer, S., Bablitz, B., Gilchrist, M., Fitzharris, P., Cheng, D., et al. (1999) Expression and translocation of Rac2 in eosinophils during superoxide generation *Immunology* **98,** 244–252.

29

Measurement of Metalloproteinases

Steven D. Shapiro, Diane Kelley, and Dale Kobayashi

1. Introduction

Matrix metalloproteinases (MMPs) *(1,2)* comprise a family of over 20 matrix degrading enzymes believed to be essential for normal development and physiologic tissue remodeling and repair. Abnormal expression of metalloproteinases has been implicated in many destructive processes, including tumor cell invasion and angiogenesis, arthritis, atherosclerosis, and arterial aneurysms. With respect to lung disease, MMPs have been associated with chronic obstructive pulmonary disease (COPD), acute lung injury, pulmonary fibrosis, and asthma. The role of MMPs in causation of pulmonary emphysema has been supported by transgenic mice overexpressing MMP-1 *(3)* and gene targeted mice lacking MMP-12 *(4)*.

MMPs are secreted as inactive proenzymes which are activated at the cell membrane surface or within the extracellular space by proteolytic cleavage of the *N*-terminal domain. Catalytic activity is dependent on coordination of a zinc ion at the active site and is specifically inhibited by members of another gene family, called tissue inhibitors of matrix metalloproteinases (TIMPs). Currently, four TIMPs have been described. Optimal activity of MMPs is around pH 7.4. MMP family members share about 40% identity at the amino acid level, and they possess common structural domains. Domains include a proenzyme domain that maintains the enzyme in its latent form, an active domain that coordinates binding of the catalytic zinc molecule, and (except for matrilysin) a C-terminal domain involved in substrate, cell, and TIMP binding. The gelatinases A and B have an additional fibronectin-like domain that mediates their high binding affinity to gelatins and elastin. Gelatinase B has one more domain with homology to type V collagen. Membrane-type MMPs (MT-MMPs 1–4 or MMP-14–17) have an additional membrane-spanning domain.

From: *Methods in Molecular Medicine, vol. 56:*
Human Airway Inflammation: Sampling Techniques and Analytical Protocols
Edited by: D. F. Rogers and L. E. Donnelly © Humana Press Inc., Totowa, NJ

Individual members of the MMP family can be loosely divided into groups based on their matrix degrading capacity. As a whole, they are able to cleave all extracellular matrix components.

1. Collagenases (MMPs-1, -8, -13) have the unique capacity to cleave native triple helical interstitial collagens. MMP-1 has a small active site pocket and restricted substrate specificity. MMP-8, and -13 are able to cleave other components of extracellular matrix (ECM), but not elastin.
2. There are two gelatinases of 72 kDa (gelatinase A, MMP-2) and 92 kDa (gelatinase B, MMP-9) which differ in their cellular origin and regulation, but share the capacity to degrade gelatins (denatured collagens), type IV collagen, elastin, and other matrix proteins.
3. Stromelysins (MMP-3, -10) have a broad spectrum of susceptible substrates, including most basement membrane components. MMP-11 is termed stromelysin-3, but has little homology to the other stromelysins and human MMP-11 has a mutation in humans making it a poor proteinase.
4. Matrilysin (MMP-7), the smallest MMP (28 kDa as a proenzyme) has broad substrate specificity of stromelysin plus it has some elastase activity. Although a potent and potentially destructive enzyme, gene targeting of MMP-7 has also demonstrated a physiological role for this MMP in tracheal wound repair *(5)* and activation of defensins *(6)*.
5. Macrophage elastase (MMP-12) also has a potent broad substrate specificity that includes elastin. MMP-12 is required for cigarette smoke-induced emphysema *(4)*.
6. Membrane-type metalloproteinases (MT-MMPs) are located at the cell surface and at least one MT-MMP, MT1-MMP, activates MMP-2. MT-MMPs also appear to directly degrade ECM proteins, but their catalytic capacities is not well-defined at present.

MMPs are active against a variety of proteins besides extracellular matrix. For example, MMPs cleave and activate latent tumor necrosis factor (TNF)-α thereby regulating inflammation, and also cleave plasminogen generating the anti-angiogenic fragment, angiostatin *(7)*. MMPs also cleave tissue factor pathway inhibitor (TFPI) augmenting tissue thrombosis (Belaaouaj and Shapiro, unpublished observations). MMPs *(8)*, particularly MMP-12 *(9)* degrade and inactivate α_1-antitrypsin, indirectly enhancing the activity of neutrophil elastase. Thus, MMPs play both direct and indirect roles in matrix-destruction associated with emphysema, and may indirectly influence cytokine release and angiogenesis that could influence the development and progression of COPD.

1.1. Cellular Expression of MMPs

1. Alveolar macrophage metalloproteinases. Alveolar macrophages are the most abundant defense cells in the lung both under normal conditions and particularly during states of chronic inflammation. Alveolar macrophages produce several MMPs including significant amounts of MMP-12, MMP-9, and smaller amounts

of MMP-3 and MMP-7. Human macrophages have the capacity to produce MMP-1, an enzyme not present in rodents. MT1-MMP (MMP-14) also appears to be a macrophage product. Expression of these MMPs is highly regulated, and under quiescent conditions, such as in normal mature lung tissue, MMPs are essentially not expressed. They are inducible, and both their production and activity are carefully controlled during normal repair and remodeling processes. With chronic inflammation, regulation of MMPs can go awry, and MMPs can be produced in excess and at inappropriate sites. A recent study demonstrated that alveolar macrophages cultured from patients with COPD express MMP-1 and MMP-9, whereas macrophages from subjects without COPD did not express these enzymes (*10*). In the latter study, MMP-12 appeared to be induced in cigarette smokers with and without COPD.

2. Neutrophil metalloproteinases. Neutrophils contain two MMPs, gelatinase B (MMP-9) and neutrophil collagenase (MMP-8). In the neutrophil these MMPs are stored in large quantities within specific granules. Neutrophil collagenase can degrade interstitial collagens, but not elastin.

3. Other Lung Cells. Many other cells in the lung have the capacity to produce MMPs. Eosinophils produce significant amounts of the MMP-9. T-lymphocytes produce MMP-2, MMP-3, and MMP-9. Various resident lung cells can produce MMPs, including fibroblasts, which are a potential prominent source of MMPs-1,-2, -3, and the MT-MMPs. Type II alveolar epithelial cells produce MMP-7 in addition to other MMPs. Endothelial cells also produce a variety of MMPs such as MMP-1, and -9. Considering the variety of lung cells capable of producing MMPs, it seems plausible that MMPs could participate in the lung destruction resulting in emphysema.

1.2. General Techniques to Assess MMP Expression

1. MMP mRNA expression. One can detect MMP mRNA in lung cells or tissue by the same techniques described in previous chapters including Northern hybridization, RNase or S1 nuclease protection, or reverse transcriptase polymerase chain reaction (RT-PCR). Because most MMPs are rapidly secreted upon production, it had been thought that *in situ* hybridization would be required to determine the cellular source of MMP production. In fact, many MMPs, even those secreted can be detected by immunohistochemistry, but *in situ* hybridization remains a valuable complementary technique.

One can apply either cell lines, bronchoalveolar lavage (BAL) cells, or lung tissue to mRNA detection. Of note, in general MMPs are 45–55% similar at the base pair level, and full-length cDNAs can be used with stringent hybridization conditions to detect individual MMPs. One exception is that stromelysin-1 (MMP-3) and stromelysin-2 (MMP-10) are 85% similar, and 3' UTR probes are best to separate these two MMPs by Northern. Use of specific S1 nuclease or PCR probes are also useful to analyze these closely related MMPs.

For nearly all known MMPs, cDNA sequence is available for human, mouse, and other species. Orthologous genes between man and mouse are generally ~75–85%. Thus, human probes could be useful to detect abundant mRNA in rodents under less stringent Northern conditions, and vice versa. However, availability of probes usually makes this unnecessary. Of note, mice and humans do have a few differences in their repertoire of MMPs. Most notably, mice do not express MMP-1, but do express the other collagenases MMP-8 and MMP-13. In addition, MMP-11 (stromelysin 2) has a mutation in humans rendering it a poorly active enzyme. Mice, however, have a functional site allowing for greater enzymatic capacity.

MMPs are detectable in various cell lines, particularly upon stimulation. For example, in fibroblasts MMP-1, MMP-2, MMP-3, and MT1-MMP are the most abundant MMPs, with marked upregulation (IL-1) in response to phorbol myristate acetate (TPA/PMA) and interleukin (IL-1). Mouse macrophage cell lines (P388D1, RAW, J777) express MMP-12 and MMP-13 most prominently, whereas human monocytic cell lines (U937 and THP-1) require PMA "differentiation" into macrophages to express MMP-1, MMP-9, and MMP-12. Human alveolar macrophages obtained from BAL have minimal MMP expression unless stimulated with lipopolysaccharide (LPS) (or to a lesser degree PMA) after which they express MMP-1, MMP-3, MMP-9, and MMP-12. MMP expression is silent in quiescent adult lung tissue. However, MMPs can be readily detected during development and in various disease states.

2. MMP Protein Expression. Most MMPs are 40–50% similar at the amino acid level. Monospecific polyclonal, peptide, and monoclonal antibodies are becoming increasingly commercially available for human MMPs. Although some antibodies may crossreact with other species, there are few commercially available antibodies directed against nonhuman MMPs. MMPs in general are secreted as inactive proenzymes. Activation occurs extracellularly by enzymatic or oxidative means resulting in loss of the *N*-terminal domain which contains a conserved cysteine that interacts with active site zinc which maintains the MMP in latent form.

To detect MMP expression in cell lines, cells are often cultured under selected conditions (i.e., expression is usually augmented in serum-containing media) and the conditioned media is assayed following sufficient time for production and secretion of MMPs. Following induction by PMA in fibroblasts, MMP mRNA can be detected within 2 h and protein secretion 4 h poststimulation. Macrophages, on the other hand, have delayed induction. Following LPS treatment, for example, MMP mRNA is readily detectable after ~8 h with significant protein detected in the conditioned media after 24 h. In culture, MMPs can be produced in the range of micrograms of protein per million cells after 24 h. To detect neutrophil MMP-8 and MMP-9, intracellular proteins can be assayed, or MMP release induced from specific granules, for example with formyl methionyl leucyl phenylalanine (fMLP). Cell lysates or membrane preparations are required to detect membrane type MMPs (MMP-14–18).

MMP protein can be detected from cell lines by standard means such as Western blotting, or enzyme-linked immunosorbent assay (ELISA) for more precise quantification. Incubation in ^{35}S-methionine labeled medium followed by immunoprecipitation provides measurement of protein biosynthesis. Zymography is one technique unique to matrix degrading proteinases and thus will be discussed in experimental detail.

Homogenates or lysates of lung tissue can be used in Western blotting, ELISA, or zymography for detection of MMPs. Immunohistochemistry can also be used to detect MMP proteins within tissues. As discussed previously, immunohistochemistry can identify the MMP-producing cell, but may also detect the site of extracellular deposition, such as the extracellular matrix (ECM), or binding to the surface of another cell type.

2. Materials
2.1. Zymography Gels

Where possible, use electrophoresis grade reagents.

1. Gelatin: store at room temperature.
2. Casein: store at 0°C.
3. Etna elastin: 4°C.
4. Trizma base, pH to 6.8 or 8.8 with concentrated HCl: store at 4°C.
5. Sodium dodecal sulphate (SDS), 10% (w/v) (wear mask when weighing powder): store at room temperature.
6. Acrylamide 30% (caution, this is a neurotoxin, wear gloves): store at room temperature.
7. Tetramethylethylenediamine (TEMED): store at room temperature in the dark.
8. Ammonium persulfate, 10% (make fresh each week): store at 4°C.
9. Recipe for mini gels (*see* **Note 1**):
a. Separating gels:

Final acrylamide %	6%	8%	9%	10%	11%	12%	15%
1.5 M Tris-HCl, pH 8.8	2.5 mL						
10% SDS	100 µL						
30% Acrylamide	2 mL	2.6	2.97	3.34	3.67	4.0	5.0
TEMED	10 µL						
DH$_2$O	5.2 mL	4.6	4.32	3.96	3.63	3.3	2.28
10% ammonium persulphate	100 µL						

For zymography, as above except for:

Distilled H$_2$O	4.8 mL	4.2	3.92	3.56	3.23	2.9	1.88
Zymographic substrate	400 µL						

b. Stacking gels:

Final acrylamide %	4.5%
0.5 M Tris-HCl, pH 6.8	2.5 mL
10% SDS	100 µL
30% Acrylamide	1.5 mL
TEMED	10 µL
Distilled H$_2$O	5.8 mL
10% ammonium persulphate	100 µL

  c. Maximum loading volume:

10 well, thin comb (0.75 mm)	27 μL
10 well, thick comb (1.5 mm)	54 μL
15 well, thin comb (0.75mm)	16 μL
15 well, thick comb (1.5 mm)	32 μL

10. Wash buffer: 2.5% Triton X-100.
11. Incubation Buffer (0.05 M Tris-HCl, pH 8.2/0.005 M CaCl$_2$/0.5 μM ZnCl$_2$): add 50 mL 1 M Tris-HCl, pH 8.2, sterile with 0.02% sodium azide (very toxic) to 5 mL 1 M CaCl$_2$ and 500 μL 1 mM ZnCl$_2$, prepared in 0.1 N HOAc. Bring volume to 1 L with distilled water.
12. Coomassie brilliant blue stain (R 250): dissolve 5 g dye in 1 L destain (*see* **step 13**). Stir overnight. Filter through Whatman #1 filter paper.
13. Destain: add 200 mL glacial acetic acid to 400 mL methanol and 3.4 L distilled water.

3. Methods

3.1. Substrate Gel Zymography

    Substrate gel zymography is performed by applying a preparation (cell lysates, conditioned media, tissue extract, or purified proteins) to gel electrophoresis in a nonreduced, nondenatured state (*see* **Notes 2** and **3**). The gel contains selected extracellular matrix substrates that are amenable to cleavage by proteinases upon prolonged incubation. Protein zymography allows the determination of whether a sample has active proteinases capable of degrading a specific substrate. The molecular mass of the proteinase can also be determined, and use of inhibitors will identify the class of proteinase(s) present.

    The basic theory is that proteins are separated by molecular mass and, upon incubation, proteinases (including zymogens) are activated. If the proteinases have the capacity to degrade the substrate within the gel, the zone of lysis will not take up the Coomassie blue stain and will remain white against a blue background.

1. Conditioned media should be serum-free and, for best results, tissue samples should contain minimal albumin.
2. If using casein or κ-elastin gels, the media to be analyzed should be dialyzed against 0.5 mM Tris-HCl, pH 7.5/0.1 mM CaCl$_2$/0.005% Brij and then lyophilized. It may then be reconstituted by adding the appropriate amount of sample buffer.
3. If using other substrates, add an equal volume of sample buffer to the media to be analysed. DO NOT add a reducing agent and DO NOT boil.
4. Run gel in the cold, or on ice, using cold running buffer. For a 0.75 mm gel, run at a constant current of 20 mA. For a 1.5 mm gel, run at 40 mA.
5. Rinse gel with 2.5% Triton X-100, followed by two washes for 15 min each in 2.5% (w/v) Triton X-100, at room temperature on a shaker.
6. Wash the gel once for 5 min in incubation buffer.

7. Cover the gel (in a "sandwich" box with lid) and incubate the buffer at 37°C for the times indicated below:
   a. Gelatin: 2–24 h.
   b. Casein: 24–48 h.
   c. κ-Elastin: 48–72 h.
8. Commassie blue staining: stain for 30 min and then destain.
9. Destain overnight with gentle shaking. Zones of lysis (clear: *see* **Subheading 3.1.**) should be visible at this time.

4. Notes

1. Substrates are prepared at 25 mg/mL in distilled water and frozen in 400 μL aliquots. The gelatin must be boiled (to get into solution), and must be heated to 37°C before use. Substitute 400 μL of substrate for the same volume of distilled water in your 10 mL separating gel recipe to get a final substrate concentration of 1 mg/mL. It is not necessary to include substrate in your stacking gel.
2. In general the precise proteinase cannot definitively identified by this technique. It is best used as a screening procedure to identify potential proteinases based on molecular mass, substrate specificity, and class of proteinase (*see* **Note 3**). For example, many MMP proenzymes migrate at ~55 kDa and can degrade casein. However, gelatinolytic activity at 92 (active 82) kDa and 72 (active 60) kDa that can be inhibited by EDTA is fairly strong evidence for MMP-9 and MMP-2, respectively. For best results, use molecular weight markers, realizing that migration under nondenatured, nonreduced conditions may not be exact. Ideally, a positive control proteinase will more precisely identify migration of the protein.
3. EDTA is used to help determine whether or not metalloproteinases or other classes of enzymes cause the zones of lysis. We use 5 mM EDTA in Tris buffer without Zn^{2+} or Ca^{2+} to inhibit metalloproteinase activity: i.e., if bands appear after EDTA incubation, then the enzymes are *not* metalloproteinases.

References

1. Parks, W. C. and Mecham, R. P. (1998) Matrix Metalloproteinases—Comprehensive and up to date reviews on many aspects of MMP biology and chemistry. Academic Press.
2. Shapiro, S. D. (1998) Biological consequences of extracellular matrix cleavage by matrix metalloproteinases in Extracellular matrix and cell-to-cell contact. *Current Opinion in Cell Biology* **10**, 602–608.
3. D'Armiento, J., Dalal, S. S., Okada, Y., Berg, R. A., Chada, K. (1992) Collagenase expression in the lungs of transgenic mice causes pulmonary emphysema. *Cell* **71**, 955–961.
4. Hautamaki, R. D., Kobayashi, D. K., Senior, R. M., Shapiro, S. D. (1997) Macrophage elastase is required for cigarette smoke-induced emphysema in mice. *Science* **277**, 2002–2004.
5. Dunsmore, S. E., Saarialho-Kere, U. K., Roby, J. D., Wilson, C. L., Matrisian, L. M., Welgus, H. G., et al. (1998) Matrilysin expression and function in airway epithelium. *J. Clin. Invest.* **102(7)**, 1321–1331.

6. Wilson, C., Ouellette, A., Satchell, D., Ayabe, T., Lopez-Boado, Y., Stratman, J., et al. (1999) Regulation of intestinal alpha-defensin activation by the metalloproteinase matrilysin in innate host defense. *Science* **286,** 113–117.
7. Cornelius, L. A., Nehring, L., Klein, B., Pierce, R., Bolinski, M., Welgus, H. G., et al. (1998) Generation of angiostatin by matrix metalloproteinases: effects on neovascularization. *J. Immunol.* **161,** 6845–6852.
8. Sires, U. I., Murphy, G., Welgus, H. G., and Senior, R. M. (1994) Matrilysin is much more efficient than other metalloproteinases in the proteolytic inactivation of alpha-1-antitrypsin. *Biophys. Biochem. Res. Comm.* **204,** 613–620.
9. Gronski, T. J., Martin, R., Kobayashi, D. K., Walsh, B. C., Holman, M. C., Van Wart, H. E., et al. (1997) Hydrolysis of a broad spectrum of extracellular matrix proteins by human macrophage elastase. *J. Biol. Chem.* **272,** 12,189–12,194.
10. Finlay, G. A., O'Driscoll, L. R., Russell, K. J., D'Arcy, E. M., Masterson, J. B., Fitzgerald, M. X., et al. (1997) Matrix metalloproteinase expression and production by alveolar macrophages in emphysema. *Am. J. Respir. Crit. Care Med.* **156,** 240–247.

30

Immunocytochemistry and Immunohistochemistry

Jochen Springer and Axel Fischer

1. Introduction

Immunohistochemistry allows the specific histochemical localization of many diverse classes of organic substances, including inflammatory markers ranging from biogenic amines to macromolecular cytokines and their receptors. Corresponding ligands and their receptors can be demonstrated simultaneously by double-labeling protocols (*1*), since the fixation and tissue processing of the two are often compatible. One can choose between monoclonal and polyclonal antibodies raised against either the purified or at least partially purified (monoclonal antibodies) (*2,3*) receptors or ligands as well as against synthetic peptides (10 to 20 amino acid residues long). The latter offers the advantage of obtaining site-specific antisera for demonstrating receptor subtypes (*4*), but the amino acid sequence corresponding to the synthetic peptide may be masked in the full protein, owing to posttranslational modifications and/or folding.

To obtain good immunohistochemical results, the fixation and tissue processing must be taken into consideration (*5,6*). When using 4% paraformaldehyde, most proteins and peptides will retain their antigenicity, yet if the antigen is of low molecular weight (e.g., biogenic amines) this mild fixative may not properly immobilize the substances. In that case either Zamboni's solution is used or 0.5% glutaraldehyde is added to the paraformaldehyde. Alternatively, 0.2% picric acid may also be added in some cases (*6*). The latter two fixation methods drastically improve the structural preservation, but in the case of protein and larger peptides it may result in a loss of antigenicity. After fixation, tissue or cells can either be embedded in paraffin or frozen in optimum cutter temperature (OCT)-compound (*7,8*). Embedding the specimens in paraffin may attenuate the antigenicity of larger antigens because of the dehydration in etha-

From: *Methods in Molecular Medicine, vol. 56:*
Human Airway Inflammation: Sampling Techniques and Analytical Protocols
Edited by: D. F. Rogers and L. E. Donnelly © Humana Press Inc., Totowa, NJ

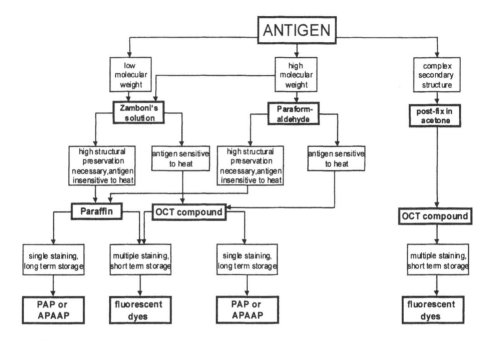

Fig. 1. Schematic overview of immunocytochemical and immunohistochemical procedures.

nol and the relatively high temperatures during the lengthy embedding process, which may be shortened to 1 d by the use of 2,2 dimethoxypropane (DMP) *(9)*. The tissue preservation of paraffin embedded tissue is usually better than that of frozen specimens, but shrinking of the tissue and therefore alterations in the relative proportions can be observed. **Figure 1** gives an overview of the immunocytochemical and immunohistochemical procedures outlined the present chapter.

2. Materials

2.1. Reagents

1. OCT compound (Miles, Elkhart, IN, USA).
2. Liquid nitrogen.

2.1.1. Fixatives

1. 4% Paraformaldehyde: add 40 g paraformaldehyde to 500 mL distilled water and heat slowly to 70°C. Drip in 2 M NaOH until solution is clear, allow to cool and add 0.2 M phosphate buffer. Adjust pH to 7.4 and filter. Prepare fresh, but aliquots may be stored at -20°C for a short period of time.
2. Zamboni´s solution: add 15% picric acid (toxic, explosive when dry) to 2% formaldehyde in 0.1 M phosphate buffer. Add 50 mL 37% formaldehyde to 500 mL 0.2 M

phosphate buffer, and add 150 mL of the saturated, filtered picric acid solution and distilled water to a final volume of 1 liter. Zamboni´s Solution is stable at 4°C.

2.1.2. Rinsing Solution

Add 9.0 g NaCl, 25 g polyvinylpyrrolidone (PVP, molecular weight 40,000; Sigma, PVP-40), 20,000 IU heparin, 5 g procaine hydrochloride to a final volume of 1 liter water. Make fresh as required.

2.1.3. Buffers

1. Phosphate buffered saline (PBS): 0.1 M NaH$_2$PO$_4$, 0.1 M Na$_2$HPO$_4$, and 0.15 M NaCl in distilled water, pH 7.4.
2. Phosphate buffer (PB) 0.2 M: 0.2 M NaH$_2$PO$_4$, 0.2 M Na$_2$HPO$_4$, adjust pH to 7.4.
3. Buffered glycerol: adjust the pH of a 0.5 M Na$_2$CO$_3$ solution to 8.6 with 0.5 M NaHCO$_3$. Add 1 part buffer to 2 parts 100% glycerol. Store at 4°C for up to 2 mo.

2.1.4. Preparation of Slides

Immerse glass-slides in chromalum/gelatin solution (0.5% gelatin powder and 0.05% potassium chromium sulfate-12-hydrate in distilled water, heat to 40°C) for 10 min, dry overnight at 40°C.

2.2. Apparatus

Only standard laboratory equipment is used in immunohistochemistry, such as microtomes, cryostats, and centrifuges (e.g., Shandon Cytospin 2, Southern Products, Runcorn, Cheshire, UK).

3. Methods

3.1. Tissue Preparation

Tissues should be as fresh as possible, for example in the case of immersion fixation they should be treated immediately upon receipt of specimens from the operating theater. The tissues should be fixed for up to 18 h at 4°C (*see* **Note 1**).

3.2. Embedding Procedure

3.2.1. Embedding in OCT Compound

1. Wash specimens in 0.1 M phosphate buffer (pH 7.4, 4 °C), changing the buffer at least 3 times in the first 4–6 h, and a final time overnight.
2. Immerse tissue in the same buffer containing 18% sucrose as cryoprotectant and store at 4°C until the tissue has sunk to the bottom. It may be necessary to change the sucrose solution, depending on the size of the specimen and the volume of sucrose buffer used.
3. Mount specimens with OCT compound on filter paper, and freeze with liquid nitrogen. They can be stored at –80°C for several years if protected from drying by wrapping them in Parafilm or Nescofilm.

4. Cut sections with a cryostat at a maximum of 10 μm and collect onto chromalum/ gelatin coated slides and air dry for 1–2 h. The sections can be stored at –20°C for up to 2 mo.

3.2.2. Embedding in Paraffin

1. Wash specimens in 0.1 *M* phosphate buffer (pH 7.4, 4°C), changing the buffer at least 3 times in the first 4–6 h.
2. Dehydrate the specimens in a graded series of alcohol, starting with 70% alcohol, overnight. The alcohol should be changed up to 4 times during that period.
3. Immerse the tissue in:

80 % alcohol,	3 times 30 min;
90 % alcohol,	3 times 30 min;
96 % alcohol,	3 times 30 min;
100 % alcohol,	3 times 30 min.

4. Transfer into the inter-medium isopropanol, 2 h.
5. Transfer into 1:1 isopropanol/paraffin, overnight at 50°C.
6. Paraffin 1 (melting point 51°C to 53°C) overnight at 55°C (removes the isopropanol).
7. Paraffin 2 (melting point 51°C to 53°C) overnight at 55°C.
8. Mount and section on a microtome.
9. Collect the sections on gelatin-coated glass slides. The sections can be stored for several years at room temperature.

3.2.3. Fast Embedding Procedure in Paraffin

1. Wash specimens in 0.1 *M* phosphate buffer (pH 7.4, 4°C), changing the buffer at least 3 times in the first 4–6 h.
2. Immerse the tissue in distilled water.
3. Dehydration :

	70% alcohol,	twice for 1 h;
	70% alcohol/DMP,	twice for 1 h;
	DMP,	twice for 1 h;
	DMP/paraffin oil,	twice for 1 h;
	Paraffin oil,	twice for 2–4 h;
	Paraffin oil/paraffin,	twice for 2–4 h;
	Paraffin,	overnight.

4. Mount and section on a microtome.
5. Collect sections on gelatin-coated glass slides.

3.3. Cytospin

Cells from lavage or blood can be investigated by concentration either on a microscope slide (*10,11*) or in a thin-walled reaction tube (*12*).

3.3.1. Microscope Slide Cytospins

1. Cells (and microorganisms) are deposited on slides by centrifuging them through a hole in a paper strip, which absorbs the supernatant fluid of the specimen by using a Shandon Cytospin 2.

2. The slides are briefly air-dried.
3. Fix in Zamboni's solution or 4% paraformaldehyde for 2–30 min and wash twice in PB.
4. Slides can be directly used or stored at –80 °C.

3.3.2. Thin-Walled Tube Cytospins

1. Pellet cells by centrifuging at 1500 rpm for 5 min in a conventional microcentrifuge.
2. Either fix or overlay with OCT compound (and subsequently postfix after sectioning).
3. The fixed pellet can be carefully embedded in OCT compound or paraffin and sectioned as described above.

3.4. Immunohistochemistry

3.4.1. Immunohistochemistry of Cryostat Sections

All steps are carried out in a moist chamber.

1. Block nonspecific binding with 0.1 *M* PBS containing 10% normal swine serum and 1% bovine serum albumin (BSA) for 30–60 min at room temperature (*see* **Notes 2** and **3**). A detergent (e.g., Tween-20, Triton-X-100, or Sapronin) should be used if the antiserum was raised against an intracellular antigen or domain.
2. Remove the blocking solution from the slides and cover the sections with the primary antibody in PBS overnight at room temperature. The appropriate dilution of polyclonal antibodies is mostly in the range of 1:200 to 1:5000; monoclonal antibodies usually have to be used in higher concentrations.
3. Wash sections in PBS 3 times for at least 10 min.
4. Remove PBS without letting the sections completely dry and apply a secondary antibody (raised against the IgG of the host animal of the primary antibody) labeled with a fluorescent dye for 1–1.5 h in the dark (*see* **Note 4**).
5. Wash sections in PBS 3 times in the dark for at least 10 min.
6. Remove PBS and mount the sections with a small volume of carbonate buffered glycerol.
7. Examine the section with an epipfluorescence microscope equipped with the appropriate filter for the chosen dye.
8. Sections can be stored for up to 6 mo at 4°C depending on the quality of the secondary antiserum.

3.4.2. Immunohistochemistry on Paraffin Sections

1. Remove paraffin in either xylene (may cause cancer) or Rotihistol twice for 10 min.
2. Rehydrate the sections in a graded series of alcohol (100%, 96%, 90%, 70% and 50%), diluted with PBS buffer for 5 min each.
3. Transfer into PBS.
4. Perform the incubation as described above.

5. Mount with carbonate buffered glycerol.
6. Alternatively, if using the peroxidase anti-peroxidase (PAP) method and DAB as substrate, dehydrate the sections in a graded series of alcohol (70%, 90%, 96%, and 100%) for 5 min each and transfer in to Rotihistol for 10 min and mount in Rotihistokit. The sections can be stored for several years at room temperature.

3.5. Controls

If not mentioned otherwise, all controls should be performed according to the protocols above (*see* **Note 5**).

1. Negative control: the primary antibody is omitted during the incubation, or if using a polyclonal antibody apply serum of the same host animal obtained before immunization (preimmune serum).
2. Preabsorption: preincubate the primary antiserum with the peptide it has been raised against overnight at 4°C. Use 20 μg to 100 μg of the antigen per mL of antiserum at its final concentration. Application of this serum for immunohistochemistry should not result in any immunolabeling. It is important to run a positive control (antiserum which has not been preabsorbed) in the same series of incubations.

3.6. Multiple Immunohistochemistry

Using more than just one antiserum on a section increases the value of the results, since more parameters can be investigated and be related to each other on one section. Primary antisera from different host species can be combined or, in the case of monoclonal antibodies from the mouse, by biotinylating one of the antibodies with a commercially available Fab fragment (e.g., ARK from DAKO). This represents a modified antimouse immunoglobulin, and subsequently a steptavidin-coupled fluorescent dye that visualizes the reaction on the section.

If using only two antisera it may prove beneficial to use a red (e.g., Texas Red) and a green [e.g., florescein isothiocyanate (FITC)] fluorescing dye, since they result in a yellow color in double exposure photography if the two antigens are present in the same location.

It is important to not only carefully select primary antisera from different species, but also the secondary antisera, as crossreactions can occur. For example, when using a primary antibody from rabbit, goat, mouse, do not use a goat antirabbit immunoglobulin secondary antiserum because it will cross-react with a secondary antiserum against the goat primary antiserum.

4. Notes

1. For a more rapid immersion fixation of whole (human) lung, fill the lung with fixative to its normal volume via the trachea. Allow to fix for up to 4 h and

transfer into phosphate buffer opening the trachea. When subjecting the tissue to cryoprotection it is important to wait until the tissue has sunk to the bottom before freezing it. The main advantage of this method is not the faster fixation, but the fact that the sucrose solution filled lung can be sectioned easily.

2. If the sections should be detached from the slides during the incubation process, alternatively collect the sections on double gelatinate-coated or poly L-lysine coated slides.

3. To simplify the incubation, the first two steps (blocking and applying the primary antiserum) can be combined, meaning the primary antibody can be diluted to its final working concentration in a modified blocking solution (5% BSA, 5% normal goat serum (NGS), 0.1% cold water fish skin gelatin in 0.1 M PBS). The blocking solution without the NGS is stable at –20 °C, after adding the NGS the solution can be stored at 4°C for 1 w.

4. To minimize background, the secondary antiserum should be briefly centrifuged and all washing steps should be performed on a tumbler.

5. If no staining or weak staining is observed, even in positive controls (i.e., tissues that are known to have the antigen that the antiserum has been raised against, e.g., different tissues or tissues from other species), it may prove beneficial to snap-freeze the tissue in iso-pentane cooled with liquid nitrogen. After cutting, postfix the sections in either –20°C acetone or –20°C acetone with 5% methanol for 10–15 min, allow to dry for 1 h. This leads very often to better staining results, but also to poorer tissue preservation.

References

1. Kummer, W. (1990) Simultaneous immunohistochemical demonstration of vasoactive intestinal polypeptide and its receptor in human colon, *Histochem. J.*, **22**, 249.
2. Pirchon, M., Hirn, J. M., Mangeat, P., and Marvaldi J. (1983) Anti-cell surface monoclonal antibodies wich antagonize the action of VIP in a human adrenocarcinoma cell line (HT29). *EMBO J.* **2**, 1017.
3. Maderspach, K., Németh, K., Simon, J., Benyhe, S., Szücs, M., and Wollemann, M. (1991) A monoclonal antibody recognizing κ- but not μ- and δ-opioid receptors. *J. Neurochem.* **56**, 1897.
4. Strader, C. D., Sigal, I. S., Blake, A. D., Cheung, A. H., Register, B. S., Rands, E., et al. (1987) The carboxyl terminus of the hamster b-adrenergic receptor expressed in mouse L cells is not required for receptor sequestration. *Cell* **49**, 855.
5. Stefanini M., de Martino, C., and Zamboni L. (1967) Fixation of ejaculated spermatozoa for electron microscopy. *Nature* **216**, 173.
6. Somogyi, P. and Tagagi, H. (1982) A note on the use of picric acid-paraformaldehyde-glutaraldehyde fixative for correlated light and electron microscopic immunocytochemistry. *Neuroscience* **7**, 1779.
7. Kummer, W., Fischer, A., Preissler, U., Couraud, J. Y., and Heym, C. (1990) Immunohistochemistry of the guinea pig trachea using an anti-idiotypic antibody recognizing substance P receptors. *Histochemistry* **93**, 541.

8. Fischer, A., Kummer, W., Couraud, J. Y., Adler, D., Branscheid, D., and Heym, C. (1992) Immunohistochemical localization of receptors for vasoactive intestinal peptide and substance P in human trachea. *Lab. Invest* **67,** 387.

9. Møller, W. and Møller, G (1994) Chemical Dehydation for Rapid Paraffin Embedding. *Biotech. and Histochem* **69, no.** 5, 289.

10. Mertens, A. H., Nagler, J. M., Galdermans, D. I., Slabbynck, H. R., Weise, B., and Coolen, D. (1998) Quality assessment of protected specimen brush samples by microscopic cell count. *Am. J. Respir. Crit. Care. Med.* **157**(4 Pt 1) 1240–1243.

11. Minshall, E. M., Schleimer, R., Cameron, L., Minnicozzi, M., Egan, R. W., Gutierrez-Ramos, J. C., Eidelman, D. H., and Hamid, Q. (1998) Interleukin-5 expression in the bone marrow of sensitized Balb/c mice after allergen challenge. *Am. J. Respir. Crit. Care. Med.* **158**(3) 951–957.

12. Fink, L., Seeger, W., Ermert, L., Hanze, J., Stahl, U., Grimminger, F., Kummer, W., and Bohle, R.M. (1998) Real-time quantitative RT-PCR after laser-assisted cell picking. *Nat. Med.* **4(11)** 1329–1333.

31

The Measurement of Cysteinyl Leukotrienes in Urine

Jay Y. Westcott and Sally E. Wenzel

1. Introduction

The cysteinyl leukotrienes, comprising leukotriene (LT) C4 and its major metabolites LTD4 and LTE4, are inflammatory lipid mediators derived from metabolism of arachidonic acid by 5-lipoxygenase. These leukotrienes have received considerable attention for their potential role in asthma and other inflammatory diseases. Since there is a potential role for these lipid mediators in both health and disease, the analysis of leukotrienes in biological fluids, especially urine, has generated significant interest.

Peptidoleukotrienes are present in many biologic fluids, although often in very low concentrations. Blood is a common fluid utilized to measure both drugs and endogenous compounds. Peptidoleukotriene concentrations are low in blood because of their rapid metabolism and clearance. In blood (ex vivo) the half-life of LTC4 is 11.5 min and LTD4 is 5 min (1). The peptidoleukotrienes are also rapidly removed from blood (in vivo) by renal and liver clearance. The calculated maximal plasma LTE4 concentration is less than 7 pg/mL (2). This rapid metabolism and clearance is a major factor why plasma LTE4 levels are not readily utilized as an index of LTC4 synthesis.

LTC4 and its metabolites are present in other fluids removed from the blood, such as tears (3), skin blister fluids (3,4), gastric fluids (5), joint fluid (6,7), middle ear fluid (8), cerebral spinal fluid (9), bile (10), and nasal fluids. Leukotriene levels in these fluids may convey information on metabolic events occurring in specific tissues at specific times. Few studies have quantified leukotrienes in these fluids and details of the methodology utilized will not be discussed here. LTC4 can also be released into the alveolar space, a compart-

From: *Methods in Molecular Medicine, vol. 56:*
Human Airway Inflammation: Sampling Techniques and Analytical Protocols
Edited by: D. F. Rogers and L. E. Donnelly © Humana Press Inc., Totowa, NJ

ment surrounded by a tight layer of epithelial cells acting as a barrier for sub-stances moving into or out of the airways *(11)*. Fiberoptic bronchoscopy coupled with bronchoalveolar lavage (BAL) has been utilized to sample fluids from the lower airways and this fluid (BALF) has been used in numerous hu-man studies to measure leukotrienes (*see* **Note 1**).

The final elimination route for much of the peptidoleukotrienes is urine. Urine has been utilized in many studies to quantify leukotriene metabo-lites *(12)* and the levels of these metabolites have been used as indices of total body leukotriene synthesis (*see* **Note 2**). It should be emphasized that a signifi-cant increase in leukotriene synthesis in a small portion of the body may be enough to cause local physiologic effects without producing a significant in-crease in urinary metabolites. Urine has three main advantages that have led to it being widely used to measure leukotrienes:

1. Easily collected noninvasively.
2. Essentially free of cells, which circumvents potential problems of ex-vivo pro-duction.
3. Has a stable metabolite (LTE4) that can be quantified by sensitive immunoas-says. LTE4 levels are typically normalized to urine creatinine for comparative quantification because of the high variability of urine volume with time.

The metabolism, elimination, and pharmacokinetics of LTE4 excretion have been well-studied *(2,13,14)*. Following the administration of leukotriene, 4–7% of the total administered leukotriene is excreted in urine within a 4 h period. Westcott et al. *(14)* compared the excretion of leukotriene metabolites in asth-matics and healthy non- asthmatics and found no significant differences. LTE4 is not *N*-acetylated in the human hepatocyte so N-acetyl LTE4 is usually a minor urinary metabolite possibly representing a product of renal metabolism *(15,16)*. LTC4 and LTD4 are not typically found in any substantial amount in human urine.

A variety of methods have been utilized for the measurement of leukotrienes in urine. It has been suggested that LTE4 can be directly quantified in urine without purification *(17)*, but this method, although providing relative differ-ences, is not accurate. High concentrations of nonleukotriene urinary contami-nants are present that interfere with quantitation by immunoassay. These contaminants stick to octadecylsilyl cartridges so purification needs to be in excess of solid-phase extraction alone. The most common methodology has utilized an initial concentration over an octadecylsilyl cartridge, high-pressure (performance) liquid chromatography (HPLC) purification, and quantitation by immunoassay. Radiolabeled LTE4 is added as an internal standard to facili-tate the detection of elution off the HPLC column and to allow for correction of losses that occur during purification. This methodology is time consuming, prone to potential errors, and a major contributor to the wide range of LTE4 levels reported. Gas chromatography mass spectrometry (GC/MS) analysis has also been utilized in a few studies, but is time consuming and requires expensive equipment *(18)*.

Recently, our laboratory has published two alternative immunologic purification methods for urinary LTE4. When combined with a sensitive immunoassay for quantitation, these methods allow for accurate measurement of LTE4 in urine quickly and easily with small volumes of urine and without using radioactivity or expensive equipment. The first method involves immunofiltration based on adding excess leukotriene antibody to urine followed by separation of bound leukotriene from unbound low molecular weight contaminants by filtration through a 10,000 molecular weight cutoff filter *(19)*. The LTE4 is dissociated from the antibody by methanol precipitation and the antibody removed after centrifugation. This purification has the disadvantage of requiring a large mass of antibody that is not commercially available.

Subsequently, a second method was developed utilizing an immunoaffinity resin containing antileukotriene antibody attached to Sepharose *(20)*. The rationale behind this assay is that LTE4 in urine will bind to the added resin containing antibody to leukotriene. Some contaminants may bind as well, but we suggest that a high percentage will not be bound. Thus, a first level of purification is achieved. By utilizing an immunoassay with a different antibody for LTE4, we also accomplish an increased specificity since the measured leukotriene will require binding to two different antibodies. This is currently the recommended method since it:

1. Utilizes reagents that are all commercially available.
2. No radioactivity required.
3. Requires only common laboratory equipment.
4. Is relatively fast and easy to perform.

2. Materials

1. Peptidoleukotriene immunoaffinity resin (Cayman Chemical, Ann Arbor, MI). The resin is utilized as a 50% dilution of resin with phosphate buffered saline containing 0.01% azide as a preservative (for storage over time). This dilution allows the resin to be distributed with a pipet.
2. Enzyme immunoassay (EIA) system (Cayman Chemical): comprised of a 96-well plate coated with mouse anti-rabbit IgG, acetylcholinesterase covalently linked to LTC4 as an enzyme tracer, standard LTE4, and antipeptidoleukotriene antibody.
3. A complete assay kit can be purchased (cysteinyl leukotriene kit) which contains all reagents necessary for performing this assay except the standard LTE4 (the kit uses an LTC4 standard). Alternatively, the reagents can be individually purchased which can be cost effective but only if numerous plates are needed.
4. The immunoassay buffers and substrate are provided in the kit.
5. "Working" EIA buffer: 0.1 *M* potassium phosphate (pH 7.4), 0.1% (v/v) bovine

serum albumin(BSA), 0.01% azide, 1 m*M* ethelynediaminetetraacetic acid (EDTA) and 0.4 *M* sodium chloride.
6. Wash buffer: 0.01 *M* potassium phosphate (pH 7.4) and 0.05% tween-20.
7. Ellman's reagent (substrate: 0.022 g/L acetylthiocholine iodide and 0.020 g/L dithiobis-2-nitro-benzoic acid in 0.1 *M* potasium phosphate buffer, pH 7.4).
8. Wash buffer (to wash the resin): 100 m*M* potassium phosphate buffer (pH 7.4) in normal saline.
9. Creatinine is measuerd using a spectrophotometric assay kit (catalog number 555-A, Sigma, St Louis, MO).

3. Methods

3.1. Binding Urinary LTE4 to the Immunoaffinity Resin

1. Thaw frozen urine at room temperature or in warm water (*see* **Note 3**).
2. Centrifuge urine at low speed (3700*g* for 3–5 min) to remove particulates.
3. Remove 1 mL from each sample and put in a 1.5 polypropylene tube containing 20μL leukotriene immunoaffinity resin diluted 1:2 (v/v) in buffer (our initial studies with urine spiked with tritiated LTE4 and unlabeled LTE4 indicated that this amount of resin could bind over 10 ng LTE4, an amount in excess of what is found in 1 mL urine).
4. The samples are allowed to mix (by rotation) at room temperature for 60 min to allow binding of LTE4 to the resin (*see* **Note 4**).
5. The resin now is bound to LTE4 from the urine and needs to be separated from the supernatant that contains an excess of interfering substances.

3.2. Removing the Resin

1. Centrifuge the samples at 10,000*g* for 5 min and carefully remove the supernatant with a 1 mL pipet. Ensure that as much of the supernatant is removed as possible.
2. Add 1 mL phosphate buffered saline (PBS) (0.9% saline in 100 m*M* potassium phosphate buffer, pH 7.4) to each tube, and mix.
3. Centrifuge the samples a second time.
4. Remove and discard wash supernatants.

3.3. Removing Bound LTE4 from the Resin

1. Add 0.5 mL methanol to each sample of resin.
2. The samples are mixed and stored at –20°C for 5–30 min, although longer times are not problematic if this works better for the investigator.
3. The samples are centrifuged again at 10,000*g* for 5 min and the methanolic supernatant is removed into a second polypropylene tube.
4. Repeat centrifugation step to ensure that all the resin is removed, and the supernatants again saved in a new tube (although the manufacturer's instructions suggest that the resin can be saved and reused, we believe that this can lead to problems and thus is not worth the possible monetary savings).

3.4. Getting the Samples Ready for Immunoassay

1. Remove the methanol using a Speed Vac concentrator on low heat (typically taking 45–60 min). The samples should not be allowed to remain in the heated concentrator for excessive times which could cause degradation.
2. Dissolve samples in 0.25–1.0 mL enzyme immunoassay (EIA) buffer. The volume used is partially dependent on the creatinine level of the urine sample. Samples with low urine creatinine (<0.5 mg/mL) are dissolved in 0.25 mL buffer, samples with 0.5–2 mg creatinine/mL in 0.5 mL buffer, and samples with high creatinine (>2 mg/mL) in 1 mL buffer. Adding different amounts of buffer maximizes the ability to measure LTE4 in the purified sample.

3.5. Quantification by Immunoassay (see Notes 5 and 6)

The immunoassay procedure is described with the assay kit.

1. Standard LTE4 (16 to 1000 pg/mL) and samples are pipeted into wells in duplicate (50 µL/well).
2. This is quickly followed by dispensing 50 µL enzyme tracer and 50 µL antibody into each well.
3. The plate is allowed to incubate at room temperature for 14–24 h.
4. Wash plate 5 times and add 200 µL substrate (Ellman's Reagent). A yellow color develops which is related to the amount of enzyme present in each well (inversely related to the amount of leukotriene present in the standard or sample).
5. When the absorbance of the zero standard (the highest absorbance) reaches 0.300 to 1.0 at 405 nm, the plate has developed sufficiently for accurate reading in the plate reader. The time for development can vary between 1–6 h.
6. When reading, the plate is blanked against substrate only, or a nonspecific binding well that contained no added antibody.
7. It is recommended that a computer be utilized to calculate a standard curve using a 4 parameter or log-log fit (alternatively, this can be done by hand).
8. The samples are compared to the standard curve and the concentrations of leukotrienes determined.
9. Concentrations are extrapolated to the original volume of urine utilized and no correction is performed for recovery (*see* **Note 7**).

3.6. Creatinine Assay

Creatinine is measured using a modification of the Sigma assay kit to allow a microassay to be used. The microassay has the advantages of using fewer reagents and is performed in a 96-well plate (flat bottom, brand not critical) which makes it easier and faster.

1. Standard (3 mg/dL standard provided), water, and samples are dispensed in duplicate (20 µL) into wells.
2. Working color reagent (a 5:1 mix of creatinine color reagent and 1*M* NaOH, both provided in the kit) is added to each well (190 µL).

3. During the next 10–30 min, the plate is read in a plate reader set to read absorbances at 490–500 nm using the wells containing water as a blank.
4. Initial absorbance of the standard and initial absorbance of the samples are determined.
5. Acid reagent (17 μL, provided with the kit) is added to each well and the plate gently shaken to mix the reagents.
6. After 20 min, the plate is again read at the same wavelength with the same blanks used and final absorbances determined.
7. The creatine (mg/mL) in a sample diluted 1:10 is calculated using the equation (initial absorbance sample – final absorbance sample)/[(initial absorbance standard – final absorbance standard)/0.3] (since 3 is the concentration of the creatinine standard in mg/dL). This calculation is also described in the kit.
8. The sample concentrations are converted to mg/mL and used in the denominator to express urine LTE4 levels (pg/mg creatinine).

4. Notes

1. In addition to urine, leukotriene metabolites have been extensively measured in BALF and their measurement in this fluid deserves additional mention. Levels of leukotrienes in BALF have been expressed as pg/mL, pg/mg protein, or pg/ug albumin and there is still much controversy on the best method to utilize *(21)*. In some studies the dilution of epithelial lining fluid that occurs during the lavaging process has been estimated by comparing urea levels in lavage fluid to that in plasma *(22)*. Absolute values of peptidoleukotrienes obtained by different laboratories are often not directly comparable due in part to differences in the methodology of lavaging and analyzing samples. When BALF samples are collected, the fluid should be put on ice until the fluid can be centrifuged to remove cells. Samples of fluid can then be aliquoted and frozen until assayed. This is easier than trying to process the fluid right away and storing fluid in a semipurified form. BALF contains a mixture of LTC4, LTD4, and LTE4, the percentage of each being dependent on the metabolism occurring in the lung as well as in isolated BALF. We previously reported that LTC4 could be metabolized to LTD4 and LTE4 in cell-free BALF *(12,14)*. Since BALF will contain a mixture of leukotriene metabolites, the preferred antibody will be one that detects all metabolites with similar crossreactivity. However, if the investigator is interested in the metabolic profile of leukotrienes, metabolism should be halted as soon as possible by either addition of methanol or (preferably) purification of BALF on an octadecylsilyl cartridge. Few detailed studies have been performed to examine the stability of leukotrienes in BALF, but as in other fluids, the peptidoleukotrienes should be relatively stable when frozen. Although there are no published studies that have extensively examined the effect of freeze-thaw on BALF leukotrienes, some degradation is likely after freeze-thaw. Peptidoleukotriene levels in BALF are typically very low. Thus, BALF is usually concentrated prior to quantitation *(14,23)*. Solid phase extraction cartridges have been utilized to concentrate BALF, with a methanolic solvent (80–100% metha-

nol) being utilized for leukotriene extraction. The methanol is subsequently removed under negative pressure. A Speed Vac concentrator works well in processing multiple samples. Some researchers commonly add [^{3}H] LTE4 to samples prior to concentration/purification. It should be stressed that this does add some mass of LTE4 to the sample (being dependent upon the specific activity of the material added) which later will be picked up by immunoassay. In addition, the tritium added as an internal standard could also interfere with the radioimmunoassay, if that is the method utilized for final quantitation. The tritiated LTE4 is also subject to degradation and may not give accurate recovery estimates. For some studies, especially those involving multiple clinical centers, it is not convenient or even possible to utilize radioactivity. For these reasons, it is generally better not to use a radiolabeled internal standard that is added to all samples. Spiking several samples with labeled or unlabeled leukotriene and determining recovery through all steps is often a better and more "user-friendly" alternative. It is important that recovery be fairly consistent in all samples and be relatively high (better than 60% in complicated purification methods).

2. There are at least two major considerations to remember when using urinary LTE4 as an index of total body LTC4 synthesis. First, an inflamed or injured kidney can directly excrete LTC4 into the urine resulting in a falsely exaggerated calculated level of total leukotrienes. This is because the normal elimination of leukotrienes synthesized outside the kidney as urinary LTE4 is only 4–7% whereas the elimination of LTC4 synthesized in the kidney could approach 100% LTE4. Second, liver function should be normal in order to use LTE4 levels as an index of total body leukotriene synthesis. Normally leukotrienes are rapidly removed from the blood by the liver. If the liver is dysfunctional, leukotrienes are not removed from the circulation as readily and kidney excretion is increased. The net result is increased levels of urinary LTE4 because of altered elimination/metabolism rather than increased synthesis.

3. Urine is often collected as spot samples for LTE4 quantitation. From these single spot urine samples information on typical leukotriene synthesis has been extrapolated. For this to be relevant, LTE4 synthesis and excretion must normally be fairly constant throughout the day. Asano et al *(24)* studied variability in urinary LTE4 excretion over several days and found that urine LTE4 levels over any 4 h period could be significantly different both in healthy subjects and asthmatics. This is surprising considering the tight range of levels reported in numerous studies with healthy subjects. More studies are needed to investigate normal daily variation in LTE4 excretion in both adults and children. It should also be noted that urine can be collected for specific time periods and the excretion of LTE4 expressed per unit of time rather than as pg/mg creatinine *(25)*. Urine is often collected at intervals following an experimental inhalation (e.g., allergen). Typically such challenges cause rapid leukotriene synthesis and since leukotrienes are quickly excreted, a 3–4 h time period following challenge is usually sufficient to detect most of the leukotrienes synthesized in response to the stimulus. Leukotriene stability is an important issue in quantitation. Leukotrienes in aque-

ous media are not very soluble and can adhere to glass or plastic in the absence of proteins. Protein helps keep leukotrienes in solution as observed with 0.1% BSA in most immunoassay buffers. Urine does not contain much protein but the presence of other unknown substances helps keep LTE4 in solution and stable. The peptidoleukotrienes are prone to becoming oxidized in aqueous solutions. This usually does not occur rapidly, but initial oxidation can lead to further and more rapid oxidation. However, LTE4 in urine appears to be fairly stable. Fauler et al *(26)* showed that [^{3}H] LTE4 in urine remained intact for at least six hours at 37°C. Westcott et al *(27)* found that 80–90% of the immunoreactive LTE4 was recovered from urine samples even after 24 h at room temperature. Despite this finding, it is best to keep urine samples cool until they are frozen. LTE4 has been shown to be stable in frozen urine samples for months without additional preservatives *(28)*. Leukotrienes in urine also appear to be stable to several freeze-thaw cycles. Partial purification of samples and storage as methanolic extracts is not beneficial for urine samples in which increased decomposition has been observed (Westcott, personal observation).

4. When starting this assay for the first time or after receiving a new lot number of resin, it is recommended that one determine that the resin is working. Several urine samples should be spiked with 0.5 ng/mL LTE4 and recovery through the assay protocol determined. One might also try several different resin amounts (10, 20, and 40 μL is reasonable) and compare recovery of the added LTE4. If the investigator has tritiated LTE4 available, the urine could be spiked with this labeled LTE4 and recovery of added tritium determined. Although the validation method using tritiated LTE4 is faster and easier, one must have relatively pure radiolabeled LTE4 that is subject to rapid degradation. It is possible to purify tritiated LTE4 from many of its degradation products by using the immunoaffinity resin to bind the LTE4. Although this procedure may not completely purify tritiated LTE4, it is much easier than HPLC purification methods.

5. Although urine samples are markedly cleaner after the purification, they likely still contain impurities that could interfere with the immunoassay if present in too high a concentration. Thus, the results could be influenced by the immunoassay utilized. In our study we chose to use a general peptidoleukotriene antibody that crossreacts well with LTC4, LTD4 and LTE4 (Cayman Chemical) and we recommend the use of this assay kit and antibody to allow for standardization in this quantitative procedure. Although it might seem more appropriate to use a more specific LTE4 antibody (i.e., one that does not crossreact with LTC4 or LTD4), it is unclear what is crossreacting with the leukotriene antibodies utilized in these assays so such an LTE4-specific antibody might actually crossreact more with other nonleukotriene urine components.

6. This assay procedure was found to provide results which correlated well with other purification methods (immunofiltration and HPLC). The method recovered LTE4 that was added to a urine extract quantitatively and it recovered 75 ± 6% of LTE4 added to urine over a range of 100–400 pg/mL. Reproducibility was evaluated by

purifying and quantifying the same sample seven separate times. The coefficient of variation was 8%. We felt that the recovery of added LTE4 to samples was sufficiently high and consistent that we would not use a radiolabeled LTE4 internal standard. We also decided not to try to correct for recovery of LTE4 present since it could vary some in samples and we would not know the exact recovery.

7. Typically, purified samples are each assayed at two dilutions (usually 1:1 and 1:2 in buffer) to ensure reproducible results. The 1/2 dilution is performed in the well itself by first adding 25 µL of buffer and then 25 µL of sample. This is both easier than making a dilution in a separate tube and saves purified sample that is often available in small volumes. If both sample dilutions are in the usable range of the standard curve, the final sample concentration is calculated using the average of the two determinations. If one of the dilutions is too high or too low, then the determination of sample concentration is obtained using the one good dilution only. If both dilutions are too high a concentration (absorbance lower than the highest standard), then the sample is said to be higher than the highest standard (for example greater than 1000 pg/mL). The sample could be repeated at a higher dilution if a more exact concentration is desired. Similarly, if the absorbance is higher than the lowest nonzero standard, then the concentration should be estimated as less than that standard (for example less than 16 pg/mL). As an additional control, it is recommended that a spiked urine sample (about 500 pg/mL) be included with every purification run (usually 10–19 samples). This is to confirm that all aspects of the purification and quantitation of LTE4 are working on any given assay. We recommend that any remaining purified sample should be frozen. If there is a problem with the total assay or any individual sample, the assay can be repeated during the next several days using these frozen samples.

References

1. Zakrzewski, J. T., Sampson, A. P., Evans, J. M., Barnes, N. C., Piper, P. J., and Costello, J. F. (1989) The biotransformation in vitro of cysteinyl leukotrienes in blood of normal and asthmatic subjects. *Prostaglandins* **37**, 425–444.
2. Maltby, N. H., Taylor, G. W., Ritter, J. M., Moore, K., Fuller, R. W., and Dollery, C. T. (1990) Leukotriene C4 elimination and metabolism in man. *J. Allergy Clin Immunol* **85**, 3–9.
3. Bisgaard, H., Ford-Hutchinson, A. W., Charleson, S., and Taudorf, E. (1985) Production of leukotrienes in human skin and conjunctival mucosa after specific allergen challenge. *Allergy* **40**, 417–423.
4. Atkins, P. C., Zweiman, B., Littman, B., Presti, C., von Allmen, C., Moskovitz, A., and Eskra, J. D. (1995) Products of arachidonic acid metabolism and the effects of cyclooxygenase inhibition on ongoing cutaneous allergic reactions in human beings. *J. Allergy Clin Immunol* **95**, 742–747.
5. Hommes, D. W., Meenan, J., de Haas, M., ten Kate, F. J., von dem Borne, A. E., Tytgat, G. N., and van Deventer, S. J. (1996) Soluble Fc gamma receptor III (CD 16) and eicosanoid concentrations in gut lavage fluid from patients with inflammatory bowel disease: reflection of mucosal inflammation. *Gut* **38**, 564–567.

6. Koshihara, Y., Isono, T., Oda, H., Karube, S., Hayashi, Y. (1988) Measurement of sulfidopeptide leukotrienes and their metabolism in human synovial fluid of patients with rheumatoid arthritis. *Prostaglandins Leukot Essent Fatty Acids* **32**, 113–119.

7. Moilanen, E. (1994) Prostanoids and leukotrienes in rheumatoid synovitis. *Pharmacol. Toxicol.* **75**, 4–8.

8. Jung, T. T. (1988) Prostaglandins, leukotrienes, and other arachidonic acid metabolites in the pathogenesis of otitis media. *Laryngoscope* **98**, 980–993.

9. Haupts, M., Smektala, K., Finkbeiner, T., Simmet, T., Gehlen, W. (1992) Immunoreactive leukotriene C4 levels in CSF of MS patients. *Acta Neurol. Scand.* **85**, 365–367.

10. Richter, L., Hesselbarth, N., Eitner, K., Bosseckert, H., and Krell, H. (1996) Increased biliary secretion of cysteinyl-leukotrienes in human bile duct obstruction. *J. Hepatology* **25**, 725–732.

11. Kilburn, K. H. (1970) Alveolar microenvironment. *Arch Intern Med* **126**, 435–49.

12. Westcott, J. Y., Taylor, I. K. (1998) Measurement of leukotrienes from human biologic fluids, in *Five Lipoxygenase Products in Asthma*. vol. 120 (eds. Drazen, J.M., Lee,T.H., Dahlen, S-E., eds.), Marcel Dekker, Inc., New York, NY, pp 245–281.

13. Orning, L., Kaijser, L., Hammarstrom, S. (1985) In vivo metabolism of leukotriene C4 in man: urinary excretion of leukotriene E4. *Biochem. Biophys. Res. Commun.* **130**, 214–220.

14. Westcott, J. Y., Voelkel, N. F., Jones, K., Wenzel, S. E. (1993) Inactivation of leukotriene C4 in the airways and subsequent urinary leukotriene E4 excretion in normal and asthmatic subjects. *Am. Rev. Respir. Dis.* **148**, 1244–1251.

15. Uemura, M., Buchholz, U., Kojima, H., Keppler, A., Hafkemeyer, P., Fukui, H., Tsujii, T., Keppler, D. (1994) Cysteinyl leukotrienes in the urine of patients with liver diseases. *Hepatology* **20**, 804–812.

16. Huber, M., Muller, J., Leier, I., Jedlitschky, G., Ball, H. A., Moore, K. P., et al. (1990) Metabolism of cysteinyl leukotrienes in monkey and man. *Eur J Biochem* **194**, 309–315.

17. Kumlin, M., Stensvad, F., Larsson, L., Dahlen, B., Dahlen, S. E. (1995) Validation and application of a new simple strategy for measurements of urinary leukotriene E4 in humans. *Clin. Exp. Allergy* **25**, 467–479.

18. Fauler, J., Tsikas, D., Holch, M., Seekamp, A., Nerlich, M. L., Sturm, J., Frolich, J. C. (1991) Enhanced urinary excretion of leukotriene E4 by patients with multiple trauma with or without adult respiratory distress syndrome. *Clin. Sci. (Colch)* **80**, 497–504.

19. Westcott, J. Y., Sloan, S., Wenzel, S. E. (1997) Immunofiltration purification for urinary leukotriene quantitation. *Anal. Biochem.* **248**, 202–210.

20. Westcott, J. Y., Maxey, K. M., MacDonald, J., and Wenzel, S. E. (1998) Immunoaffinity resin for purification of urinary leukotriene E-4. *Prostaglandins & Other Lipid Mediators* **55**, 301–321.

21. Walters, E. H. and Gardiner, P. V. (1991) Bronchoalveolar lavage as a research tool. *Thorax* **46**, 613–618.

22. Rennard, S. I., Basset, G., Lecossier, D., O'Donnell, K. M., Pinkston, P., Martin, P. G., Crystal, R. G. (1986) Estimation of volume of epithelial lining fluid recovered by lavage using urea as marker of dilution. *J. Appl. Physiol.* **60,** 532–538.

23. Westcott, J. Y., Johnston, K., Batt, R. A., Wenzel, S. E., Voelkel, N. F. (1990) Measurement of peptidoleukotrienes in biological fluids. *J. Appl. Physiol.* **68,** 2640–2648.

24. Asano, K., Lilly, C. M., O'Donnell, W. J., Israel, E., Fischer, A., Ransil, B. J., Drazen, J. M. (1995) Diurnal variation of urinary leukotriene E4 and histamine excretion rates in normal subjects and patients with mild-to-moderate asthma. *J. Allergy Clin. Immunol.* **96,** 643–651.

25. Westcott, J. Y., Smith, H. R., Wenzel, S. E., Larsen, G. L., Thomas, R. B., Felsien, D., Voelkel, N. F. (1991) Urinary leukotriene E4 in patients with asthma. Effect of airways reactivity and sodium cromoglycate. *Am. Rev. Respir. Dis.* **143,** 1322–1328.

26. Fauler, J., Neumann, C., Tsikas, D., Frolich, J. (1993) Enhanced synthesis of cysteinyl leukotrienes in atopic dermatitis. *Br. J. Dermatol.* **128,** 627–630.

27. Westcott, J. Y., Sloan, S., Wenzel, S. E. (1997) Immunofiltration purification for urinary leukotriene E4 quantitation. *Anal Biochem* **248,** 202–210.

28. Kumlin, M. (1996) Analytical methods for the measurement of leukotrienes and other eicosanoids in biologic samples from asthmatic subjects. *J. Chromatog. A* **725,** 29–40.

32

Quantitative Analysis of Cyclooxygenase Metabolites of Arachidonic Acid

Ryszard Dworski, James R. Sheller, and Brian W. Christman

1. Introduction

Metabolism of arachidonic acid results in a host of biologically active compounds with profound effects on airway inflammation (1). After activation of cellular phospholipases and release of free arachidonic acid, catalyzed insertion of oxygen occurs enzymatically via action of one of the two known cyclooxygenase isoenzymes (COX-1 and COX-2). The unstable bicyclic intermediate, PGH_2, undergoes subsequent metabolism to form prostaglandins (PG), thromboxane (Tx), and leukotrienes (LT) (see **Fig. 1**). In addition, free radicals can oxygenate arachidonate although it is bound to the diacylglycerol backbone of membrane phospholipids. The family of compounds formed in this way, known as isoprostanes, are stereochemically different and incorporate a large number of regioisomeric compounds that may confound measurement of PG (2–5; and see Chapter 33). Arachidonic acid can also be metabolized by specific cytochrome P_{450} enzymes to regioisomeric epoxides and stereospecific hydroxyeicosatetraenoic (HETE) acids (6).

The prostanoids have potent and diverse effects on vascular and airway smooth muscle. For example, TxA_2 is a powerful constrictor of smooth muscle; PGI_2 (prostacyclin), by elevating intracellular cAMP after engagement of IP receptors, tends to relax smooth muscle. The emphasis on smooth muscle effects (probably because this effect can be easily measured) has tended to obscure the potentially more important effects of prostanoids on processes as diverse as mast cell activation, gene transcription, neovascularization, and modulation of inflammation. It is important to avoid ascribing exclusively pro- or antiinflammatory roles to these autacoids. For instance, excess prostacyclin

From: *Methods in Molecular Medicine, vol. 56:*
Human Airway Inflammation: Sampling Techniques and Analytical Protocols
Edited by: D. F. Rogers and L. E. Donnelly © Humana Press Inc., Totowa, NJ

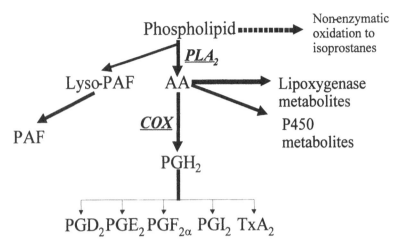

Fig. 1. Overview of pathways of metabolism of arachidonic acid during airway inflammation. Following activation of cellular phospholipases, arachidonic acid is cleaved from membrane phospholipids. It is undergoing dioxygenation catalyzed by cyclooxygenase (either COX-1 or COX-2 isoforms) to form the unstable endoperoxide intermediate PGH2. Specific isomerases with varied cellular distribution further metabolize PGH2 to bioactive prostaglandins and thromboxanes.

production in inflamed regions of the lung may deleteriously maintain blood flow, allowing for enhanced influx of phagocytes and exuberant edema formation.

Since the complement of specific enzymes necessary for conversion of PGH_2 into specific bisenoic prostaglandins differs between cells, activation of certain cell types can be inferred by the appearance of certain PG (*see* **Table 1**). For example, the discovery of PGD_2 in the bronchoalveolar lavage of asthmatics provided direct evidence of mast cell activation, since the mast cell is a principal source for PGD_2 in the airway *(7)*. Likewise the appearance of TX metabolites in the urine after allergen inhalation in atopic asthmatics suggested platelet activation, especially when the increased excretion of 2,3-dinor-TxB_2 was blocked by low doses of aspirin *(8)*.

Prostanoids were first measured using biological assays, with contraction of isolated smooth muscle strips being a popular methodology. These techniques are now used primarily to document biological effects of newly discovered compounds and to explore receptor pharmacology. Physicochemical methods of measurement, such as high performance liquid chromatography (HPLC), remain important for in vitro experiments, and can add to the accuracy of antibody and mass spectrometry methods by improving purification of samples. HPLC methods are often not sensitive enough for detection of prostanoids in biological samples. Today the most widespread method for measuring

Table 1
Spectrum of Cyclooxygenase Metabolites of Arachidonic Acid Produced by Common Cell Types Present in the Airway Environment

Cell type	PGD_2	PGE_2	PGF_2	PGI_2	TxA_2
Macrophages	4+	3+	1+	0	4+
Epithelium	1+	4+	2+	0	0
Endothelium	0	4+ (micro.)	1+	4+(macro.)	2+ (micro.)
Smooth muscle	0	4+	2+	3+	1+
Mast Cells	4+	2+	1+	0	+
Eosinophils	2+	1+	0	0	1+
Fibroblasts	1+	4+	1+	0	1+

Extent of production of autocoids by each cell type ranges from 0 (not produced) to 4+ (major producer or predominant metabolite). Both mast cells and eosinophils produce more lipoxygenase metabolites, such as LTC_4, than cyclooxygenase products.

eicosanoids are immunoassay techniques. These methods employ antibodies raised to prostanoids linked to larger haptens, and are used in a variety of ways to quantify mediators. Most primary prostanoids, and many of their main urinary metabolites, can be measured using commercially available kits. Although these methods are relatively straightforward to perform, the data must be interpreted with caution when complex biological fluids are assayed.

Although extremely valuable, immunoassays of prostanoids can yield confusing data. For example, although crossreactivity with other compounds is listed as being trivial, sometimes such substances, such as free fatty acids, are present in such high amounts that even a small percentage crossreaction with the antibody results in a large error. Also, in many competitive immunoassays, concentrations are determined by displacement of labeled tracer, presumably by endogenous eicosanoids, from the immobilized antibody. Such failure of tracer binding can also occur because of solvent impurities, alterations in pH, and changes in ionic strength of buffers. In almost every instance when immunoassays are compared with more specific chemical methods, such as stable isotope dilution methods combined with gas chromatography mass spectrometry (GC/MS) methods (see **steps 1–3**), the concentrations determined by immunoassay are much greater than those measured by GC/MS. The source of this error is unclear, but could result from metabolites of the compound of interest or crossreacting materials, such as isoprostanes. This caution does not preclude the use of immunoassays, but when knowledge of the absolute amounts of prostanoids is critical, a confirmatory physicochemical method of analysis should be considered. Our bias has been to rely heavily on GC/MS methods because of the rigorously quantitative nature of the data that is generated. The drawbacks to use of GC/MS methods include:

1. Analysis is labor intensive.
2. GC/MS requires use of specialized equipment that is expensive to maintain.
3. Trained personnel are necessary to perform and troubleshoot the assays.

Because reduced interassay variability tends to decrease the number of analyses required to confirm or refute the experimental hypothesis; the overall expense to the individual investigator may not be significantly greater than using commercially available assay kits.

2. Materials

2.1. Reagents

1. Organic solvents, including ethyl acetate, methanol, and hexane are obtained from Baxter Healthcare (Burdick and Jackson Brand, McGaw Park, IL). HPLC grade is recommended.
2. Analytes in aqueous solutions (plasma, urine, or culture media) are purified with octadecylsilyl (C18) Sep-Pak cartridges obtained from Waters Associates (Milford, MA).
3. Reagents to derivatize functional groups: methoxyamine hydrochloride, pentafluorobenzyl bromide, and *N, N*-diisopropylethylamine are obtained from Sigma Chemical Co. (St. Louis, MO, USA). N, O-*bis*-(trimethylsilyl) trifluoroacetamide (BSTFA) is purchased from Supelco (Bellefonte, PA).
4. Dimethylformamide and undecane are obtained from Aldrich Chemical Co. (Milwaukee, WI).
5. LK6DF Silica Gel 60A thin layer chromatography (TLC) plates are obtained from Whatman (Clinton, NJ).
6. Many heavy isotope labeled internal standards are available from Cayman Chemical (Ann Arbor, MI) or Biomol Research Laboratories, Inc. (Plymouth Meeting, PA), for example deuterium labeled PGF_{2a}, 6-keto-PGF_{1a} (the major metabolite of PGI_2), TXB_2, PGE_2, and PGD_2.
7. Fused silica capillary columns for gas chromatography: 15 m DB 1701 (J & W Scientific Inc., Folsom, CA) or 10 m SPB 1 (Supelco; Bellefonte, PA).

2.2. Apparatus

1. C_{18} Sep-Pak column (Waters Associates, Milford, MA).
2. Standard benchtop microcentrifuges.
3. Analytical sample concentrator: Speed-Vac (Savant Inc., Farmingdale, New York) for reduced pressure concentrating (recommended) or with a continuous stream of dry nitrogen.

4. Effective fume hood to scavenge volatile organic solvents.
5. Automated thin layer chromatography radiomatic detector (Bioscan, Washington, DC) (optional).
6. 3–4 thin layer chromatography chambers.
7. Gas chromatograph: Varian Vista 6000 GC (Sunnyvale, CA).
8. GC columns: 15 m DB 1701 fused silica capillary columns (J and W Scientific Inc., Folsom, CA) or 10 m SPB1 fused capillary column (Supelco Inc., Bellefonte, PA).
9. Mass Spectrometer: Nermag R-1010C (Fairfield, NJ) or a Hewlett-Packard 5982A interfaced with an IBM Pentium grade computer system.

3. Methods

3.1. Mass Spectrometric Quantification of Cyclooxygenase Metabolites of Arachidonic Acid in (bronchoalveolar lavage) BAL Fluid

Analysis of cyclooxygenase metabolites by gas chromatography/negative-ion chemical ionization mass spectrometry (GC/NICI-MS) is extremely sensitive with a lower limit of detection in the range 1–5 pg when employing deuterated internal standards with a blank of less than 5 parts per thousand. The following assay procedure, summarized in **Fig. 2**, is the method utilized for analysis of prostanoids in BAL fluid (*see* **Notes 1** and **2**). However, the method is adaptable to other biological fluids such as sputum and cell culture media. These methods evolved from those published over the last decade (*9–12*).

3.1.1. Handling and Storage of BAL Fluid

1. Filter BAL fluid through sterile loose gauze and place container on melting ice.
2. Centrifuge the sample at 400*g* for 10 min.
3. Divide the cell-free supernatant into smaller aliquots and store at −70°C until analysis is performed (*see* **Note 5**)

3.1.2. Purification and Derivatization of Primary Eicosanoids

1. Acidify 2 mL BAL fluid to pH 3 with 1 *N* HCl.
2. Add 200 pg deuterium labeled internal standards (*see* **Notes 2** and **3**).
3. Vortex the sample and equilibrate for 30 min at room temperature.
4. Apply to a C_{18} Sep-Pak column preconditioned with 5 mL methanol and 5 mL water (pH 3) (*see* **Note 4**).
5. Rinse the cartridge sequentially with 10 mL water (pH 3) and 10 mL heptane.
6. Elute the prostanoids with 10 mL ethyl acetate/heptane (50:50, v/v).
7. Evaporate the ethyl acetate/heptane elute from the C_{18} Sep-Pak under a stream of nitrogen. The procedure can be expedited by a gentle pumping or using a vacuum manifold. Other types of octadecyl-silyl bonded columns work well, too; minor modifications of eluting solvents may be necessary.

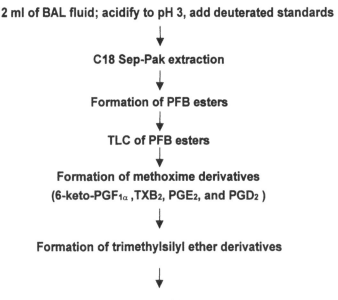

Fig. 2. Outline of the procedures used for the mass spectrometric analysis of prostanoids in BAL fluid.

8. The prostanoids are converted to pentafluorobenzyl (PFB) esters by treatment with 20 mL 12.5% 2,3,4,5,6 pentafluorobenzyl bromide in acetonitrile and 10 mL *N,N*-diisopropylethylamine at room temperature for 30 min.

9. Dry the reagents under nitrogen and reconstitute the sample in 40 mL methanol.

10. Apply the sample to LK6D silica gel 60A TLC plates using the solvent ethyl acetate/methanol (98:2, v/v).

11. Chromatograph ~5 μg PGF_{2a}, 6-keto-PGF_{1a}, TXB_2, PGE_2, and PGD_2 standard PFB derivatives on a separate plate and visualize by spraying with a 10% solution of phosphomolybdic acid in ethanol followed by heating (*see* **Notes 7** and **8**). Appropriate silica segments containing the analytes are removed after plate development (*see* **Note 6**). The compounds migrating in the regions of the appropriate PFB ester standards are carefully scraped, placed in microcentrifuge tubes, and 1 mL of ethyl acetate is added together with 1 drop of water. The samples are vigorously vortexed and spun at high speed for 5 min. The supernatant is transferred to new tubes and evaporated under nitrogen. The PFB ester of PGD_2 is well-isolated from the other compounds of interest, and can be isolated individually. However, the PFB esters of PGE_2 and TXB_2 are poorly separated from each other, and therefore they need to be extracted collectively. Likewise, PGF_{2a} and 6-keto-PGF_{1a} are also scraped and extracted jointly.

12. The methoxime derivatives of 6-keto-PGF_{1a}, TXB_2, PGE_2, and PGD_2 are then made by adding 20 mL of 0.5% methoxyamine hydrochloride in pyridine, vortexing, centrifuging, and incubating for at 37°C for 1 h (overnight incubation at room temperature works well, too).

13. Dry the reagents under nitrogen and add 1 mL ethyl acetate together with 3–4 drops of water and vortex vigorously.
14. Centrifuge, remove ethyl acetate removed and dry under nitrogen.
15. The prostanoids are then converted to trimethylsilyl ether derivatives by adding 10 mL BSTFA and 10 mL pyridine, and incubating at room temperature for 15–20 min.
16. The reagents are dried under nitrogen and the compounds redissolved in 20 mL undecane for final analysis by GC/MS.

3.2. Analysis of Eicosanoid Major Urinary Metabolites

Although analysis of prostanoids in BAL fluid is an important tool for studying the involvement of these compounds in airway inflammation, there are disadvantages and limitations associated with this approach. This is because bronchoscopy to obtain BAL fluid for analysis is:
1. Invasive.
2. Not amenable to large clinical projects.
3. Cannot be safely performed when airway function is severely compromised.

Measuring the urinary excretion of prostanoid metabolites can circumvent some of these shortcomings. Collection of urine is noninvasive and thus suitable for clinical studies involving even severely ill patients. Moreover, this approach may offer some important advantages:

1. Analysis of urine collected over a period of several hours can provide an integrated index of prostanoid production over extended periods of time.
2. Analysis of individually voided urines can provide an index of prostanoid formation over shorter periods of time.

It is important to emphasize, however, that only analysis of urinary metabolites of prostanoids provides a reliable index of systemic production of prostanoids. This is because levels of unmetabolized cyclooxygenase products (e.g., PGE_2) in urine are not exclusively derived from filtration from the circulation but in part arise from the formation in the kidney. Metabolism of eicosanoids occurs predominantly in extrarenal tissues. Analysis of other compounds in urine such as histamine and unmetabolized isoprostanes has caused the same difficulties in interpretation. **Table 2** shows the urinary metabolites of the major prostanoids and F_2-isoprostanes. Stable isotope dilution mass spectrometric assays for these compounds are available. As an example, a method for the analysis of 2,3-dinor-6-keto-PGF1α (PGI-M), the stable urinary metabolite of prostacyclin, by stable isotope dilution methods in conjunction with GC/MS is described below (*13*):

1. Add 3 mL pH 3.0 water to 15-mL conical bottom polypropylene tubes containing 1 ng tetradeuterated PGI-M (*see* **Notes 3** and **5**).

Table 2
Listing of Major, Stable Urinary Metabolites of Prostaglandins

Parent prostanoid	Major urinary metabolite
$PGF_2\alpha$	$9\alpha,11\alpha$-dihydroxy-15-oxo-2,3,4,5-tetranor-prostan-1,20-dioic acid (PGF-M)
PGE_2	9,15-dioxo-11α-hydroxy-2,3,4,5-tetranor-prostan-1,20-dioic acid (PGE-M)
PGD_2	$9\alpha,11\beta$-dihydroxy-15-oxo-2,3,18,19-tetranor-prost-5-ene-1,20-dioic acid (PGD-M)
PGI_2	6-oxo-$9\alpha,11\alpha$,15S-trihydroxy-2,3-dinor-prost-13E-en-1-oic acid (2,3-dinor-6-keto $PGF_1\alpha$)
TxB_2	9α,11,15S-trihydroxy-2,3-dinor-thromba-5Z,13E-dien-1-oic acid (2,3-dinor TXB_2)
8iso-$PGF_2\alpha$	2,3-dinor-5,6-dihydro-8-iso-prostaglandin $F_2\alpha$ (F_2-IsoP-M)

2. Add 1-mL urine sample to each tube, adjust pH to 3.0, and allow to equilibrate at room temperature for 30 min.

3. Each sample is then applied by gravity filtration to a C-18 Prep-Seps preconditioned with 5 mL methanol, then 5 mL water (pH 3.0).

4. Wash columns with 10 mL water and 7 mL hexane.

5. Elute analytes with 4 mL ethyl acetate into 4.5 mL conical bottom tubes, and evaporate to dryness in an analytical concentrator.

6. Add 1 mL dichloromethane and wash samples twice with 2 mL 50 mM sodium borate buffer (pH 8.1), discarding the aqueous layer each time (i.e., the PGI-M exists in a lactone form and does not easily extract into the aqueous phase, allowing for differential extraction of nonlactonized fatty acids).

7. Evaporate the organic phase to dryness, reconstitute in 50 µL acetonitrile, and vortex with 200 µL of 3% methoxyamine HCl in water.

8. Incubate for 1 h at room temperature to open the lactone ring and convert the free keto group to the corresponding O-methyloxime.

9. Extract samples with 2 mL dichloromethane (discard acqueous layer) and evaporate to dryness under vacuum.

10. Carboxyl functions are derivatized by addition of 20 µL acetonitrile, 15 µL of 25% pentafluorobenzyl bromide in acetonitrile, and 10 µL diisopropylethylamine and incubation at room temperature for 30 min.

11. Dry under vacuum, reconstitute in 25 µL methanol, and apply to the preadsorbent zone of LK6DF silica TLC plates. Using a solvent system of ethyl acetate: methanol (98:2, v/v), plates are developed to the top with ascending technique (*see* **Note 8**).

12. In a *separate* tank, chromatograph a 5 µg standard of derivatized MOX-PFB of PGI-M in a similar way. This allows sample localization by spraying only this plate with phosphomolybdic acid, followed by heating. Two bands, corresponding to the syn- and antimethyloxime isomers will appear with an R_F of approx 0.25 (*see* **Note 7**).

13. Silica extending from 0.7–1.0 cm above the upper band to 0.7–1.9=0 cm below the lower band is scraped into polypropylene microfuge tubes and eluted with 1.3 mL ethyl acetate (*see* **Note 6**).

14. Vortex samples, allow to stand for 5 min, centrifuge and remove solvent by evaporation to dryness under vacuum.

15. Samples are converted to the trimethylsilyl ether derivatives by addition of 15 μL BSTFA and 10 μL pyridine.

16. Samples are incubated at 60°C for 15 min, followed by 45 min at room temperature.

17. After drying under vacuum, dissolve samples in 20 μL undecane in preparation for GC/MS.

3.3. Quantification of Endogenous Metabolites by Negative Ion Gas Chromatographic-Mass Spectrometry

For analysis of PGF_{2a}, 6-keto-PGF_{1a}, TXB_2, PGE_2, and PGD_2, we ordinarily use a Nermag R10-10C coupled to a Varian Vista 6000 gas chromatograph or Hewlett-Packard 5982A mass spectrometer interfaced with an IBM Pentium computer system. The compounds are chromatographed on a 15 m DB1701 fused silica capillary column or 10 m SPB1 fused capillary column according to the following parameters:

1. The column temperature is programmed from 190 to 300°C at 20°C/min.

2. Methane is used as the carrier gas for negative ion chemical ionization at a flow rate of 1 mL/min.

3. Ion source temperature is 250°C, electron energy is 70 eV.

4. The filament current is 0.25 mA.

5. A quantitative analysis of the metabolites is accomplished by selected ion monitoring. The following mass-to-charge ratio (m/z) ions are observed for the endogenous metabolite and for the heavy isotope labeled internal standard, respectively:

    a. $PGF_{2\alpha}$ 569 and 573.
    b. 6-keto-$PGF_{1\alpha}$ 614 and 618.
    c. PGE_2, 524 and 528.
    d. TXB_2 614 and 618.
    e. PGD_2 524 and 528.

The TLC separation of compounds having the same m/z values (for example PGE_2 and PGD_2) makes their analysis by GC/MS feasible. For analysis of the urinary metabolite of prostacyclin, selected ions monitored include m/z 586 (endogenously generated PGI-M) and 590 (heavy isotope standard), each representing the carboxylate anion resulting from loss of the pentafluorobenzyl group during negative ion chemical ionization MS. Comparison of the peak intensity area of the endogenous compound to that of the heavy isotope internal standard allows for rigorous quantification (*see* **Notes 9** and **10**).

4. Notes

1. It is best to combine "workable" amounts of samples to be assayed at one time, such as one patient or one experiment. The number of samples that can be successfully assayed varies with experience, but about 40 samples is usually the maximum.

2. The first step when performing a new assay is the generation of clear selected ion current profiles with good signal/noise ratios. Next, a standard curve with fixed amount of internal standard and increasing amounts of eicosanoid should result in a linear increase in the ratio of peak area intensities.

3. Most stable isotope dilution assays begin by combining a known amount of internal standard with the endogenous sample. Using a microsyringe, add the known amount of internal standard to aqueous media that does not contain any unlabeled eicosanoid. This prevents contamination of the standard syringe and carryover effects between samples. To further avoid contaminating the stock of internal standards, label a specific Hamilton syringe and use exclusively for each heavy isotope standard. Precise introduction of internal standard volume is critical to successful quantitative analysis.

4. For efficiency, use "repipet" dispensers for adding solvents in greater than 1 mL volumes. An example would be when preconditioning the silica and reverse phase minicolumns with methanol and water. For volumes of 1 mL or less, an adjustable hand held pipetor is used.

5. The use of polypropylene tubes is strongly advised. Some other polymers used in test tubes are not adequately organic solvent resistant and may generate interfering peaks in the GC trace. Tubes are available with conical bottoms in a variety of sizes (i.e., microcentrifuge, 4.5 mL and 15 mL). The conical shape allows for reconstitution and sample transfer with small volumes of organic solvent.

6. For removing analytes from silica segments of TLC plates, we recommend using an X-Acto straight, beveled point artist's knife to score the silica lane. Silica is scraped onto creased, gelatin-coated paper ordinarily used with analytical balances, then emptied into conical polypropylene vial for elution of the analyte.

7. It is very important to either isolate unlabeled standards used for localization of analytes on TLC in a separate tank, or to use a heterologous standard with an identical R_F that will not contaminate the other lanes. Minimal leeching of a microgram concentration standard into the solvent will radically alter the reliability of measurements of picogram amounts of PG in the samples.

8. TLC plates must be kept dry and free of impurities prior to use. Occasionally, prerunning the plates in an organic solvent to remove contaminating lipids can eliminate interfering peaks in the GC trace.

9. Extensive interfering peaks on the GC tracings likely indicates the need for more extensive preparative work to purify the compound of interest. Alternatives include alteration of the GC temperature gradient program to isolate the peak corresponding to the analyte (e.g., by adding another TLC purification after solid phase extraction), or changing the assay procedure entirely and moving to LC/MS.

10. Inspection of the selected ion current profiles that are generated is important before accepting computer-generated peak areas. Occasionally, an incompletely resolving interfering peak is included in the integration program and, if undetected, will adversely affect the validity of measurement.

References

1. Peters-Golden, M. (1997) Lipid mediator syntheis by lung macrophages, in *Lung Macrophages and Dendritic Cells in Health and Disease* (Lipscomb, M. F. and Russell, S. W., ed.) **102,** 151–182.

2. Roberts, L. J., 2nd., Brame, C. J., Chen, Y., and Morrow, J. D. (1999) Novel eicosanoids. Isoprostanes and related compounds. *Methods in Mol. Bio.* **120,** 257–285.

3. Roberts, L. J., 2nd., Salomon, R. G., Morrow, J. D., and Brame, C. J. (1999) New developments in the isoprostane pathway: identification of novel highly reactive gamma-ketoaldehydes (isolevuglandins) and characterization of their protein adducts. *FASEB Journal.* **13,** 1157–1168.

4. Morrow, J. D. and Roberts, L. J. 2nd. (1999) Mass spectrometric quantification of F2-isoprostanes in biological fluids and tissues as measure of oxidant stress. *Methods in Enzymology.* **300,** 3–12.

5. Dworski, R., Murray, J. J, Roberts, L. J., II, Oates, J. A., Morrow, J. D., Fisher, L., and Sheller, J. R. (1999) Allergen-induced Synthesis of F2-Isoprostanes in Atopic Asthmatics Evidence for Oxidant Stress *Am. J. Respir. Crit. Care Med.* **160,** 1947–1951.

6. Capdevila, J., Falck, J., and Estabrook, R. (1992) Cytochrome P450 and the arachidonate cascade. *FASEB J* **6,** 731–736.

7. Murray, J. J., Tonnel, A. B., Brash, A. R., Roberts, L. J., 2nd, and Gosset, P. (1986) Workman R. Capron A. Oates JA. Release of prostaglandin D2 into human airways during acute antigen challenge. *N. Engl. J. of Med.* **315,** 800–804.

8. Luppinetti, M. D., Sheller, J. R., Catella, F., FitzGerald, G. A. (1989) Thromboxane biosynthesis in allergen induced bronchospasm: evidence for platelet activation. *Am. Rev. Respir. Dis.* **140,** 932–935.

9. Christman, B. W., Gay, J. C., Christman, J. W., Prakash, C., Blair, I. A. (1991) Analysis of effector cell-derived lyso platelet activating factor by electron capture negative ion mass spectrometry. *Biol. Mass Spectrom.* **20,** 545–552.

10. Christman, B. W., Christman, J. W., Dworski, R., Blair, I. A., Prakash, C. (1993) PGE$_2$ limits arachidonic acid availability and inhibits LTB$_4$ synthesis in alveolar macrophages by a nonphospholipase A$_2$ mechanism. *J. Immunol.* **151,** 2096–2104.

11. Sebaldt, R., Sheller, J., Oates, J., Roberts, L. J., II, and Fitzgerald, G. (1990) Inhibition of eicosanoid biosynthesis by glucocorticoids in humans. *Proc. Natl. Acad. Sci. USA* **87,** 6974–6978.

12. Morrow, J. D., Prakash, C., Awad, J. A., Duckworth, T. A., Zackert, W. E., Blair, I. A., Oates, J. A., and Roberts, L. J., II. (1991) Quantification of the major urinary metabolite of prostaglandin D2 by a stable isotope dilution mass spectrometric assay. *Analyt. Biochem.* **193,** 142–148.

13. Daniel, V. C., Minton, T. A., Brown, N. J., Nadequ, J. H., and Morrow, J. D. (1994) Simplified assay for the quantification of 2,3-dinor-6-keto-prostaglandin F1α by gas chromatography-mass spectrometry. *J. Chromatography B: Biomedical Applications* **653(2),**117–122.

33

Quantitative Analysis of F$_2$ Isoprostanes

Ryszard Dworski, Brian W. Christman, and James R. Sheller

1. Introduction

The discoveries by Jack Roberts and Jason Morrow of the nonenzymatic oxidation of cell membrane phospholipids to form isoprostanes has revolutionized the field of eicosanoids (1). Prior to their discoveries, it was dogma that the important biologically active eicosanoids were formed by enzymes acting on arachidonic acid that had been cleaved from phospholipids by the action of phospholipases. Their research has clearly shown that important biologically active fatty acid metabolites are formed in a variety of inflammatory conditions from the action of oxygen radicals on arachidonic acid, while it is still present in complex phospholipids. These oxidized compounds may alter cell structure and signaling, and when released by the action of phospholipases, are immediately available to bind to receptors to modulate cell activity. The free radical attack on arachidonate yields an endoperoxide which can then be transformed nonenzymatically to F, D, E ring prostaglandins. Thus, each enzymatically formed eicosanoid appears to have its own class of isoprostanes, including isothromboxanes (2,3). Likewise, the isoleukotrienes have been described. In addition, compounds such as the hydroxyeicosatetraenoic acids (HETEs) can also be formed in this fashion (4,5). The biologic activity of these compounds is only now being examined.

Because the isoprostanes are formed by oxidant reactions, their presence has been used as a measure of oxidant stress (6), and it is in this situation that they have been used to document oxidant based inflammation in asthma and other airway inflammatory disorders. For example, we have shown elevation of F$_2$-isoprostanes (F$_2$-IsoPs) in the airways of asthmatic individuals 24 h after an allergic reaction (7). Others have shown elevation of F$_2$-IsoPs in interstitial lung disease (8).

From: *Methods in Molecular Medicine, vol. 56:*
Human Airway Inflammation: Sampling Techniques and Analytical Protocols
Edited by: D. F. Rogers and L. E. Donnelly © Humana Press Inc., Totowa, NJ

To examine the formation of isoprostanes in the airway, bronchoalveolar lavage (BAL) fluid seems the most straightforward medium to analyze. Because the isoprostanes are formed intitially in membrane phospholipids, it may also be important to measure these compounds, by extracting them and then following the analytical procedures for free isoprostanes. Sputum and airway biopsies are amenable to assay, as is urine and blood for compounds presumably formed in the lung and released into the circulation. Since ex vivo formation of the compounds is often quite substantial, care must be taken to extract the materials quickly.

There are commercial sources for enzyme linked immunoassay kits for analysis of F_2-IsoPs. The antibodies are likely to have difficulty in distinguishing between enzymatically formed F_2 compounds and will have even more difficulty in distinguishing among the 64 compounds comprising the class of F_2-IsoPs. However, this may convey an advantage in some experimental strategies, since the antibody may assay for the total amounts of F_2-IsoPs, instead of only one or two of the isomers formed (but see *9*). As mentioned in the previous chapter, immunoassays have distinct advantages over the physiochemical methods described here, but suffer from cross reactivity and lack of quantitative accuracy. When it is critical to know the exact amounts of compound present, gas chromatography mass spectrometry (GC/MS) appears to have the advantage.

The chemical quantification of F_2-IsoPs is conducted by chemical derivitization of the products of interest to make them amenable to MS. Then a series of separation steps based on molecular mobility is carried out, first with thin layer chromatography (TLC) followed by GC, leading directly to analysis of selected ion fragments of the molecule of interest. Internal standards of a higher molecular weight than the compound of interest are synthesized using heavy hydrogen (deuterium) or isotopes of oxygen. Thus, a known amount of the compound is carried through the entire process of extraction, derivitization, and chromatography and its ion current is compared to that of the compound of interest. This yields remarkably sensitive and specific results, with lower limits of detection in the range of 1–5 pg.

2. Materials

2.1. Reagents

1. Butylated hydroxytoluene (BHT) and triphenylphosphine (Sigma Chemical Company, St. Louis, MO).
2. Deterium labeled 8-iso-PGF$_{2\alpha}$ (8-iso-PGF$_{2\alpha}$-d$_4$) and methyl ester PGF$_{2\alpha}$ (Cayman Chemical, Ann Arbor, MI).

3. Derivatization reagents (derivatization grade): Pentafluorobenzyl (PFB) bromide and *N,N*-Diisopropylethylamine (Aldrich Chemical Company, Milwaukee, WI), *N,O-bis*(trimethylsilyl)trifluoroacetamide (BSTFA) (Supelco Inc., Bellefonte, PA).

4. Organic solvents (HPLC grade); methanol, ethyl acetate, heptane, ethanol, chloroform, and acetonitrile (Fisher Scientific Company, Pittsburgh, PA), pyridine and undecane (Aldrich).

5. Solid phase extraction C_{18} Sep-Pak cartridges and silica Sep-Pak cartridges (Waters Associates, Milford, MA).

6. LK6D silica gel 60A TLC plates (Whatman Inc., Clifton, NJ).

7. Phosphomolybdic acid (Aldrich).

8. Microliter syringes (Hamilton Company, Reno, Nevada).

9. Polypropylene tubes.

2.2. Apparatus

1. Standard benchtop microcentrifuge

2. Effective fume hood to scavenge volatile organic solvents

3. The Mayer analytical evaporator (N-EVAP) (Organomation Associates Inc., South Berlin, MA) or Speed-Vac (Savant Inc., Farmingdale, New York) for reduced pressure concentrating or with a continuous stream of nitrogen.

4. Glass rectangular tank with flat glass lid for development of TLC plates (Fisher).

5. Hotplate (Fisher).

6. Channel/adsorbent scraper (Altech Associates, Inc., Deerfield, IL).

7. Nermag R10-10C (Fairfield, NJ) or Hewlett-Packard 5982A (Palo Alto, CA) mass spectrometer with coupled gas chromatograph (Varian Vista 6000GC, Sunnyvale CA).

8. 15 m DB1701 fused silica capillary column (J and W Scientific Inc., Folsom, CA).

3. Methods

3.1. Handling and Storage of Samples for Mass Spectrometric Quantification of F₂ Isoprostanes

Spontaneous formation of F_2-IsoPs has been described at room temperature and at $-20°C$ in specimens containing arachidonyl lipids. To avoid ex vivo generation of F_2-IsoPs, samples need to be processed immediately after collection or alternatively, frozen in liquid nitrogen and stored at $-70°C$. This is particularly important when tissue and plasma F_2-IsoPs are analyzed. BAL samples and especially urine samples are more amenable to rapid freezing for later analysis. Urine and BAL fluids can be analyzed directly; tissue and lipids containing esterified F_2-IsoPs such as plasma require extraction of bound isoprostanes. (We have found that extraction of BAL fluid does not improve the quantification of isoprostanes) (*see* **Note 1**).

3.2. Extraction and Hydrolysis of F₂-IsoPs Esterified to Tissue Phospholipids

1. The tissue is weighed, and added to a mortar placed on ice together with 1 mL ice-cold Folch solution (chloroform/methanol, 2:1, v/v) containing 0.005% BHT (a free radical scavenger), and homogenized by careful grinding.
2. The solution is then transferred to 15-mL conical polypropylene tubes (*see* **Note 2**). The mortar is eluted twice more with 1-mL cold Folch solution to ensure that no homogenate has been left on the mortar.
3. The tube is purged of air with nitrogen, vortexed, and the sample incubated at room temperature for 30 min, with vortexing every 10 min.
4. One mL of physiological saline is then added and the solution is vortexed and centrifuged at 800*g* for 10 min. The upper aqueous layer is discarded and the organic layer containing the extracted phospholipids is carefully transferred to a new tube containing the internal standard.
5. The sample is dried down to 0.5 mL under nitrogen and 0.5 mL of 15% KOH is then added and incubated at 37oC for 30 min.
6. The mixture is then acidified to pH 3 with 1 *N* HCl and diluted to 10 mL with pH 3 water (the concentration of methanol in the sample needs to be adjusted to 5% or less before the extraction on a C_{18} Sep-Pak column). The method continues as in **Subheading 3.4.3**.

3.3. Extraction of F₂-IsoPs in Plasma

1. A Folch-solution containing both 0.005% BHT (Sigma) and 0.025% triphenylphosphine (a reducing agent) is used. The mixture of 1 mL plasma and 20 mL Folch-solution is shaken for 2 min.
2. Then 10 mL of 0.043 % $MgCl_2$ in water is added. The sample is shaken again for 2 min and is then centrifuged at 800*g* for 10 min.
3. The organic layer is dried under a stream of nitrogen and the residue hydrolyzed according to the procedure delineated for tissue phospholipids as given in **Subheading 3.2.4**.

3.4. Derivitization of F₂-IsoPs

1. 4 mL BAL fluid, 3 mL plasma, or 0.2 mL centrifuged urine is acidified to pH 3 with 1 *N* HCl and the internal standard is added.
2. Typically BAL fluid is spiked with 400 pg, plasma with 200–1000 pg, and urine with 1000 pg deuterium labeled isoprostane [$^2H_4$]8-iso-PGF$_{2\alpha}$.
3. The sample is vortexed and applied to a C_{18} Sep-Pak column preconditioned with 5 mL methanol followed by 5 mL water (pH 3).
4. The cartridge is then rinsed sequentially with 10 mL water (pH 3) and 10 mL heptane (if urine is analyzed the column is additionally washed with 5 mL of 10% (v/v) acetonotrile in water (pH 3.0) prior to heptane).
5. The sample is eluted with 10 mL ethyl acetate/heptane (50:50, v/v). A further purification of plasma and urine is necessary using a silica Sep-Pak, although this step can be omitted if BAL fluid is assayed.

6. The ethyl acetate/heptane eluate from C_{18} Sep-Pak is dried over anhydrous sodium sulphate.

7. The dried eluate is then applied to a silica Sep-Pak previously prewashed with 5 mL methanol and 5 mL ethyl acetate.

8. The column is then washed with 5 mL ethyl acetate and the F_2-IsoPs are eluted with 5 mL ethyl acetate/methanol (50:50, v/v).

9. The eluate is dried under nitrogen and converted to (PFB) ester by treatment with 20 µL of 12.5% 2,3,4,5,6 (PFB) bromide in acetonitrile and 10 µL *N,N*-diisopropylethylamine at room temperature for 30 min.

10. The solution is then evaporated under nitrogen and the residue reconstituted in 40 µL methanol.

11. The sample is then subjected to TLC using the solvent chloroform/ethanol (93:7 v/v) (*see* **Note 3**).

12. Approximately 5 µg methyl ester of $PGF_{2\alpha}$ is chromatographed on a separate lane and visualized by spraying with a 10% solution of phosphomolybdic acid in ethanol followed by heating. The methyl ester of $PGF_{2\alpha}$ instead of the 8-isoPGF$_{2\alpha}$ PFB ester is preferred as the TLC standard because this technique prevents contamination of the analyzed samples which would result in falsely elevated levels of 8-iso-PGF$_{2\alpha}$.

13. Compounds migrating in the area of the methyl ester of $PGF_{2\alpha}$ and the neighboring zones 1 cm above and below are scraped to weighing paper (Fisher) using a scraper, placed in microcentrifuge tube, and extracted with ethyl acetate (*see* **Note 4**).

14. The ethyl acetate is evaporated under nitrogen and the F_2-IsoPs are then converted to trimethylsilyl ether derivatives by adding 10 µL BSTFA and 10 µL pyridine, and incubating for 20 min at room temperature.

15. The reagents are then dried under nitrogen and the F_2-IsoPs are redissolved in 20 µL undecane.

3.5. Mass Spectrometric Quantification of F_2-IsoPs

The GC/NICI-MS is accomplished using a Nermag R10-10C (Fairfield, NJ) coupled to a Varian Vista 6000 gas chromatograph (Sunnyvale, CA) or Hewlett-Packard 5982A mass spectrometer, and a 15 m DB1701 fused silica capillary column (J and W Scientific Inc., Folsom, CA).

1. The column temperature is programmed from 190 to 300°C at 20°C/min. Helium is used as the carrier gas (*see* **Notes 5** and **6**).

2. Ions are monitored at a mass-to-charge ratio (m/z) of 569 for endogenous F_2-IsoPs and at m/z 573 for the $[^2H_4]$8-iso-PGF$_{2\alpha}$. The m/z 569 selected ion current chromatogram contains a series of peaks representing different endogenous F_2-IsoPs (*see* **Fig. 1**). However, for the most precise and accurate quantification of F_2-IsoPs, only a single peak, which coelutes with the 8-iso-PGF$_{2\alpha}$ internal standard is measured (*see* **Note 7**).

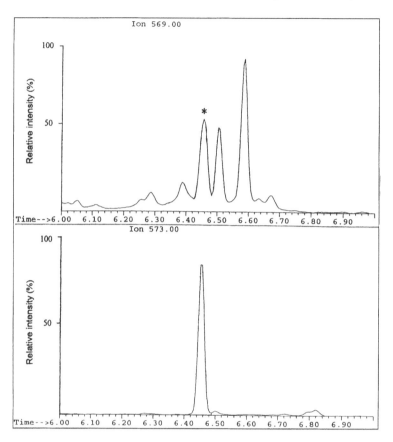

Fig. 1. Analysis of F_2-IsoPs in BAL fluid obtained from a human asthmatic subject 24 h after local allergen challenge. Quantification of the F_2-IsoPs is accomplished by measuring the peak in the upper chromatogram marked by an asterisk. Other peaks probably represent other isomers of F_2-IsoPs. Even the peak indicated by the asterisk probably consists of at least two and possibly 3 F_2-IsoPs.

4. Notes

1. It is best to combine a "workable" amount of samples to be assayed at one time, such as one patient or one experiment. The number of samples that can be successfully assayed varies with experience, but about 30–40 samples is usually the maximum.
2. The use of polypropylene tubes is strongly advised. Some other polymers used in test tubes are not adequately organic solvent resistant and may generate interfering peaks in the GC trace. Conical shaped tubes allow reconstitution and sample transfer with small volumes of organic solvent.
3. TLC plates must be kept dry and free of impurities prior to use. Occasionally, prerunning the plates in an organic solvent to remove contaminating lipids can eliminate interfering peaks in the GC trace.

4. For removing analytes from silica segments of TLC plates, it is scraped onto creased, gelatin-coated weighing paper ordinarily used with analytical balances, then emptied into conical polypropylene vial for elution of the analyte.

5. The first step when performing a new assay is the generation of clear selected ion current profiles with good signal/noise ratios. Next, a standard curve with a fixed amount of internal standard and increasing amounts of 8-iso-PGF$_{2\alpha}$ should result in a linear increase in the ratio of peak area intensities.

6. Most stable isotope dilution assays begin by combining a known amount of internal standard with the endogenous sample. Using a microsyringe, add the known amount of internal standard to aqueous media that does not contain any unlabeled eicosanoid. This prevents contamination of the standard syringe and carryover effects between samples. To further avoid contaminating the stock of internal standard, label a specific Hamilton syringe and use it exclusively for the heavy isotope standard.

7. Visual inspection of the selected ion monitoring peaks is important to insure that contaminating peaks are not present. As shown in Fig. 1, this is especially important with the measurement of F$_2$-IsoPs.

References

1. Liu, T., Stern, A., Roberts, L. J., and Morrow J. D. (1999) The isoprostanes: novel prostaglandin-like products of the free radical-catalyzed peroxidation of arachidonic acid *J. Biomed. Science* **6,** 226–235.

2. Morrow, J. D., Roberts, L. J., Daniel, V. C., Awad, J. A., Mirochnitchenko, O., Swift L. L., and Burk, R. F. (1998) Comparison of formation of D2/E2-isoprostanes and F2-isoprostanes in vitro and in vivo—effects of oxygen tension and glutathione. *Arch. Biochem. Biophysi.* **53,** 160–171.

3. Taber, D. F., Morrow, J. D., and Roberts, L. J. II. (1997) A nomenclature system for the isoprostanes. *Prostaglandins* **53,** 63–67.

4. Mallat, Z., Nakamura, T., Ohan, J., Leseche, G., Tedgui, A., Maclouf, J., and Murphy, R. C. (1999) The relationship of hydroxyeicosatetraenoic acids and F2-isoprostanes to plaque instability in human carotid atherosclerosis. *J. Clin. Invest.* **103,** 421–427.

5. Murphy, R. C., Khaselev, N., Nakamura, T., and Hall, L. M. (1999) Oxidation of glycerophospholipids from biological membranes by reactive oxygen species: liquid chromatographic-mass spectrometric analysis of eicosanoid products. J. Chromat., *Biomed. Sciences & Applications.* **731,** 59–71.

6. Morrow, J. D., and Roberts, L. J. II (1999) Mass spectrometric quantification of F2-isoprostanes in biological fluids and tissues as measure of oxidant stress. *Methods in Enzymology* **300,** 3–12.

7. Dworski, R., Murray, J. J., Roberts, L. J. II, Oates, J. A., Morrow, J. D., Fisher, L, and Sheller, J. R. (1999) Allergen-induced synthesis of F2-Isoprostanes in atopic asthmatics: evidence for oxidant stress. *Am. J. Respir. Crit. Care Med.* **160,** 1947–1951.

8. Montuschi, P., Ciabattoni, G., Paredi, P., Pantelidis, P., du Bois, R. M., Kharitonov, S. A., and Barnes, P. J. (1998) 8-Isoprostane as a biomarker of oxidative stress in interstitial lung diseases. *Am. J. Respir. Crit. Care Med.* **158,** 1524–1527.

9. Proudfoot, J., Barden, A., Mori, T. A., Burke, V., Croft, K. D., Beilin, L. J., and Puddey, I. B. (1999) Measurement of urinary F_2-isoprostanes as markers of in vivo lipid peroxidarion — A comparison of enzyme immunoassay with 995 chromarography/mass spectrometry. *Analytical Biochemistry* **272,** 209.

Index

Lightning Source UK Ltd.
Milton Keynes UK
UKOW06n1319310315

248843UK00001B/6/P

9 780896 039230